Energy Balance and Cancer

Volume 3

Series Editor
Nathan A. Berger,
Case Western Reserve University,
Cleveland, OH, USA

For further volumes:
http://www.springer.com/series/8282

Anne McTiernan
Editor

Physical Activity, Dietary Calorie Restriction, and Cancer

Springer

Editor
Anne McTiernan
Fred Hutchinson Cancer Research Center
1100 Fairview Ave. N.
Seattle, WA 98109-1024, USA

ISBN 978-1-4419-7550-8 e-ISBN 978-1-4419-7551-5
DOI 10.1007/978-1-4419-7551-5
Springer New York Dordrecht Heidelberg London

Printed on acid-free paper

Springer is part of Springer Science+Business Media (www.springer.com)

Contents

Contributors

Rachel Ballard-Barbash Applied Research Program, Division of Cancer Control and Population Sciences, National Cancer Institute, Bethesda, MD 6130, USA, barbashr@dcpcepn.nci.nih.gov

Lisa H. Colbert Department of Kinesiology, University of Wisconsin, Madison, WI, USA, lhcolbert@education.wisc.edu

Catherine Duggan Division of Public Health Sciences, Fred Hutchinson Cancer Research Center, Seattle, WA 98109-1024, USA, cduggan@fhcrc.org

Stephen D. Hursting Department of Nutritional Sciences, University of Texas at Austin, Austin, TX, USA, shursting@mail.utexas.edu

Ikuyo Imayama Division of Public Health Sciences, Fred Hutchinson Cancer Research Center, Seattle, WA 98109-1024, USA, iimayama@fhcrc.org

Melinda L. Irwin Epidemiology and Public Health Yale, School of Medicine, New Haven, CT 06520-8034, USA, melinda.irwin@yale.edu

Weiqin Jiang Cancer Prevention Laboratory, Colorado State University, Fort Collins, CO 80523, USA, weiqin.jiang@colostate.edu

I.-Min Lee Department of Epidemiology, Harvard School of Public Health, Boston, MA 02215, USA, ilee@rics.bwh.harvard.edu

Caitlin Mason Division of Public Health Sciences, Fred Hutchinson Cancer Research Center, Seattle, WA 98109-1024, USA, cmason@fhcrc.org

Anne McTiernan Division of Public Health Sciences, Fred Hutchinson Cancer Research Center, Seattle, WA 98109, USA, amctiern@fhcrc.org

Linda Nebeling Behavioral Research Program, Division of Cancer Control and Population Sciences, National Cancer Institute, Bethesda, MD 6130, USA, nebelinl@mail.nih.gov

Susan N. Perkins Department of Nutritional Sciences, University of Texas at Austin, Austin, TX, USA, susan.ciolino@nih.gov

Andrew G. Renehan School of Cancer, Enabling Sciences and Technology, Manchester Academic Health Science Centre, University of Manchester, Manchester M13 9PL, UK; Department of Surgery, The Christie NHS Foundation Trust, Manchester M13 9PL, UK, arenehan@picr.man.ac.uk

Connie J. Rogers Department of Nutritional Sciences, Pennsylvania State University, University Park, PA, USA, cjr102@psu.edu

Andrew Rundle Department of Epidemiology, Mailman School of Public Health, Columbia University, New York, NY, USA, agr3@columbia.edu

Kathryn H. Schmitz Division of Clinical Epidemiology, Department of Clinical Epidemiology and Biostatistics, University of Pennsylvania School of Medicine, Philadelphia, PA 19104-6021, USA, schmitz@mail.med.upenn.edu

Rebecca M. Speck Division of Clinical Epidemiology, Department of Biostatistics and Epidemiology, University of Pennsylvania School of Medicine, Philadelphia, PA 19104-6021, USA, speckr@mail.med.upenn.edu

Henry J. Thompson Cancer Prevention Laboratory, Colorado State University, Fort Collins, CO 80523, USA, henry.thompson@colostate.edu; thomph@lamar.colostate.edu

Zongjian Zhu Cancer Prevention Laboratory, Colorado State University, Fort Collins, CO 80523, USA, zongjian.zhu@colostate.edu

Chapter 1
Introduction

Anne McTiernan, Linda Nebeling, and Rachel Ballard-Barbash

Abstract An increasing body of literature has linked overweight, obesity, and a sedentary lifestyle to increased risk for several types of cancers. These lifestyle factors have also been associated with prognosis of several types of cancers. This volume provides a review of the state of the science on the role of energy balance, physical activity, and cancer incidence and prognosis, as well as mechanisms that may underlie associations of energy balance with cancer risk and prognosis. The epidemic of overweight and obesity and the increasing sedentary lifestyles will impact the magnitude and quality of the cancer problem globally. Increasing the knowledge of scientists, clinicians, and policy experts will aid in defining new prevention and treatment methods, to reduce the impact of energy balance on cancer, with the goal to eventually reduce the burden of cancer.

An increasing body of literature has linked overweight, obesity, and a sedentary lifestyle to increased risk for several types of cancers. These lifestyle factors have also been associated with prognosis of several types of cancers. This is an important public health problem, because cancer is a common disease (one in two men and one in three women will develop cancer in their lifetime), and because overweight/obesity and sedentariness are extremely common and becoming more so (two third of American adults are overweight or obese, and the great majority do not meet the minimal recommendations for 150 min of moderate-to-vigorous intensity aerobic activity per week) [1, 2]. It is an important clinical issue since a marked increase in prevalence of a cancer risk factor will result in an increase in number of cancer cases unless some other widespread prevention factor negates this effect. In addition, treating oncologists and other health care providers will need to develop new and better therapies to counteract the adverse effects of overweight, obesity, and lack of physical activity on prognosis. The American Cancer Society estimates that a third of all cancer deaths could be prevented through avoidance of obesity

A. McTiernan (✉)
Division of Public Health Sciences, Fred Hutchinson Cancer Research Center, Seattle, WA 98109, USA
e-mail: amctiern@fhcrc.org

A. McTiernan (ed.), *Physical Activity, Dietary Calorie Restriction, and Cancer*,
Energy Balance and Cancer 3, DOI 10.1007/978-1-4419-7551-5_1,

and sedentary lifestyles [3]. The World Health Organization's International Agency for Research on Cancer estimates that 25–30% of several cancers could be prevented if individuals avoided lifetime weight gain and obesity and participated in regular physical activity [4]. The US Department of Health and Human Services commissioned an advisory committee to develop a report on health effects of physical activity, including the associations of physical activity with risks for cancers and with prognosis in persons with cancer. The resulting report found that increased physical activity was associated with reduced risk for several cancers including breast, colon, and lung [1]. It further found that among individuals with cancer, survival was prolonged and quality of life increased in those who were physically active, with most data available for persons diagnosed with breast or colon cancer.

There is great need for a definitive textbook that provides the scientific background and evidence supporting the relationships between these lifestyle factors and cancer risk and prognosis. This volume provides a review of the state of the science on the role of energy balance, physical activity, and cancer incidence and prognosis. Given the rapid expansion of research in this area, evidence is evolving rapidly. One example of the expansion of evidence is a recent review undertaken by the American College of Sports Medicine in June 2009 on the role of physical activity and cancer survivorship and survival. This review will form the basis for the development of a set of practice guidelines for exercise therapists in working with cancer patients and survivors.

We are very fortunate to have a world-class group of authors for this text. The individuals writing chapters have been chosen because they are the top researchers in the field of obesity, physical activity, and cancer. Chapters 2 is a review of the epidemiology of overweight/obesity and cancer risk by Dr. Andrew Renehan of the University of Manchester England. Chapter 3 summarizes the epidemiology of physical activity and cancer risk, drawing on the experience of Drs. Lee (Harvard University), Schmitz (University of Pennsylvania), Speck (University of Pennsylvania), and McTiernan (Fred Hutchinson Cancer Research Center, Seattle) in preparing the cancer chapter of the US DHHS Physical Activity Guidelines Advisory Committee report [1]. Chapter 4 updates the state of the science of animal models of dietary energy restriction, exercise, and mammary carcinogenesis by Dr. Henry Thompson of Colorado State University. The interplay of dietary energy restriction, exercise, and colon carcinogenesis is the subject of Chapter 5 written by Dr. Stephen Hursting of the University of Texas. Drs. Catherine Duggan, Ikuyo Imayama, and Caitlin Mason of the Fred Hutchinson Cancer Research Center in Seattle describe the potential mechanisms linking obesity to cancer risk in humans in Chapter 6. Mechanisms linking physical activity to cancer risk in humans are the topic of Chapter 7, written by Dr. Andrew Rundle of Columbia University. The increasing body of knowledge on physical activity, weight control, and cancer prognosis is summarized by Drs. Schmitz and Speck (University of Pennsylvania) and Irwin (Yale University) in Chapter 8.

This book focuses on how obesity and sedentary lifestyles adversely affect cancer risk and survival for individuals as well as mechanisms that may underlie those associations. However, evidence is accumulating rapidly on the cost of obesity and sedentary lifestyles to society. For example, obesity is estimated to lead to costs of $147 billion in the United States [5]. While research on individual level interventions for weight loss and increasing physical activity have identified efficacious approaches, these changes in behavior are not maintained by many in the current environments in the United States and worldwide that promote weight gain and inactivity. Research on environmental and policy approaches for addressing these problems at the societal level is needed [6, 7] and is a major component of the President's Report on Childhood Obesity released in April 2010.

The epidemic of overweight and obesity and the increasing sedentary lifestyles will impact the magnitude and quality of the cancer problem globally. Increasing the knowledge of scientists, clinicians, and policy experts will aid in defining new prevention and treatment methods to reduce the impact of energy balance on cancer, with the goal to eventually reduce the burden of cancer. Hopefully, this knowledge can be translated into incentives for the general public, persons at high risk, and cancer patients and survivors to increase physical activity, reduce excess weight, and maintain energy balance lifelong.

References

1. Physical Activity Guidelines Advisory Committee (2008) Physical activity guidelines advisory committee report, 2008. Department of Health and Human Services, Washington, DC
2. Carlson SA, Densmore D, Fulton JE, Yore MM, Kohl HW 3rd (2009) Differences in physical activity prevalence and trends from 3 U.S. surveillance systems: NHIS, NHANES, and BRFSS. J Phys Act Health 6(Suppl 1):S18–S27
3. Kushi LH, Byers T, Doyle C et al (2006) American Cancer Society guidelines on nutrition and physical activity for cancer prevention: reducing the risk of cancer with healthy food choices and physical activity. CA Cancer J Clin 56(5):254–281quiz 313–314
4. IARC Working Group (2002) Evaluation of cancer-preventive strategies weight control and physical activity. IARC Press, Lyon
5. Finkelstein EA, Trogdon JG, Cohen JW, Dietz W (2009) Annual medical spending attributable to obesity: payer-and service-specific estimates. Health Aff (Millwood) 28(5):w822–w831
6. McKinnon RA, Orleans CT, Kumanyika SK et al (2009) Considerations for an obesity policy research agenda. Am J Prev Med 36(4):351–357
7. Abdel-Hamid T (2009) Thinking in circles about obesity: applying systems thinking to weight management. Springer, New York, NY

Chapter 2
Epidemiology of Overweight/Obesity and Cancer Risk

Andrew G. Renehan

Abstract Increased body adiposity is an established risk factor for cancer development. In a large standardized meta-analysis of prospective observational studies, the author and collaborators quantified the risk associated with body mass index (BMI) in 20 cancer types and demonstrated that associations are often sex- and site-specific; exist for a wider range of malignancies than previously thought; and are broadly consistent across geographic populations. Given the biological plausibility, the consistency of associations, the sufficiently long latency times between BMI measurement and cancer occurrence and the recent observations of apparent cancer risk protection in grossly obese patients following bariatric surgery, these associations are probably causal. Further analyses are now revealing that other major cancer risk factors may effect associations between BMI and cancer risk in a site-specific manner – for example hormonal replacement therapy usage and risk of breast and endometrial cancers. These observations point to a diversity of potential processes operating for different cancer types, such that it is unlikely that there is a 'one system fits all' mechanism. As the obesity epidemic continues, incidences of obesity-related cancers may rise. There is a need to better understand the biological and molecular mechanisms underpinning the link between obesity and different cancers, so that targeted-based strategies are developed to integrate with population-based weight control policies.

1 Introduction

Increased adiposity has long been recognized as an important risk factor for cardiovascular disease and type 2 diabetes. While a link between obesity and cancer risk had been postulated in the nutritional literature dating back to the classical animal

A.G. Renehan (✉)
School of Cancer and Enabling Sciences, Manchester Academic Health Science Centre, University of Manchester, Manchester M20 4BX, UK; Department of Surgery, The Christie NHS Foundation Trust, Manchester M20 4BX
e-mail: arenehan@picr.man.ac.uk

A. McTiernan (ed.), *Physical Activity, Dietary Calorie Restriction, and Cancer*, Energy Balance and Cancer 3, DOI 10.1007/978-1-4419-7551-5_2,

experiments in the 1940s from Tennenbaum [1], this association has only recently been highlighted in the epidemiology literature.

The amount of body adiposity may be approximated by a number of anthropometric measures, including body mass index (BMI: expressed in kg/m^2), waist circumference (expressed in cm) and waist–hip ratio. By far the most commonly reported index in the literature is BMI, and this will be the main focus of this review. Using this metric, there is a well-established World Health Organization classification of four broad categories as follows: underweight, BMI <18.5 kg/m^2; normal weight, BMI 18.5–24.9 kg/m^2; overweight, BMI 25.0–29.9 kg/m^2; and obese, BMI $\geq$30 kg/m^2. Combining overweight and obesity may be expressed as excess body weight. Limitations of using BMI to express risk are recognized in the context of diseases such as cardiovascular disease – for example, central obesity determined by waist circumference or waist–hip ratio may be a most sensitive disease predictor – but it is unclear whether this is the case in the context of cancer risk.

This review updates the epidemiology of excess body weight and cancer risk focusing mainly of the large volume of association data linking BMI with several cancer types. The smaller volume of data linking waist circumference or waist–hip ratio and cancer risk will also be discussed. In support of these associations, the review also includes sections on ecological observations, biological mechanisms, causal associations (critiqued against the Bradford-Hill criteria) and attributable risk. Additionally, it has emerged that associations between excess body weight and cancer risk at specific sites may be considerably modified in the presence of other risk factors – and examples will be discussed. As a prelude to these discussions, some key aspects of the epidemiology of excess body weight are summarized.

2 Epidemiology of Excess Body Weight

To estimate the global prevalence of overweight and obesity in the world (2005), Kelly and colleagues [2] pooled sex- and age-specific prevalences in representative population samples from 106 countries and found the following: overall, 23.2% of the world's adult population was overweight (24.0% in men:22.4% in women) and 9.8% was obese (7.7% in men:11.9% in women). The estimated total numbers of overweight and obese adults were 937 million and 396 million, respectively. These values have been adopted by the World Health Organization. In many westernized countries, over a fifth of adult populations are obese – for example, 24.2% in men and 23.5% in women in the United States (2005) [3] and 21.9% in men and 24.4% in women in the United Kingdom (2007) [4] – but obesity is also prevalent in developing world countries. There are complex inter-relationships between socio-educational stratifications and excess body weight prevalence; but in general, outside the context of very low-income populations, obesity is more prevalent among lower socio-educational classes [5].

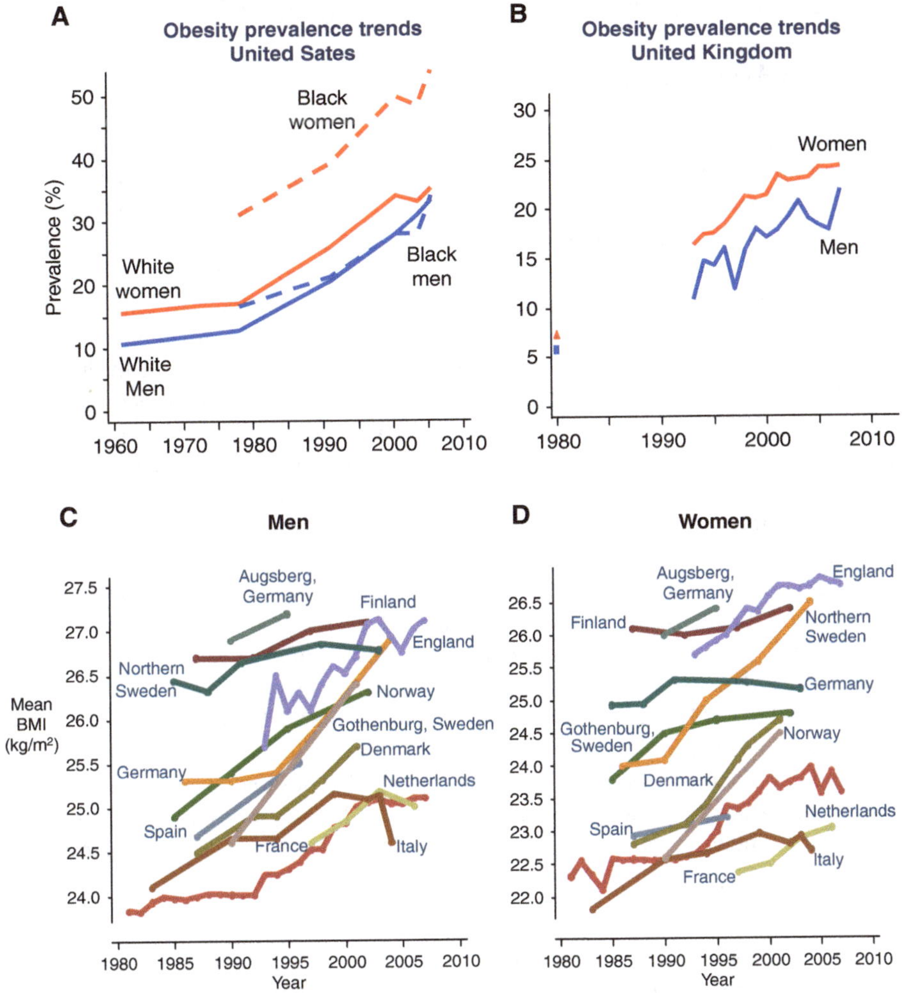

Fig. 2.1 Epidemiology of overweight and obesity (**a**) Trends in sex-specific obesity prevalences for Whites and Blacks in the United States (*Source*: National Health and Nutrition Examination Surveys). (**b**) Trends in sex-specific obesity prevalences in the United Kingdom (taken as equivalent to England and Wales) (*Source*: Office of National Statistics Health Survey for England). (**c** and **d**) Trends for means of BMI distributions for 12 populations across 10 European countries. References for studies are cited in the supplemental material of ref. [42] or available from author. Trends are all increasing and generally linear, with some countries demonstrating plateau effects. Note: different *y*-axis ranges for men and women

In countries where there have been robust nationally representative historical data, trends in BMI distributions have been increasing since the 1980s, though from different starting points and at different rates as shown in Fig. 2.1a–d. Trend increases have generally been linear, but there are signals from some countries (England, Netherlands, Italy) of 'tail off' in the past 5 years.

3 Associations Between Adiposity and Cancer Risk

3.1 Body Mass Index (BMI)

Epidemiological studies in the last three decades of the twentieth century often focused on associations between cancer risk and dietary macro- and micro-constituents and food processing, with less emphasis on the composite endpoints of nutrition, such as anthropometric measures and physical activity [6]. In 2002, the International Agency for Research into Cancer (IACR) [7] concluded, from a semi-quantitative review of the literature, that excess body weight is associated with increased risk of developing cancers of the post-menopausal breast, colorectum, endometrium, kidney and oesophageal adenocarcinoma. In 2007, the World Cancer Research Fund [8] used a more standardized approach to review the literature and reported that the evidence that body fatness is associated with increased risk of oesophageal adenocarcinoma, and with cancers of the pancreas, colorectum, post-menopausal breast, endometrium and kidney is 'convincing' and that a 'probable' association exists between body fatness and risk of gall bladder cancer.

In parallel with the World Cancer Research Fund report, the author together with collaborators from the University of Bern, Switzerland, reported in the *Lancet* [9] a systematic review and standardized meta-analysis of prospective observational studies (221 datasets including 281,137 incident cases) quantifying associations with a 5 kg/m^2 BMI increase and risk of incident cancer for 20 cancer types. The summary of the risk estimates by gender is shown in Table 2.1. By using the standardized approach across a large number of cancer types and an updated literature search (to December 2007, capturing several studies from Asia-Pacific populations not included in previous meta-analyses), we were able to demonstrate that associations

- are sex- and site-specific – for example, associations are consistently stronger for colon versus rectal cancer; in turn, within these cancer types, associations are stronger for men than women;
- exist for a wider range of malignancies than previously thought – 'new' obesity-related cancers added to the list were thyroid cancer, malignant melanoma in men, multiple myeloma, leukaemia and non-Hodgkin lymphoma;
- are broadly consistent across geographic populations, namely North American, European and Australian and Asia-Pacific;
- may be ranked per given change in BMI across the cancer types by gender;
- with excess body weight are significant for several cancer types conventionally considered non-smoking-related malignancies.

  In addition, we identified that for some cancer types, such as gastric cancer (based on reasonable study numbers), there are null associations, where earlier studies had raised possibilities that positive associations existed.

Table 2.1 Gender-specific estimated risk ratios by cancer types

	Men			Women		
	n^{a}	Risk ratio (95% CIs)	I^2 (%)	n^{a}	Risk ratio (95% CIs)	I^2 (%)
Colorectal cancer						
Colon	22	1.24 (1.20, 1.28)	21	19	1.09 (1.05, 1.13)	39
Rectum	18	1.09 (1.06, 1.12)	3	14	1.02 (1.00, 1.05)	0
Gall bladder cancer		No association		2	1.59 (1.02, 2.47)	67
Leukaemia	7	1.08 (1.02, 1.14)	0	7	1.17 (1.04, 1.32)	80
Malignant melanoma	6	1.17 (1.05, 1.30)	44		No association	
Multiple myeloma	7	1.11 (1.05, 1.18)	7	6	1.11 (1.07, 1.15)	0
Non-Hodgkin lymphoma	6	1.06 (1.03, 1.09)	0	7	1.07 (1.00, 1.14)	47
Oesophageal adenocarcinoma	5	1.52 (1.33, 1.74)	24	3	1.51 (1.31, 1.74)	0
Pancreatic cancer		No association		11	1.12 (1.02, 1.22)	43
Renal cancer	11	1.24 (1.15, 1.34)	21	12	1.34 (1.25, 1.43)	45
Thyroid cancer	4	1.33 (1.04, 1.70)	77	3	1.14 (1.06, 1.23)	5
Prostate cancer	27	1.03 (1.00, 1.09)	0		NA	
Post-menopausal breast cancer		NA		31	1.12 (1.08, 1.16)	43
Endometrial cancer		NA		19	1.59 (1.50, 1.68)	77

Risk estimates are per increase in 5 kg/m^2 BMI (body mass index)
All risk estimates are taken from meta-analyses of the previously published meta-analysis [9]
Only risk estimates for cancer types with a significant positive association with BMI are shown
[a]Number of studies
NA Not applicable

3.2 Other Adiposity-Related Anthropometric Measures

Body adiposity is often sub-classified as subcutaneous adipose tissue and visceral adipose tissue (VAT) – waist–hip ratio and waist circumference measurements are thought to better reflect central adiposity or VAT, whereas BMI reflects total body fatness (combined subcutaneous adipose tissue and visceral adipose tissue). Waist–hip ratio or waist circumference might therefore be better measures of adiposity than BMI in terms of cancer risk, as is the case for cardiovascular risk [10], but the number of cohort studies relating these parameters to subsequent cancer development is small.

Two previous meta-analyses [11, 12], both including case–control and cohort studies, examined the cumulative evidence linking waist–hip ratio and breast cancer risk. For pre-menopausal breast cancer risk, both analyses arrived at the same conclusion: namely that adiposity determined by waist–hip ratio reverses the inverse association noted with BMI to either a null or positive association. For post-menopausal breast cancer risk, the findings were less straightforward: the analysis by Connolly and colleagues [11] suggested that waist–hip ratio may have a stronger positive association than BMI, whereas the analysis by Harvie and colleagues [12], having adjusted for BMI, found a null association for waist–hip ratio.

For colorectal cancer, two meta-analyses [13, 14] addressed associations with waist–hip ratio and/or waist circumference, both limiting their inclusions to cohort studies. Dai and colleagues [13] concluded that indices of abdominal obesity are more sensitive than BMI for predicting cancer risk, but this conclusion was based on analyses of uppermost categories versus lowermost categories of distributions for BMI, waist–hip ratio and waist circumference – however, these may not be directly comparable categories. The analysis reported by Moghaddam and colleagues [14] used a dose–response approach and arrived at a more cautious conclusion – namely that for a 2 kg/m^2 increase in BMI, the risk of colorectal cancer increased by 7%, and for a 2 cm increase in waist circumference, the risk increased by 4%. Here again, however, it is unclear whether a 2 kg/m^2 increase in BMI and a 2 cm increase in waist circumference equate to equivalent quantities of adipose tissue.

The European Prospective Investigation into Cancer and Nutrition have recently examined this question for oesophageal cancer recognizing that two main histological types exist – oesophageal adenocarcinoma and oesophageal squamous cell carcinoma – and that associations with BMI are positive for oesophageal adenocarcinoma, yet negative for oesophageal squamous cell carcinoma [15]. The European Prospective Investigation into Cancer and Nutrition analysis found that where waist–hip ratio was the anthropometric measure of adiposity, the negative associations with oesophageal squamous cell carcinoma disappeared.

In summary, in at least two examples where BMI is inversely associated with cancer risk (pre-menopausal breast and oesophageal squamous cell carcinoma), indices of central adiposity probably provide a more appropriate measure, i.e. the true relationship with adiposity is probably a null association. However, where indices of central adiposity are 'more sensitive', measures of risk association is far from conclusive. In all of these analyses, one needs to be cautious in the interpretation of risk estimates derived from multivariate models due to potential problems of overfitting and collinearity between covariates.

4 Ecological Observations

If the associations between BMI and risk of several cancer types were causal (and the likelihood is that they are – see later), and given the rising trends of obesity in many populations, one may expect to observe parallel temporal trends in some obesity-related certain cancers. For example, in the United Kingdom, the incidence of endometrial cancer was relatively stable for two-and-half decades after the commencement of national cancer registrations in the early 1970s. However, after 1996, there have been clear increases – these may be attributable to the parallel increases in obesity in the United Kingdom population (Fig. 2.2a), but equally may reflect changes in other major risk factors, such as hormonal replacement therapy usage. By contrast, the incidence of endometrial cancer is little changed in White women in the United States (despite the increasing prevalence of obesity in this population over the time period 1975–2006), though there have been modest increases among Black women (Fig. 2.2b).

In a similar manner, there are well-documented increases in the incidences of oesophageal adenocarcinoma in countries such as the United Kingdom over the past decades (Fig. 2.2c) [16]. These may in part be attributable to the parallel rises in levels of obesity in that country. However, on deeper examination, it is clear that the rises in incidence of oesophageal adenocarcinoma predated the rises in obesity prevalence. Furthermore, for this cancer type, the incidence rates are considerably higher in men compared with women, despite the near identical risk estimates per 5 kg/m^2 increment in BMI for each gender. Taken together, increased prevalence of obesity in a population is likely to be only one of several 'drivers' of cancer incidence for that population. This contrasts with cigarette smoking prevalence in a population that does 'track' incidences of lung cancer-related mortality (albeit with a lag period of 30–40 years) [17]. For the exposure of excess body weight and cancer risk, associations are more modest (1.2–1.6 per shift from one World Health Organization BMI category to the next) compared with those of smoking and lung cancer (risk estimates from 12- to 20-fold for ever versus never smokers) [18], and there are several other factors determining rates of incident obesity-related cancers (e.g. mammographic, colorectal and prostate-specific antigen screening, hormone replacement therapy usage).

5 Biological Mechanisms

The mechanisms linking excess body weight and cancer risk are not fully understood (Table 2.2), though three hormonal systems – insulin and insulin-like growth factor (IGF) axis, sex steroids and adipokines – are the most studied candidates. Extensive reviews may be found elsewhere [19–22]. While all three systems are interlinked through insulin, their roles may vary between cancer sites. The

Table 2.2 Candidate mechanisms linking obesity and cancer risk

Most studied biological mechanisms	
	Insulin and insulin-like growth factors (IGFs)
	Sex steroids and sex steroid binding globulin
	Adipokines (e.g. adiponectin and leptin)
Hypoxia and angiogenesis	
Shared genetic susceptibility	
Migrating adipose stromal cells	
Other biological mechanisms	
	Obesity-related inflammatory cytokines
	Nuclear factor κβ system
	Altered immune response
Mechanical mechanisms	
	Hypertension and renal cancer
	Acid reflux and oesophageal adenocarcinoma
	Increased iodine uptake and thyroid cancer

Source: See ref. [20] for full details

Fig. 2.2 Ecological observations: trends in obesity and cancer risk. (**a**) Trends for endometrial cancer incidence in the United Kingdom (UK: for these purposes taken as equivalent to England and Wales). Endometrial cancer is an obesity-related malignancy ranked highest BMI–cancer association among women ([9]). For the United Kingdom, secular trends increased in the past decade consistent with the corresponding increasing trends in prevalence of obesity. (**b**) By contrast, secular trends for endometrial cancer incidence in the United States have remained essentially constant in Whites and risen only slightly among Blacks (source: SEER 9 areas http://seer.cancer.gov/). (**c**) Sex-specific secular trends for oesophageal adenocarcinoma incidences in the United Kingdom (*Source*: Ref. [16]). *Standardized against European standard population. †Standardized against US standard population

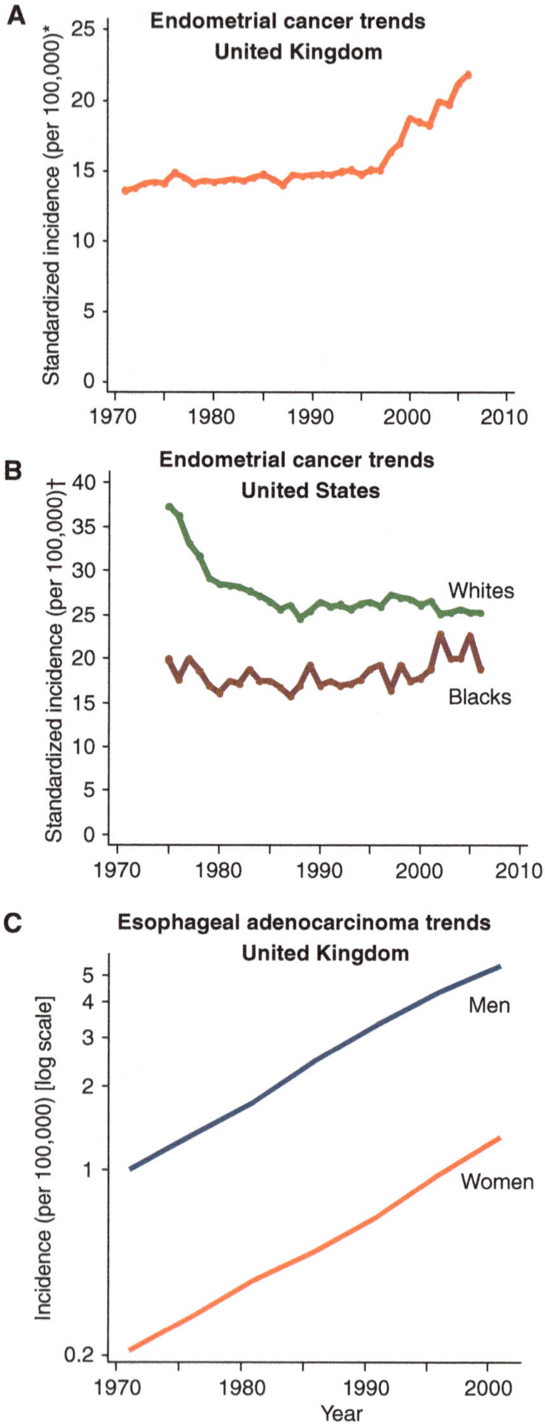

insulin-IGF hypothesis postulates that chronic hyperinsulinaemia decreases concentrations of IGF binding proteins-1 and -2, leading to increased bio-available or free IGF-I with concomitant changes in the cellular environment (IGF-I increases mitosis; is anti-apoptotic, pro-angiogenic; and increases cell motility) favouring tumour formation [23]. Circulating total IGF-I, a major determinant of free IGF-I concentrations, is also consistently associated with increased risk of prostate, colorectal and pre-menopausal breast cancers [24], and in some studies of post-menopausal breast cancer [25, 26]. Mean circulating concentrations of total IGF-I are higher in men than women [27], which may in part explain some observed differences, for instance, in colorectal cancer risk are greater in men compared with women. However, the insulin-IGF hypothesis has two fundamental inconsistencies – first, levels of total IGF-I increase linearly with increasing BMI but only to a pivotal point around 27 kg/m^2, thereafter declining with increasing weight [23]; second, in overweight/obese individuals who intentionally lose weight (a presumed cancer-protective behaviour), total IGF-I concentrations tend to increase (a conceptually 'bad' environment for cancer risk) [28].

For post-menopausal breast cancer, the increase in risk might be explained by the higher rates of conversion of androgenic precursors to oestradiol through increased aromatase enzyme activity in adipose tissue. In endometrial cancer, there may be more than one system involved: Increased oestradiol levels not only increase endometrial cell proliferation and inhibit apoptosis but might also stimulate the local synthesis of IGF-I in endometrial tissue [21]. Furthermore, chronic hyperinsulinaemia may promote tumourigenesis in oestrogen-sensitive tissues by reducing blood concentrations of sex hormone binding globulin, which in turn increases bio-available oestrogen [21]. Adiposity is inversely related to testosterone concentrations in men [29], but positively related in women [30], which may be relevant to gender differences in the relationship of BMI and cancer risk.

Adiponectin is the most abundant adipokine, secreted mainly from VAT, and is inversely correlated with BMI. In terms of tumour development, this insulin-sensitizing agent is anti-inflammatory, anti-angiogenic and inhibits tumour growth in animal models [31]. Beyond these mechanisms, other candidate systems include mutual genetic susceptibility, obesity-related inflammatory cytokines, altered immune response, oxidative stresses, obesity-related hypoxia, adipocyte-secreted pro-angiogenic factors, the nuclear factor κβ system [23], hypertension and lipid peroxidation for renal cancer [32] and acid reflux for oesophageal adenocarcinoma [33, 34]. The mechanisms linking adiposity and less common malignancies are speculative.

6 Causal Association and Attributable Risk

While the syntheses from others [8] and our review [9] demonstrated associations between BMI and cancer risks, a key question (not least for the development of cancer prevention strategies) is whether these associations are causally related. We recently addressed this in a review testing the data from our systematic review against the nine Bradford-Hill criteria [35, 36] for judging causal association. The review [37] argued that the available data support strength of association, consistency, specificity, temporality, biological gradient, plausibility, coherence and probably analogy, suggesting that many of the observed associations are probably causal. Additionally, recent studies with long-term follow-up of patients undergoing bariatric surgery for morbid obesity point to a reduction in cancer incidence (albeit this reduction seems limited to women) associated with sustained weight loss [38, 39], and in turn, add further support to a causal association between obesity and cancer risk. Furthermore, investigators have argued that additional criteria for assessing causality should include adjustment for available confounding factors, evaluation of measurement error and study design and assessment of residual confounding [40] – these too were evaluated in our review [37] and we found lack of alternative explanations.

Given the likely causal association, it seems reasonable to ask the question, what proportion of cancers in a population are attributable to excess body weight, as this in turn relates to the potential number of avoidable incident cancers. The media often highlight that obesity is linked to 20% of all cancer deaths in women and 14% in men, quoting the large US Cancer Prevention Study II [41]. Using the risk estimates derived from our meta-analysis [9], we recently estimated more conservative population attributable risks for incident cancers of 3.2% in men and 8.6% in women [42]. Nonetheless, across 30 European countries, this amounts to over 124,000 avoidable cancer cases per year; and importantly, this analysis showed that as the prevalence of hormonal replacement therapy usage declines (hormonal replacement therapy tends to attenuate the relative effect of BMI – see later) and BMI distributions in populations are 'skewed to the right', these numbers may climb considerably in the future.

7 Confounding and Effect Modifications

7.1 Hormonal Replacement Therapy and Breast Cancer

Evidence from randomized controlled trials [43] and observational studies [44] have shown that women taking hormonal replacement therapy for menopause are at increased risk of breast cancer, a risk that is greater with the use of combined oestrogen–progesterone than oestrogen-only preparations. As hyperoestrogenaemia secondary to increased aromatase activity in peripheral adipose tissue is relevant to the development of obesity-related post-menopausal breast cancer, it is reasonable to hypothesize that the use of hormonal replacement therapy may effect the association between BMI and breast cancer risk. This hypothesis has been tested in at least five cohort studies [45–49] where risk estimates were reported stratified by hormonal replacement therapy status. Table 2.3 summarizes these studies and demonstrates that hormonal replacement therapy is an effect modifier for the associations between BMI and post-menopausal breast cancer, namely risk estimates per 5 kg/m^2 increase in BMI are higher among never users compared with ever users.

Table 2.3 Associations between BMI and post-menopausal breast cancer risk stratified by HRT usage

	Total cohort		Never users		Ever users		
	n[a]	Risk ratio (95% CIs)	n[a]	Risk ratio (95% CIs)	HRT type	n[a]	Risk ratio (95% CIs)
Morimoto et al. [45]	1030	1.11 (0.83, 1.50)	319	1.34 (1.18, 1.52)	HRT, NOS	711	1.00 (0.91, 1.10)
Feigelson et al. [46]	1934	1.08 (0.98, 1.19)	1182	1.22 (1.14, 1.30)	EO and EP combined[b]	752	0.94 (0.85, 1.03)
Lahmann et al. [47]	1402	1.05 (0.86, 1.28)	911	1.14 (1.04, 1.26)	HRT, NOS	494	0.88 (0.77, 1.01)
Mellemkjaer et al. [48]	633	1.02 (0.93, 1.12)	217	1.08 (0.93, 1.24)	HRT, NOS	416	0.98 (0.86, 1.11)
Ahn et al. [49]	2087	1.10 (0.95, 1.28)[c]	925	1.19 (1.13, 1.27)	HRT, NOS	1162	1.02 (0.95, 1.09)

Risk estimates are per increase in 5 kg/m^2 BMI (body mass index) as per methods used in ref. [9]

CI confidence intervals, *HRT* hormonal replacement therapy, *NOS* not otherwise specified

[a]Number of cases

[b]*EO* (oestrogen only) and *EP* (oestrogen and progesterone) reported together as 'risk ratio estimates were similar in the two groups'

[c]This risk estimate is not reported directly in the paper – instead this has been calculated combining the estimates for never and ever HRT (random-effects)

Indeed, associations in ever users are generally null: The mechanistic implication is that the 'excess' oestrogen environment associated with hormonal replacement therapy (of the order of a 10-fold increase compared with normal physiological ranges) dilutes the association seen between BMI and post-menopausal breast cancer risk. These observations are consistent with the findings of the Million Women Study [50] and other studies (seven studies cited in ref. [48]) where the increase risk associated with use of oestrogen-only or combined oestrogen–progesterone is attenuated with increasing BMI category. The observations are also consistent with the findings from the pooled analysis of the Hormonal Breast Collaborative that the increase in breast cancer risk associated with BMI is largely accounted for by circulating oestrogen levels [30].

A further dimension to the association between BMI and breast cancer risk is mammographic density, the latter being negatively correlated with BMI. Where there is adjustment of mammographic density, BMI–cancer risk estimates increase [51].

7.2 Hormonal Replacement Therapy and Endometrial Cancer

Similar to breast cancer risk, evidence from randomized controlled trials [52] and observational studies [53] have shown that post-menopausal women taking hormonal replacement therapy are at increased risk of endometrial cancer, but in contrast, the risk is greater with the use of oestrogen-only compared with combined oestrogen–progesterone, as the inclusion of progesterone is thought to offer some protection. Here again, it is reasonable to hypothesize that the use of hormonal replacement therapy may effect the association between BMI and endometrial cancer risk. Three cohort studies [54–56] have reported risk estimates stratified by hormonal replacement therapy status, and similar findings to those for breast cancer emerge (Table 2.4); namely, the risk estimates per 5 kg/m^2 increase BMI are higher among never users compared with ever users. When these data are taken together with the findings from the Million Women Study [57] (which only reported on the interaction between BMI, hormonal replacement therapy and endometrial cancer risk among hormonal replacement therapy ever users), it appears that the risk estimates per 5 kg/m^2 for cyclical combined hormonal replacement therapy were similar to those for oestrogen-only (approximately 1.20) and only return a null association for continuous combined hormonal replacement therapy, suggesting that the effect of progesterone is dependent on the numbers of days per cycle exposure. Furthermore, in the example of endometrial cancer, obesity is predominantly a risk factor for type I endometrioid tumours (accounting for 70% of endometrial cancers), which is linked with hyperoestrogenic states [58].

7.3 BMI, Smoking and Cancer Risk

In our meta-analysis [9], we noted three cancer types in which the association between BMI and risk was inverse, namely pre-menopausal breast cancer,

Table 2.4 Associations between BMI and endometrial cancer risk stratified by HRT usage

	Total cohort		Never users		Ever users		
	n^a	Risk ratio (95% CIs)	n^a	Risk ratio (95% CIs)	HRT type	n^a	Risk ratio (95% CIs)
Chang et al. [54]	677	1.40 (1.17, 167)	358	2.26 (1.87, 2.73)	EO	34	1.19 (0.93, 1.53)
Chang et al. [54]	NA		NA		EP, NOS	242	1.25 (1.05, 1.47)
Friedenreich et al. [55]	567	1.34 (1.22, 1.47)	151	1.61 (1.151, 1.85)	HRT, NOS	186	1.10 (0.88,1.38)
McCullough et al. [56]	318	1.89 (1.64, 2.17)	207	1.93 (1.64, 2.28)	EP, NOS	186	1.29 (0.82, 2.01)
Beral et al. [57]	NA		NA		EP continuous	73	1.02 (0.73, 1.42)
Beral et al. [57]	NA		NA		EP cyclic	242	1.25 (1.05, 1.47)

Risk estimates are per increase in 5 kg/m^2 BMI (body mass index) as per methods used in ref. [9]

CI confidence intervals, *NA* not applicable, *EO* oestrogen only, *EP* oestrogen and progesterone combined, *HRT, NOS* hormonal replacement therapy, not otherwise specified

[a]Number of cases

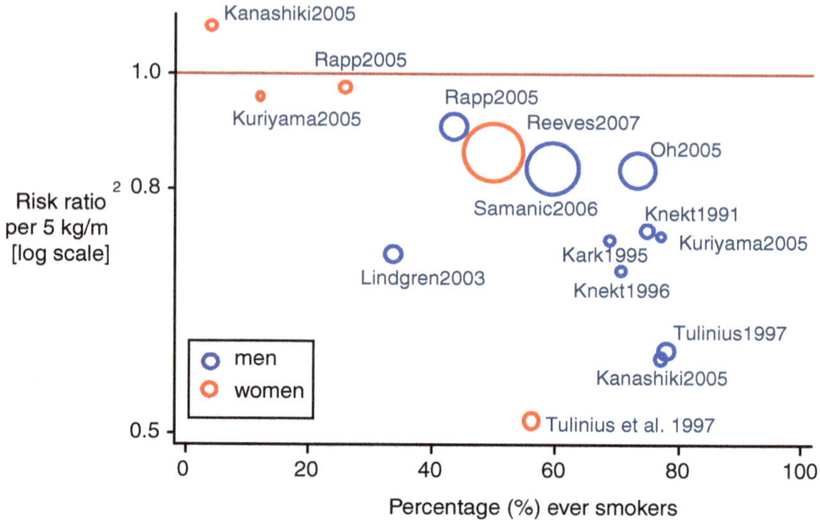

Fig. 2.3 BMI, smoking and lung cancer risk. Plot of sex-specific risk ratios per 5 kg/m^2 increment increase in BMI (i.e. 'slopes') for cohort studies of lung cancer risk versus percentage ever smokers per study. The references for the studies are available from the supplemental file of ref. [9] and author. The size of each circle is proportional to the sample size of each cohort. The plot demonstrates that as the percentage of ever smokers increases, the 'study–slope' or BMI–cancer association becomes more negative

oesophageal squamous cell carcinoma and lung cancer (in the latter two, these inverse relationships were in both genders). Clearly, the public health message here is not one that if a population is overweight and obese, they are at less risk of these cancers. As pointed out in an earlier section, the associations between adiposity and pre-menopausal breast cancer and oesophageal squamous cell carcinoma may be better expressed using indices of central obesity. For lung cancer, given the well-recognized observation that smokers consistently have a lower mean BMI [59] and the strong association between smoking and lung cancer risk, it is reasonable to hypothesize that smoking may be an effect modifier in the relationship between BMI and lung cancer risk. This indeed seems to be the case (Fig. 2.3) – when sex-specific risk estimates per 5 kg/m^2 (derived from the analysis in ref. [9]) are plotted against the prevalence of smoking in the sex-specific populations of each study, the greater the percentage ever smokers, the greater the inverse association. In the absence of smoking, it appears that the association between BMI and lung cancer risk is null.

Interestingly, when the European Prospective Investigation into Cancer and Nutrition investigators [15] recently examined the question of the relationship between adiposity and oesophageal cancer risk recognizing that two main histological types exist – oesophageal adenocarcinoma and oesophageal squamous cell carcinoma – they found, as in our meta-analysis [9], a strong association between BMI and oesophageal adenocarcinoma. This was essentially unaffected when the data were analysed by smokers and non-smokers. In sharp contrast, the association between BMI and oesophageal squamous cell carcinoma, which was significantly inverse among smokers (risk estimate for uppermost quintile versus lowermost quintile: 0.09, 0.03–0.29) was null among non-smokers (0.68, 0.11–4.10).

7.4 PSA Screening and Prostate Cancer Risk

Initial epidemiologic data appeared to suggest that increasing BMI was positively associated with prostate cancer risk. For all invasive prostate cancers, when we meta-analysed risk estimates across 27 cohort studies [9], the summary estimate was only very modestly positive (1.03, 1.00–1.07). However, there was considerable heterogeneity judged by the heterogeneity statistic I^2 value of 73%. A variety of commentaries [60–62] suggest that BMI is associated with high-grade and/or aggressive histological types of prostate cancer (and possibly a reduced risk of low-grade/less aggressive prostate cancer). Supporting this posit, obesity is consistently associated with an increased rate of prostate cancer progression and mortality [62]. In turn, the proportion of high-grade/aggressive histology prostate cancers in a cohort reflects the level of prostate-specific antigen screening in that population and hence the high level of heterogeneity noted may be partly explained by the level of prostate-specific antigen screening. This would appear to be true – Fig. 2.4 shows risk ratios per 5 kg/m^2 increment increases in BMI per study plotted against the

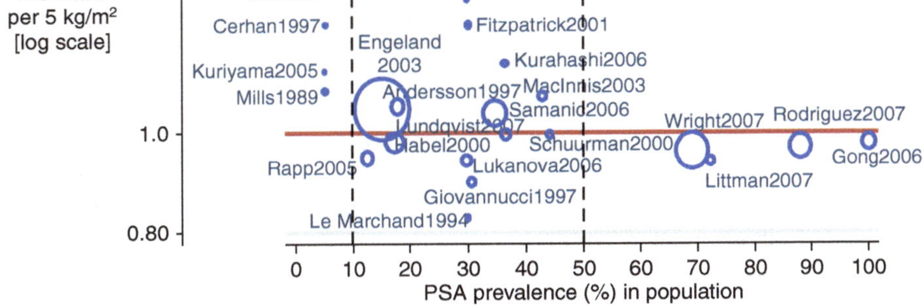

Fig. 2.4 BMI, PSA screening and prostate cancer risk. Plot of sex-specific risk ratios per 5 kg/m^2 increment increase in BMI (i.e. 'slopes') for cohort studies of prostate cancer risk versus prevalence of PSA screening per study. The references for the studies are available from the supplemental file of ref. [9] and author. The size of each circle is proportional to the sample size of each cohort. Where exact prevalence was not reported in each paper, the prevalence was allotted to the mid-point of respective categories: 'no routine PSA screening or very low prevalence'; 'moderate level of PSA screening'; or 'widespread PSA screening'. The plot demonstrates that as the level or prevalence of PSA screening in a population increases, the 'study–slope' or BMI–cancer association approaches one or 'null'

prevalence of prostate-specific antigen screening. In recent studies with large sample sizes and greater than 50% prevalence of prostate-specific antigen screening in the populations, the associations between overall prostate cancer risk and BMI are essentially null.

There are a number of site-specific mechanisms that need to be considered in the interpretation of associations between obesity and prostate cancer risk as follows:

- increasing BMI is correlated with a reduction in mean serum prostate-specific antigen concentrations;
- there is an inherent bias in a clinician's ability to detect prostate cancer in obese men as larger sized prostates make biopsy less accurate for finding an existing cancer;
- obesity (and type 2 diabetes) is associated with lower testosterone mean levels compared with normal weight men;
- recent genetic studies have highlighted a potential genetic link between insulin resistance and prostate cancer: One study identified an allele in the *HNF1B* (also known as *TCF2*) gene that predisposes to type 2 diabetes, while also protecting men from prostate cancer; another study identified different variants in the *JAZF1* gene, one associated with insulin resistance, another associated with prostate cancer [63].

8 Future Directions

Important questions remain in relation to the cumulative effects of excess body weight over several decades, the effect of key weight change periods in the life-course of individuals and interactions with other risk factors [64]. Other unresolved questions relate to the most appropriate measure of adiposity in terms of cancer risk, the mechanisms underpinning the observed gender differences and whether there are differences across ethnicities. Finally, while public health policies aimed at curbing the underlying causes of the obesity epidemic are being implemented, there is a parallel need to better understand the biological processes linking obesity and cancer as a pre-requisite to the development of new approaches to the prevention and treatment of obesity-related cancers.

References

1. Simopoulos AP (1987) Obesity and carcinogenesis: historical perspective. Am J Clin Nutr 45(1 Suppl):271–276
2. Kelly T, Yang W, Chen CS, Reynolds K, He J (2008) Global burden of obesity in 2005 and projections to 2030. Int J Obes (London) 32(9):1431–1437
3. CDC (2006) State-specific prevalence of obesity among adults – United States, 2005. MMWR wkly 55(36):985–988.

4. Health Survey for England 2007 Latest trends (2007) http://www.ic.nhs.uk/statistics-and-data-collections/health-and-lifestyles-related-surveys/health-survey-for-england/health-survey-for-england-2007-latest-trends-%5Bns%5D (accessed August 2009)
5. Canoy D, Buchan I (2007) Challenges in obesity epidemiology. Obes Rev 8(Suppl 1):1–11
6. WCRF (1997) World Cancer Research Fund. Food, nutrition and the prevention of cancer: a global perspective. American Institute for Cancer Research, Washington, DC
7. IARC (2002) International agency for research in cancer. In: Vainio H, Bianchini F (eds) Weight control and physical activity. IARC Press, Lyon
8. WCRF (2007) World Cancer Research Fund. Food, Nutrition, Physical Activity, and the Prevention of Cancer: a Global Perspective, 2nd edn. American Institute for Cancer Research, Washington
9. Renehan A, Tyson M, Egger M, Heller RF, Zwahlen M (2008) Body mass index and incidence of cancer: a systematic review and meta-analysis of prospective observational studies. Lancet 371(9612):569–578
10. Yusuf S, Hawken S, Ounpuu S, Bautista L, Franzosi MG, Commerford P et al (2005) Obesity and the risk of myocardial infarction in 27,000 participants from 52 countries: a case-control study. Lancet 366(9497):1640–1649
11. Connolly BS, Barnett C, Vogt KN, Li T, Stone J, Boyd NF (2003) A meta-analysis of published literature on waist-to-hip ratio and risk of breast cancer. Nutr Cancer 44(2): 127–138
12. Harvie M, Hooper L, Howell AH (2003) Central obesity and breast cancer risk: a systematic review. Obes Rev 4(3):157–173
13. Dai Z, Xu YC, Niu L (2007) Obesity and colorectal cancer risk: a meta-analysis of cohort studies. World J Gastroenterol 13(31):4199–4206
14. Moghaddam AA, Woodward M, Huxley R (2007) Obesity and risk of colorectal cancer: a meta-analysis of 31 studies with 70,000 events. Cancer Epidemiol Biomarkers Prev 16(12):2533–2547
15. Steffen A, Schulze MB, Pischon T, Dietrich T, Molina E, Chirlaque MD et al (2009) Anthropometry and esophageal cancer risk in the European prospective investigation into cancer and nutrition. Cancer Epidemiol Biomarkers Prev 18(7):2079–2089
16. Lepage C, Rachet B, Jooste V, Faivre J, Coleman MP (2008) Continuing rapid increase in esophageal adenocarcinoma in England and Wales. Am J Gastroenterol 103(11): 2694–2699
17. Peto R, Darby S, Deo H, Silcocks P, Whitley E, Doll R (2000) Smoking, smoking cessation, and lung cancer in the UK since 1950: combination of national statistics with two case-control studies. Bmj 321(7257):323–329
18. IARC (2004) IARC monographs on the evaluation of carcinogenic risks to humans. Tobacco Smoke and Involuntary Smoking, vol 83. WHO/IARC, Lyon
19. Renehan AG, Roberts DL, Dive C (2008) Obesity and cancer: pathophysiological and biological mechanisms. Arch Physiol Biochem 114(1):71–83
20. Roberts DL, Dive C, Renehan AG (2009) Biological Mechanisms linking obesity and cancer risk: new perspectives. Ann Rev Med 61:301–316
21. Calle EE, Kaaks R (2004) Overweight, obesity and cancer: epidemiological evidence and proposed mechanisms. Nat Rev Cancer 4(8):579–591
22. van Kruijsdijk RC, van der Wall E, Visseren FL (2009) Obesity and cancer: the role of dysfunctional adipose tissue. Cancer Epidemiol Biomarkers Prev 18(10):2569–2578
23. Renehan AG, Frystyk J, Flyvbjerg A (2006) Obesity and cancer risk: the role of the insulin-IGF axis. Trends Endocrinol Metab 17(8):328–336
24. Renehan AG, Zwahlen M, Minder C, O'Dwyer ST, Shalet SM, Egger M (2004) Insulin-like growth factor (IGF)-I, IGF binding protein-3, and cancer risk: systematic review and meta-regression analysis. Lancet 363:1346–1353
25. Rinaldi S, Peeters PH, Berrino F, Dossus L, Biessy C, Olsen A, et al. (2006) IGF-I, IGFBP-3 and breast cancer risk in women: The European Prospective Investigation into Cancer and Nutrition (EPIC. Endocr Relat Cancer 13(2):593–605

26. Baglietto L, English DR, Hopper JL, Morris HA, Tilley WD, Giles GG (2007) Circulating insulin-like growth factor-I and binding protein-3 and the risk of breast cancer. Cancer Epidemiol Biomarkers Prev 16(4):763–768
27. Juul A, Bang P, Hertel NT, Main K, Dalgaard P, Jorgensen K, et al. (1994) Serum insulin-like growth factor-I in 1030 healthy children, adolescents, and adults: relation to age, sex, stage of puberty, testicular size, and body mass index. J Clin Endocrinol Metab 78(3):744–752
28. Harvie M, Renehan AG, Frystyk J, Flyvbjerg A, Mercer T, Malik R et al (2010) Paradoxical increases in serum total IGF-I and maintenance of free IGF-I levels following 12 months of intentional weight loss in pre-menopausal women at increased risk of breast cancer. BMC Open J Obes doi:10.2174/1876823701002020063
29. Derby CA, Zilber S, Brambilla D, Morales KH, McKinlay JB (2006) Body mass index, waist circumference and waist to hip ratio and change in sex steroid hormones: the Massachusetts Male Ageing Study. Clin Endocrinol (Oxf) 65(1):125–131
30. Key TJ, Appleby PN, Reeves GK, Roddam A, Dorgan JF, Longcope C et al (2003) Body mass index, serum sex hormones, and breast cancer risk in postmenopausal women. J Natl Cancer Inst 95(16):1218–1226
31. Rose DP, Komninou D, Stephenson GD (2004) Obesity, adipocytokines, and insulin resistance in breast cancer. Obes Rev 5(3):153–165
32. Gago-Dominguez M, Castelao JE, Yuan JM, Ross RK, Yu MC (2002) Lipid peroxidation: a novel and unifying concept of the etiology of renal cell carcinoma (United States). Cancer Causes Control 13(3):287–293
33. Whiteman DC, Sadeghi S, Pandeya N, Smithers BM, Gotley DC, Bain CJ et al (2008) Combined effects of obesity, acid reflux and smoking on the risk of adenocarcinomas of the oesophagus. Gut 57(2):173–180
34. Jacobson BC, Chan AT, Giovannucci EL, Fuchs CS (2009) Body mass index and Barrett's oesophagus in women. Gut 58(11):1460–1466
35. Hill AB (1965) The environment and disease: association or causation? Proc Royal Soc Med (London) 88:295–300
36. Hofler M (2005) The Bradford Hill considerations on causality: a counterfactual perspective. Emerg Themes Epidemiol 2:11
37. Renehan AG, Egger M, Zwahlen M (2010) Body mass index and cancer risk: the evidence for causal association. BMC Open J Obesity doi:10.2174/1876823701002020012
38. Sjostrom L, Gunmmessson A, Sjostrom CD, Narbro K, Peltonen M, Wedel H et al (2009) Effects of bariatric surgery on cancer incidences in Sweden (Swedish Obese Subjects): a prospective, controlled intervention trial. Lancet Oncol 10(7):653–662
39. Renehan AG (2009) Bariatric surgery, weight reduction and cancer prevention. Lancet Oncol 10:640–641
40. Lawlor DA, Davey Smith G, Bruckdorfer KR, Kundu D, Ebrahim S (2004) Those confounding vitamins: what can we learn from the differences between observational versus randomised trial evidence?. Lancet 363:1724–1727
41. Calle EE, Rodriguez C, Walker-Thurmond K, Thun MJ (2003) Overweight, obesity, and mortality from cancer in a prospectively studied cohort of U.S. adults. N Engl J Med 348(17):1625–1638
42. Renehan AG, Soerjomataram I, Tyson M, Egger M, Zwahlen M, Coebergh JW, et al. (2010) Incident cancer burden attributable to excess body mass index in 30 European countries. Int J Cancer 126(3):692–702
43. Nelson HD, Humphrey LL, Nygren P, Teutsch SM, Allan JD (2002) Postmenopausal hormone replacement therapy: scientific review. JAMA 288(7):872–881
44. Beral V (2003) Breast cancer and hormone-replacement therapy in the Million Women Study. Lancet 362(9382):419–427
45. Morimoto LM, White E, Chen Z, Chlebowski RT, Hays J, Kuller L et al (2002) Obesity, body size, and risk of postmenopausal breast cancer: the Women's Health Initiative (United States). Cancer Causes Control 13(8):741–751

46. Feigelson HS, Jonas CR, Teras LR, Thun MJ, Calle EE (2004) Weight gain, body mass index, hormone replacement therapy, and postmenopausal breast cancer in a large prospective study. Cancer Epidemiol Biomarkers Prev 13(2):220–224
47. Lahmann PH, Hoffmann K, Allen N, Van G CH, Khaw KT, Tehard B et al (2004) Body size and breast cancer risk: findings from the European Prospective Investigation into Cancer and Nutrition (EPIC). International Journal of Cancer 111(5):762–771
48. Mellemkjaer L, Bigaard J, Tjonneland A, Christensen J, Thomsen B, Johansen C et al (2006) Body composition and breast cancer in postmenopausal women: a Danish prospective cohort study. Obesity (Silver Spring) 14(10):1854–1862
49. Ahn J, Schatzkin A, Lacey JV Jr, Albanes D, Ballard-Barbash R, Adams KF et al (2007) Adiposity, adult weight change, and postmenopausal breast cancer risk. Arch Intern Med 167(19):2091–2102
50. Reeves GK, Beral V, Green J, Gathani T, Bull D (2006) Hormonal therapy for menopause and breast-cancer risk by histological type: a cohort study and meta-analysis. Lancet Oncol 7(11):910–918
51. Boyd NF, Martin LJ, Sun L, Guo H, Chiarelli A, Hislop G et al (2006) Body size, mammographic density, and breast cancer risk. Cancer Epidemiol Biomarkers Prev 15(11):2086–2092
52. Hulley SB, Grady D (2004) The WHI estrogen-alone trial – do things look any better?. JAMA 291(14):1769–1771
53. Grady D, Gebretsadik T, Kerlikowske K, Ernster V, Petitti D (1995) Hormone replacement therapy and endometrial cancer risk: a meta-analysis. Obstet Gynecol 85(2):304–313
54. Chang SC, Lacey JV Jr., Brinton LA, Hartge P, Adams K, Mouw T, et al. (2007) Lifetime weight history and endometrial cancer risk by type of menopausal hormone use in the NIH-AARP diet and health study. Cancer Epidemiol Biomarkers Prev 16(4):723–730
55. Friedenreich C, Cust A, Lahmann PH, Steindorf K, Boutron-Ruault MC, Clavel-Chapelon F et al (2007) Anthropometric factors and risk of endometrial cancer: the European prospective investigation into cancer and nutrition. Cancer Causes Control 18(4):399–413
56. McCullough ML, Patel AV, Patel R, Rodriguez C, Feigelson HS, Bandera EV et al (2008) Body mass and endometrial cancer risk by hormone replacement therapy and cancer subtype. Cancer Epidemiol Biomarkers Prev 17(1):73–79
57. Beral V, Bull D, Reeves G (2005) Endometrial cancer and hormone-replacement therapy in the Million Women Study. Lancet 365(9470):1543–1551
58. Bokhman JV (1983) Two pathogenetic types of endometrial carcinoma. Gynecol Oncol 15(1):10–17
59. Prospective Studies C (2009) Body-mass index and cause-specific mortality in 900 000 adults: collaborative analyses of 57 prospective studies. Lancet 373(9669):1083–1096
60. Freedland SJ, Giovannucci E, Platz EA (2006) Are findings from studies of obesity and prostate cancer really in conflict?. Cancer Causes Control 17(1):5–9
61. Freedland SJ, Platz EA (2007) Obesity and prostate cancer: making sense out of apparently conflicting data. Epidemiol Rev 29:88–97
62. Hsing AW, Sakoda LC, Chua S Jr (2007) Obesity, metabolic syndrome, and prostate cancer. Am J Clin Nutr 86(3):s843–s857
63. Frayling TM, Colhoun H, Florez JC (2008) A genetic link between type 2 diabetes and prostate cancer. Diabetologia 51(10):1757–1760
64. Ben-Shlomo Y, Kuh D (2002) A life course approach to chronic disease epidemiology: conceptual models, empirical challenges and interdisciplinary perspectives. Int J Epidemiol 31(2):285–293

Chapter 3
Epidemiology of Physical Activity and Cancer Risk

Rebecca M. Speck, Kathryn H. Schmitz, I.-Min Lee, and Anne McTiernan

Abstract There is a large amount of epidemiological data derived from cohort and case–control studies regarding the association between physical activity and risk of developing cancer. Most of the evidence is available for breast and colon cancers. In summarizing the research to date, the effect of physical activity on colon cancer is a reduction in risk of 25% for men and women. The reduced risk of breast cancer across studies is a median 20%. A body of evidence is growing that supports a protective effect of physical activity for lung and endometrial cancers as well. Many studies have evaluated physical activity and prostate cancer risk; the evidence has been inconsistent. Physical fitness has been evaluated in cohort studies for its association with cancer mortality. Findings suggest that increased levels of physical fitness decrease the risk of cancer mortality by more than 50% in men. Evidence as to the association in women is limited, and additional research is needed in this area.

1 Introduction

In the United States, the likelihood of an individual developing cancer within their lifetime is 44% for men and 37% for women, translating to projections of 1,479,350 new cancer cases and 562,340 deaths in the United States for 2009 [1]. However, those estimates are based on general population data and may be an overestimate or underestimate of individual risk as a result of variation in genetic predisposition and environmental factors. It is estimated that 10–15% of cancer is due to genetic susceptibility [2], and the remainder a result of environmental and lifestyle factors that are not inherited [3]. Evidence suggests that one third of cancer deaths may be due to diet and physical activity habits, and that maintaining a healthy weight and staying physically active or adopting an active lifestyle can reduce an individual's lifetime risk of developing cancer [4, 5].

R.M. Speck (✉)
Division of Clinical Epidemiology, Department of Biostatistics and Epidemiology, University of Pennsylvania, School of Medicine, Philadelphia, PA 19104-6021, USA
e-mail: speckr@mail.med.upenn.edu

A. McTiernan (ed.), *Physical Activity, Dietary Calorie Restriction, and Cancer*, Energy Balance and Cancer 3, DOI 10.1007/978-1-4419-7551-5_3,

Of all cancer sites, the association between increased physical activity and reduced risk of cancer development has been observed most consistently for breast and colon cancers. There is increasing evidence supporting a reduced risk of endometrial and lung cancers in physically active versus sedentary persons. Numerous studies have examined the association between physical activity and prostate cancer, and have found no association between physical activity and risk of prostate cancer. Unfortunately, there are too few data available to determine whether physical activity affects the risk of developing cancer at other sites.

1.1 Physical Activity and Cancer Incidence

Much research has been conducted in order to understand the association between physical activity and the risk of developing various types of cancer. Epidemiologic data providing direct evidence of the association of physical activity and cancer have been derived from observational studies (cohort and case–control designs), while randomized controlled trials (RCTs) have yielded indirect evidence through examining the association of physical activity with markers of cancer risk, such as circulating levels of sex hormones, insulin, and cytokines. An important consideration in summarizing and interpreting epidemiologic data is the variation in methods and means by which physical activity information is assessed and presented from study to study.

Observational data from cohort and case–control studies supporting a moderate, inverse relationship between physical activity and the risk of development of cancer are the most consistent for colon and breast cancer. Individuals engaging in aerobic physical activity for approximately 3–4 h/week at moderate or greater levels of intensity have on average a 30% reduction in colon cancer risk and a 20–40% lower risk of breast cancer, compared with those who are sedentary. The risk decreases at higher levels of physical activity, indicating a dose–response relation. However, little information exists as to what additional amount and intensity of physical activity is associated with further risk reductions, as well as what magnitude the additional decreases in risk may be. The available evidence suggests that at least 30–60 min per day of moderate to vigorous intensity physical activity is required to significantly lower the risk of colon and breast cancer.

In comparison to sedentary people, epidemiologic data suggest that active people have approximately 20–30% reductions in risk of lung, endometrial, and ovarian cancers. Overall, the data do not support associations of physical activity and prostate or rectal cancers. Further, too few data exist in other site-specific cancers to frame conclusions.

1.1.1 Methods and Study Design

Assessing physical activity in relation to cancer can be challenging. There are study design and methodologic issues that need to be considered in order to properly assess physical activity, adjust for potential confounding variables, and account for and interpret a meaningful temporal relationship. These common research challenges demand knowledge of epidemiologic study design and methods when interpreting and summarizing the findings observed between studies.

The goal in assessing physical activity is to quantify the intensity, frequency, and duration of recreational, occupational, and household activity, though this is complex and usually not feasible [6]. Depending on the study design and sample size, certain methods of data collection can be costly and inconvenient. Further, assessment should take place at multiple time points because a single response does not accurately reflect the patterns of physical activity that may occur in the lifetime of an individual.

Investigators have measured physical activity via multiple methods including:

- self-report questionnaire
- participation in high school or college athletics
- occupational status
- objectively measured fitness levels

Each method has its advantages depending on the target population and research resources available. However, the common limitation of all methods is the potential inaccuracy that results from inferring patterned or lifetime physical activity behavior based on the data collected at minimal time points or with narrow scope.

The study designs responsible for providing the direct evidence of a physical activity and cancer association are case–control and cohort study designs. The known limitation of case–control designs is the real potential for bias in the recall of physical activity. Recall bias may be a result of recall being poor in general or a differentiation in recall between cases and controls [7]. Conversely, prospective cohort designs are not limited by recall bias, because activity level is assessed before cancer diagnosis or the endpoint of interest. Unfortunately, cohort studies consume time and financial resources and require larger sample sizes [8]. Regardless of study design, confounding factors that may enhance or diminish the observable association must be controlled for. When studying physical activity, it is imperative to account for other positive health behaviors, such as abstinence from smoking and alcohol and maintenance of a balanced diet.

1.1.2 Body of Evidence by Cancer Site

Breast Cancer

Over thirty prospective cohort studies [9, 10, 11, 12, 13, 14, 15, 16, 17, 18, 19, 20, 21, 22, 23, 24, 25, 26, 27, 28, 29, 30, 31, 32, 33, 34, 35, 36, 37, 38, 39] and even more population-based case–control studies [40, 41, 42, 43, 44, 45, 46, 47, 48, 49–51, 52, 53, 54, 55, 56, 57–60, 61, 62, 63, 64, 65, 66, 67, 68, 69, 70, 71, 72, 73, 74, 75, 76, 77–79, 80, 81, 82, 83, 84] have examined the relation between physical activity and breast cancer risk. The majority of studies have assessed the role of recreational or leisure-time physical activity, in particular, on breast cancer risk. Overall, most studies suggest that physically active women have a lower risk of developing breast cancer than sedentary women. The majority of cohort studies [10, 11, 12, 13, 15, 16,

17, 18, 19, 20, 24, 25, 28, 29, 30, 31, 32, 34, 36, 37, 38, 39] have reported a reduction in risk with physical activity ranging from 13 to 80%, and a number of population-based case–control studies [41, 42, 43, 44, 48, 49, 53, 56, 57, 58, 60, 66, 67, 68, 71, 72, 73, 74, 75, 76, 77, 78, 82, 83, 84] have reported reduction in risk ranging from 20 to 70%. An extensive systematic review of recreational activity and breast cancer risk was completed, which included 19 cohort and 29 case–control studies [85]. The review determined that evidence for the inverse relation of physical activity and postmenopausal breast cancer risk ranged from a reduced risk of 20–80%. Further, for each additional hour of physical activity per week, the risk of breast cancer was reduced by 6% (95% CI 3–8%). They concluded that the effect of physical activity on premenopausal breast cancer risk was much smaller, being a 15–20% reduction.

The periods of life that may be the most crucial for potentially benefiting from the protective effects of physical activity on breast cancer risk are not established. Lifetime recreational physical activity [42, 44, 50, 58, 72, 73], adolescent physical activity [16, 24, 25, 39, 42, 66, 67, 76], and physical activity at various points in life [12, 16, 17, 20, 24, 25, 29, 32, 34, 38, 44, 53, 54, 67, 68, 73,] have been associated with lower breast cancer risk in multiple studies. Studies that have examined risk by specific decades of life have observed an inverse association with some or all examined time periods [25, 63, 69, 73, 76]. Further, physical activity after menopause has been found to reduce breast cancer risk [12, 25, 29, 30, 74]. Other studies that have looked at physical activity during various life periods have not observed a reduced risk of breast cancer with physical activity at any time [23].

To date, one cohort study [86] and two case–control studies [87, 88] have examined physical activity as a risk factor for male breast cancer. Results were split on the significant inverse relation of physical activity level with breast cancer. One case–control study [88] found an approximately 50% reduction in breast cancer risk for the highest versus lowest categories of combined moderate to strenuous recreational and occupational physical activity; the other study found no association. The cohort study [86] reported no association in current or adolescent physical activity level, though observed a 50% reduction in breast cancer risk for those with a physically active routine (lifting light to heavy loads and walking or climbing frequently versus sitting most or all of the day).

Subgroup Associations

Investigators have researched the relation of physical activity and breast cancer risk within subgroups for demographic or health factors such as age, race/ethnicity, BMI, or other elements of energy balance, finding some consistent evidence. Associations between increased physical activity and decreased breast cancer risk have been observed in multiethnic populations in the United States [25, 43, 77]. Similar observations have also been made for specific racial and ethnic populations, including black [41, 43], Hispanic [53, 77], and Asian American women [84].

Some studies have had large enough subgroup populations that the association of physical activity in women with or without a family history of breast cancer has been able to be evaluated. Results suggest that the association with physical activity may be stronger in women without a family history of breast cancer than in those with a family history [15, 29, 44, 73, 78]. Other large studies have found that both women with and without a family history of breast cancer had reduced risk of breast cancer with increasing physical activity [25, 30, 37]. Multiple studies have reported a greater reduction in risk with higher physical activity among parous compared to nulliparous women [15, 42]. However, other studies have observed converse findings with risk reduction greater in nulliparous women [24, 37, 71], or have observed parity to not be an effect modifier [25]. A few studies have found that physical activity may be more strongly associated with reduced risk of postmenopausal breast cancer in women who do not use menopausal hormones [18, 29, 30, 77]. However, other studies observed that the effect of physical activity did not alter by menopausal hormone use [25, 27, 37, 50, 52].

Five studies have examined effect modification by adult weight gain [16, 32, 75, 76, 89]. One study reported a greater reduction in risk among women who had less than a 17% increase in adult weight [89]. Several studies have observed a greater risk reduction among leaner compared to heavier women [24, 25, 38, 44, 71]. However, other studies have found that physical activity reduced the risk of breast cancer in women of varying body mass index (BMI) [15, 37]. One study found that women with a BMI >25 had a statistically significant dose–response trend to physical activity level, as well as a statistically significant greater reduction in risk compared to women with a BMI <25 [73].

Two cohort studies and one case–control study have addressed the effect of physical activity on breast cancer risk within the context of other variables related to energy balance, specifically adiposity (or body size) and dietary energy intake. One cohort study observed that premenopausal women who did not participate in vigorous activity were overweight or obese (BMI greater than 25 kg/m), and had a caloric intake just under 2,000 kcal/d (measured via self-report food frequency questionnaire), experienced a statistically significant 60% increased risk of breast cancer compared with active, normal weight women with lower calorie intake [35]. The other cohort study found that women with energy intake in the highest quartile, were obese, and participated in less than 4 h/week of vigorous physical activity had a RR of 2.1 (95% CI 1.27–3.45) compared with normal or overweight, active women in the lowest quartile of calorie intake [13]. The case–control study observed that women with a high waist-to-hip ratio and low total physical activity level (<10.9 MET h/d) had the highest risk of breast cancer with an OR of 2.7 (95% CI 1.4–4.9) for postmenopausal and OR of 2.1 (95% CI 1.5–3.1) for premenopausal women, as compared to the women with low waist-to-hip ratios who were highly active [75].

Dose–Response Pattern

Quantifying the level of physical activity necessary to decrease the risk of breast cancer has been the aim of numerous studies. Multiple levels of exercise have been reported by investigators as statistically significantly lowering the rates of breast cancer by 20–40%. The various levels include: exercising at least 1 h/week [32]; exercising at least 3.8 h/week (primarily vigorous exercise) [42]; exercising to keep fit at least 4 h/week [38]; and exercising vigorously at least 7 h/week [41]; expending at least 1,500 kcal/week [20] (approximately 4 h/week of moderate–intensity activity); at least 15.3 metabolic equivalent (MET)-hours per week (approximately 4 h/week of moderate–intensity activity) [82]; and at least 17.6 MET-hours per week (4–5 h/week of moderate–intensity activity) [89]. Finally, in a study where total physical activity over the lifetime was assessed, significantly lower breast cancer rates were seen in women who expended at least 47.5 MET-hours per week per year in total activity [49]. Some studies that have looked specifically at dose–response have not found an effect of exercise dose on breast cancer risk [26, 33]. Overall, evidence suggests that at least 4–7 h/week of moderate to vigorous intensity physical activity is necessary in order to yield a statistically significant reduction in risk. Some evidence indicates a greater reduction in risk with greater amount of activity.

Tumor Characteristics

The prevalence of screening greatly influences the incidence of in situ breast cancer, thus it is essential to examine the effects of physical activity on invasive breast cancer separately from that of in situ breast cancer. Furthermore, there are unique biological subtypes of breast cancers that are more strongly related to prognosis. These cancers may differ in etiology including tumor responsiveness to hormones (i.e., estrogen and progesterone receptor [ER/PR] status) and other tumor characteristics like Her2neu receptor status.

Two cohort studies [21, 30] and one case–control study [74] have recently examined physical activity effects separately in hormone receptor positive or negative tumors. The case–control study and one of the cohort studies have also examined the tumor grade and histology (i.e., ductal and lobular). In the case–control study, postmenopausal breast cancer risk was found to be reduced by nearly 30% with higher levels of physical activity after age 50 in individuals with ER+/PR+ tumors [74]. One of the cohort studies observed a significant dose–response trend with increased physical activity and a greater than 20% reduction of breast cancer risk in individuals with ER-/PR- hormone receptor status [30]. Three studies have reported risk ratios separately for ER/PR positive and negative tumors, finding no difference in risk by ER/PR subtype [20, 21, 90]. A recent cohort study found that women who reported high versus low levels of physical activity at enrollment had a 13, 33, and 20% decreased risk of developing ER+/PR+, ER+/PR−, and ER−/PR− breast cancer, respectively [10].

In one study, researchers examined the association between physical activity and breast cancer stratified by stage of disease and found risk reduction to be greater for localized invasive disease compared to either in situ or regional/distant breast cancer [72]. One cohort study found a significantly moderate reduction in breast cancer risk and significant dose–response trend in invasive breast cancer (RR 0.78, *P* for trend 0.0071), and a suggested increase in risk for in situ (RR 1.31, 95% CI 0.82–2.10) [74]. Conversely, a recent large cohort study found a greater risk reduction for in situ (RR 0.69, *P* for trend 0.04) than for invasive breast cancer (RR 0.80, *P* for trend 0.02) [15]. One case–control study focusing specifically on in situ breast cancer found that risk of this stage of breast cancer was approximately 35% lower in women reporting any lifetime exercise activity compared to women who were sedentary [72]. Another large cohort study found the greatest risk reduction from increased physical activity for ER−/PR− breast cancer [15]. Most other studies have included too few women with hormone receptor negative disease to be able to assess the association of physical activity with risk of this subtype of breast cancer. Only one case–control study has evaluated HER2neu tumor status [74]. Investigators reported an OR of 0.74 (95% CI 0.56–0.98) for the highest quintile of leisure-time physical activity and a nonsignificant test for trend.

Type of Physical Activity

An association of sedentary occupations with increased risk of breast cancer has been documented in reports from some prospective cohort studies [16, 31, 38]. Published reports from some [46, 49, 56, 67, 75, 83], but not other [47, 71, 80, 82, 84], population-based case–control studies also document an inverse association between occupational physical activity and breast cancer risk.

The effect of low-intensity or nonvigorous activity (such as household activities, gardening, dancing, leisurely walking, or other activities with a MET score below 4) on breast cancer risk is still unclear. These activities may be of importance for postmenopausal breast cancer, as a large portion of activity among postmenopausal and elderly women is not vigorous. However, the Breast Cancer Detection Demonstration Project Follow-Up Study specifically evaluated nonvigorous activity and found no association by quintiles of activity for relative risk of postmenopausal breast cancer [21]. Few studies have included the effects of other low-intensity activities, such as gardening, housework, or shopping, in their calculation of leisure-time physical activity, which may lead to an underestimation of true energy expenditure, especially among groups of women who do not have access to or participate in recreational or sports activities. Interested in the role of household activity, a large European cohort study found that women in the highest versus lowest household activity quartile experienced reduced risks for postmenopausal and premenopausal breast cancer (19%, P for trend = 0.0001; and 29%, P for trend = 0.0003, respectively) [19].

Prostate Cancer

In the past 25 years, numerous epidemiologic studies have examined physical activity and prostate cancer risk [33, 91, 92, 93, 94, 95, 96, 97, 98, 99, 100, 101, 102, 103, 104, 105, 106, 107, 108, 109, 110, 111, 112, 113, 114, 115–117, 118, 119, 120, 121, 122, 123, 124, 125–129, 130, 131, 132, 133, 134, 135, 136, 137, 138, 139, 140, 141, 142, 143–145], including over two dozen cohort studies [33, 95, 96, 97, 101, 103, 104, 106, 114, 115–117, 118, 119, 120, 121, 122, 124, 127–129, 131, 132, 135, 136, 138, 144, 145] and 20 case–control studies [92, 93, 94, 98, 99, 100, 107, 108, 109, 110, 111, 125, 130, 133, 134, 137, 139, 141, 142, 143]. Several of the cohort studies [101, 118, 122, 124, 127, 136] included prostate cancer mortality or advanced or metastatic prostate cancer as at least one endpoint. One study [121] also examined the association between cardiopulmonary fitness and risk of prostate cancer.

The evidence is split as to the relation of physical activity and reduced risk of prostate cancer development. Findings from 22 studies suggest an inverse relation between physical activity and prostate cancer [92, 93, 94, 96, 97, 100, 101, 103, 108, 117, 119, 120, 121, 122, 124, 132, 133, 135, 136, 137, 138, 143]. No overall association between physical activity and prostate cancer has been found in 14 studies [33, 98, 99, 104, 109, 110, 111, 114, 115, 116, 118, 128, 129, 130, 131, 141, 144, 145]. Some studies found an increased risk of prostate cancer among the most physically active men [95, 127, 134, 139, 142]. The size of association ranged from an 80% reduction in prostate cancer risk for the highest physical activity levels [93] to a 220% increased risk in one study [134].

Subgroup Associations

Any relation of physical activity and prostate cancer risk has yet to be consistently defined by subgroups for demographic or health factors such as age, race/ethnicity, or BMI. One recent study found that, among men with a family history of prostate cancer, risk for those in the highest quartile of physical activity was reduced by 52% compared to that for those in the lowest quartile of physical activity. Those without a family history had no risk reduction [99].

Many subgroups of the population could be defined by chronic disease state. As such, there is interest in the relation of chronic diseases and risk of prostate cancer and the role physical activity may play in the association. For example, history of diabetes has been shown to be associated with decreased risk of developing prostate cancer [146], though the role of physical activity is unknown. Two studies have examined the relationship between history of diabetes and prostate cancer risk in relation to physical activity level [147, 148]. Both studies found history of diabetes to be associated with decreased risk of prostate cancer, but only one study observed a significantly reduced risk in the more versus less active individuals [147].

Dose–Response Pattern

Many studies have attempted to decipher a dose–response association of prostate cancer risk with level of physical activity [92, 93, 94, 95, 98, 99, 101, 103, 104, 107, 109, 111, 114, 115–117, 118, 119, 120, 121, 124, 125, 129, 131, 135, 137, 138, 141, 143]. A statistically significant trend toward decreasing prostate cancer risk with increasing physical activity level has been observed in several studies [93, 94, 101, 103, 107, 119, 120, 135, 143]. One study observed a 74% reduction in prostate cancer risk in the highest compared to the lowest quartile of fitness level [121].

Type of Physical Activity

Occupational activity was associated with a decreased risk of prostate cancer in several studies [93, 94, 96, 100, 103, 108, 122, 125, 133, 136], and recreational activity decreased risk of either overall or advanced prostate cancer in several additional studies [99, 101, 103, 117, 121, 124, 138, 143]. In two studies, nonsignificant risk decreases were found for occupational activity, but an increased risk was observed for household activity [99, 142]. No study differentiated between types of recreational activity (aerobic or resistance exercise) or to the specific activity (running, walking, cycling, playing sport, etc.). Activities were typically combined into measures of MET-hours per day or week, or to measures of frequency or total duration of activity per day or week.

Considerations

One consideration regarding the observed association of prostate cancer risk and occupational physical activity is the method by which the physical activity data was collected. The majority of studies collected physical activity data with a survey or self-report instrument, some focusing on lifetime, current, or specific time points of employment. However, some studies collected occupational physical activity based on the career or occupation reported by the participant and made inferences as to the level of activity that person would perform in that job [110, 133]. It is important to consider not just the type of physical activity (occupational, recreational, household, lifetime, etc.) but also the means by which it was collected.

Another consideration for prostate cancer is the effect of screening. Prostate-specific antigen (PSA) screening for early detection became common practice in the United States in the 1990s. One may hypothesize that if physically active men also are more health conscious (i.e., they are more likely to be screened for prostate cancer), higher rates of prostate cancer may be observed among these men because of increased detection. This hypothesis is supported by several cohort studies [101, 119, 124], which identified a reduction in risk of aggressive, metastatic, or fatal prostate cancer with increased physical activity level. Conversely, an investigation of physical activity and prostate cancer, diagnosed in 1988 or earlier (before PSA screening was more commonly available), found nearly half the prostate cancer incidence rates among men aged 70 years or older who expended at least 4,000 kcal/week in physical activity versus those expending less than 1,000 kcal/week [112]. However, in the published updated analysis of these men, which examined prostate cancer diagnosed after 1988, the earlier observations were not supported [114]. These inconsistent findings may have been a result of bias arising from increased screening for prostate cancer among the most active men.

Colon Cancer

To date, there have been nearly three dozen prospective cohort studies [33, 94, 98, 106, 113, 128, 144, 149, 150, 151, 152, 153, 154, 155, 156, 157, 158, 159, 160, 161, 162, 163, 164, 165, 166, 167, 168, 169, 131, 170, 171, 172, 173] and two dozen case–control studies [174, 175, 176, 177, 178, 179, 180, 181, 182, 183, 184, 185, 186, 187, 188–192, 193, 194, 195, 196, 197, 198, 199, 200] that have examined the association of physical activity and colon cancer risk. Studies have been conducted in the United States [150, 151, 158, 159, 163, 166, 167, 173, 189–192, 197, 200], Europe (Denmark) [33], Finland [128, 152], Italy [194], Norway [169, 171],

Sweden [161, 168], Switzerland [186], and Turkey [98], and Asia (China) [180], Japan [106, 164, 170, 181], Taiwan [193], and Korea [144]).

Overall, studies have consistently observed an inverse association between physical activity and the risk of developing colon cancer. Findings of a recent meta-analysis on physical activity and colon cancer risk, including studies published as early as 1984, found similar results for gender, but varied in the degree of protective effect between cohort and case–control studies [201]. When comparing the most versus least active individuals across all studies, there was a 24% reduced risk of colon cancer (RR=0.76). The magnitude was smaller for cohort studies (RR=0.83, 95% CI 0.78–0.88) compared to case–control design (0.69, 95% CI 0.65–0.74). Results were similar for men (RR=0.76, 95% CI 0.71–0.82) and women (RR=0.79, 95% CI: 0.71–0.88).

Subgroup Associations

Several studies have examined whether the association between physical activity and decreased colon cancer risk varies, depending on use of menopausal hormone therapy [150, 166], various aspects of diet [144, 150, 191], or BMI [150, 161, 164, 180, 190, 200]. Overall, the findings have been largely inconsistent, but suggest that higher levels of physical activity may amend the adverse impact of high BMI on colon cancer risk [180, 190, 200].

Several studies also have examined whether physical activity has a different association with colon cancers occurring at different subsites of the colon. The data have been equivocal, with some studies suggesting a larger magnitude of association for cancers occurring in the proximal colon [164, 168, 186, 200] while others have reported greater associations for cancers of the distal colon [161, 167, 173]. Most studies, however, have observed equivalent associations or unclear differences across proximal and distal sites of the colon [150, 151, 166, 171, 181, 192, 194]. One study has assessed the association of recreational physical activity with cancer risk in anatomically defined segments of the colon [169]. Significant reduced risk of colon cancer (>50%) with increased physical activity was observed in the transverse and sigmoid colon sites.

Dose–Response Pattern

With few exceptions [128, 144] most studies categorized subjects according to at least three levels of physical activity, allowing dose–response to be assessed. The majority of cohort studies with at least three physical activity levels reported significant, inverse trends between physical activity and colon cancer risk [106, 151, 152, 158, 159, 161, 164, 167, 168, 169, 170, 171]. Half of the case–control studies observed significant, inverse trends between activity level and colon cancer risk [180, 186, 193, 194]. Given the evidence, a dose–response relation appears likely. However, due to the multiple and variable methods used to assess and categorize physical activity in these studies, it is difficult to determine the shape of the dose–response curve.

Types and Amount of Physical Activity

Most studies have assessed recreational or leisure-time and/or occupational physical activity, only one study having assessed active commuting (walking or bicycling to work) [180]. Due to the variation of questionnaires and methods utilized in assessing physical activity and the different categories used to group study participants, generalizing the findings across studies is challenging. In addition, most studies presented their findings according to overall volume of energy expended, and not by specific type of activity as it relates to decreased colon cancer risk.

Evidence specific to the amount of activity needed for reduced risk of colon cancer exists for recreational or leisure-time physical activity (in order of approximate ascending doses of physical activity).

–At least twice a week for at least 10 min duration [200]
–At least 4 h/week of moderate-to-vigorous intensity [166]
–At least 20 MET-hours per week [193]
–More than 21 MET-hours per week [167]
–7 or more hours per week [151]
–A median of 35.25 MET-hours per week [164]
–A median of 46.8 MET-hours per week [158]

Additionally, results of a case–control study suggest that physical activity needs to be vigorous in intensity to reduce colon cancer risk [189–192]. In summary, these data suggest that 30–60 min per day of moderate-to-vigorous intensity physical activity may be necessary to significantly reduce the risk of developing colon cancer.

Considerations

Any misclassification of physical activity is likely to be random in a prospective cohort study, given that recall bias is unlikely since physical activity is assessed prior to the development of cancer. Random misclassification would dilute associations rather than cause erroneous inverse relations. Results are likely not confounded by other factors associated with colon cancer risk because many studies adjust their findings for several factors, including BMI, smoking, alcohol, diet (e.g., energy intake, intake of calcium and folate, intake of fiber, vegetables, and meat), use of aspirin, screening, menopausal status and use of menopausal hormone therapy, and family history of colon cancer. Though the data on physical activity and risk of developing colon cancer are based on observational epidemiologic studies, the inverse associations indicated by these studies are consistent and likely to be real.

Rectal Cancer

Unlike the associations found between physical activity and colon cancer, there is more disagreement in the data on physical activity and risk of developing rectal cancer. More than half of the studies have reported no significant associations [106,

128, 151, 164, 168, 170, 171, 193,194, 202,], with the remaining studies observing significantly lower risks (or of borderline significance) with higher levels of physical activity [152, 159, 161, 181, 186, 192].

Additional Cancer Sites

There is less evidence available regarding the association of physical activity with reduced risk of lung, endometrial, ovarian, pancreatic, and other cancers. The remainder of Section 1 provides a general overview for each cancer.

Lung Cancer

The association of physical activity and lung cancer risk was included within a chapter on physical activity in a book published in 2006 titled, "*Cancer Epidemiology and Prevention*" [203]. At the time of that review, 15 cohort studies and six case–control studies had been published, with an overall median of 20% reduced risk for lung cancer in the highest versus lowest active individuals. Similar to the findings in that review, results to date indicate a 23% median reduction of lung cancer risk for the most versus least active subjects [106, 138, 144, 204, 205, 206, 207–210, 211, 212, 213, 214, 215, 216, 217]. Further, as with the prior review, the reduction of risk is more apparent in case–control studies (median RR over four studies = 0.62) [207, 209, 210, 213] than in cohort studies (median RR over 12 studies = 0.77) [106, 138, 144, 204, 205, 206, 211, 212, 214, 215, 216, 217]. Evidence indicates the inverse relation of physical activity with lung cancer risk is similar for men and women: a 25% reduced risk of cancer development.

Most of the studies evaluating the association of physical activity and lung cancer have adjusted for cigarette smoking. However, even given this adjustment, the potential for residual confounding is high. Some studies have reported risk reductions specifically for current smokers, former smokers, or never smokers ([144, 208, 211, 212, 214, 215]. The risk reduction in these studies is more similar for current and former smokers (median RR of 0.65 [208, 211, 212, 214] and 0.63 [211, 212, 214], respectively) than for never smokers (median RR of 1.03 for three studies reporting for this subgroup) [208, 212, 214]. To date, there is too little evidence to conclude that the reduction of lung cancer risk by physical activity is limited to current and former smokers.

Exploration of the association of physical activity with lung cancer in never smokers and evaluation of the consistency of the association in subtypes of lung cancer have enabled researchers to deal with the issue of residual confounding. There is evidence that smoking is more clearly linked to certain histologic types of lung cancer. Given that evidence, researchers have been able to explore residual confounding by smoking status through evaluation of whether the association of physical activity and reduced lung cancer risk is present for all histologic subtypes. Four studies to date have examined whether the association of physical activity is similar across most lung cancer histologic subtypes [212, 213, 216, 217]. Evidence suggests that the physical activity association is present across histologic subtypes, including adenocarcinoma. As stated, another approach in determining whether the association of physical activity and lung cancer is attributable to residual confounding by smoking is through the study of nonsmokers. The reported RR (or odds radio) for nonsmokers was 1.32 and 1.02 in the cohort studies and 0.74 and 0.64 in two case–control studies [208, 210, 212, 214].

Endometrial Cancer

A review of the association of physical activity and endometrial cancer risk was published in a book chapter in 2006 [203]. Included in that review were 4 cohort studies and 11 case control studies. The review indicated an overall median relative risk of 0.70 for the highest versus lowest categorized activity level of subjects. Of the more recent studies (nine cohort studies and eight case–control) [218, 219, 220, 221, 222, 223, 224, 225, 226, 227, 228, 229, 230, 231, 232, 233, 234], five included relative risks that were adjusted for multiple variables but not for BMI [218, 219, 227, 228, 234]. Prior to adjustment for BMI, the median RR was 0.73. In those studies adjusting for BMI, the RR was 0.79. Body weight has been hypothesized to confound, mediate, or act as an intermediary in the relationship between physical activity and endometrial cancer. Some studies conclude that BMI attenuates the inverse relationship, while others have not found that same result [222].

Menopausal hormone therapy use is another potential confounder (or moderator) of the association of physical activity and endometrial cancer. There is a strong link between use of unopposed estrogen therapy and increased risk of endometrial cancer. Some studies have accounted for hormone therapy use through elimination of estrogen-only hormone therapy replacement or hormone therapy users of unknown type from the study population [231], while others have adjusted for hormone therapy use in the analyses. The median RR from the three case–control studies and one cohort study that adjusted for menopausal hormone therapy was 0.76 [222, 225, 226, 229] compared to a median RR of 0.68 for the studies that did not adjust for menopausal hormone therapy [218, 219, 220, 221, 224, 227, 228, 232, 233, 234].

Overall, evidence from reviewed studies indicates an inverse association between physical activity and incidence of endometrial cancer. However, the borderline change in the median relative risks for studies that did versus did not adjust for BMI or menopausal hormone therapy suggest that further research is needed in order to better understand whether the association is mediated through or moderated by obesity or exogenous hormonal exposure.

Ovarian Cancer

The association of physical activity with risk of ovarian cancer development was examined in a meta-analysis and systematic review published in 2007 (Olsen et al. 2007). The review concluded there was a modest inverse association with recreational physical activity and incidence of ovarian cancer, with a weighted pooled RR of 0.81 (95% confidence interval was 0.72–0.92). Sensitivity analyses were conducted to determine whether there was a difference in findings when studies did versus did not adjust for BMI or exogenous hormone use (oral contraceptives), and no difference in findings was observed. Since the 2007 review, one cohort study

[236] and one case–control study [237] have been conducted. The case–control study reported an inverse association between occupational physical activity and ovarian cancer risk, with no heterogeneity across histologic subtypes (OR = 0.7 for serous, and 0.5 for mucinous and endometrioid). The cohort study found no association in total, recreational, household, or occupational physical activity and risk for overall or histologic subtypes of ovarian cancer and no dose–response trends. Sensitivity analyses for BMI, menopausal status, and hormone replacement therapy use found no differences in subgroup results.

Pancreatic Cancer

The relation between physical activity and pancreatic cancer risk was examined in a systematic review published in 2008 [238]. Authors reviewed 16 prospective cohort studies, 1 nested case–control study, and 2 retrospective case–control studies. The individual study relative risks ranged from 0.42 to 1.24, while the pooled relative risk was 0.76 (0.53–1.09). Since that review was published, three additional cohort studies have been conducted [106, 239, 240]. At time of diagnosis for pancreatic cancer, patients often have advanced disease and may be experiencing cachexia, which may make case–control studies in pancreatic cancer more susceptible to bias from unmeasured adiposity levels prior to the onset of the cancer illness. The two case–control studies did not adjust for BMI in women subjects and the average odds ratio for the two studies was 0.82 [241, 242]. The average odds ratio for men in the two studies was 0.66, one adjusted for BMI [242] and the other did not [241]. Half of the cohort studies examining physical activity and pancreatic cancer adjusted for BMI in multivariate models. In the five cohort studies that did not adjust for BMI [243, 244, 245, 246, 247], the median relative risk for the association of physical activity with pancreatic cancer incidence was 1.21. The median RR for all studies was 1.0. Though the evidence is not consistent, it is possible that there is a level of physical activity that may be associated with reduced incidence of pancreatic cancer.

Other Cancers

The association between physical activity and risk for other cancers (e.g., thyroid, kidney, bladder, stomach, and hematopoietic) has been investigated in a small number of studies. Reviews of these cancers are not included here because the data are much more limited in both the total number of studies as well as the number of subjects and identified cases within each trial. As a result, it is more challenging to draw conclusions regarding a potential relation with physical activity and risk of these other cancers.

1.1.3 Conclusions

There is a large amount of epidemiologic data available regarding the association of physical activity and the risk of developing various types of cancer. Evidence supporting an association of increased physical activity with reduced risk of cancer development is greatest for breast and colon cancers. The magnitude of the protective effect of physical activity on breast cancer development varies by individual characteristics (menopausal status, parity, BMI) with a median effect of roughly 20% across studies. Findings from over 50 studies indicate the reduced risk of colon cancer development to be nearly 25%, which is consistent for both men and women. Data suggest that 30–60 min/d of moderate-to-vigorous intensity physical activity is likely necessary in order to significantly decrease the risk of developing breast and colon cancers. A growing body of research suggests a protective effect of physical activity for lung and endometrial cancers as well. Increased physical activity is associated with a median 23% reduced risk of lung cancer development, while the reduced risk of endometrial cancer is estimated at 20–30%, depending on the decision of investigators to adjust for BMI or menopausal hormone therapy use. Though numerous studies have examined physical activity and prostate cancer risk, the evidence is inconsistent as to whether the relation is positive, negative, or nonexistent.

Observational data from cohort and case–control studies are the primary sources of evidence on the association of physical activity and risk of cancer development. Study design, methods of data collection, and type of physical activity being collected (recreational or leisure-time, occupational, household, lifetime, etc.) vary by study. These factors should be considered when interpreting individual study results and making general conclusions.

1.2 Physical Fitness and Cancer

1.2.1 Background

Physical fitness is a term often used to define an individual's ability or state of physical activity performance. Physical fitness can be measured by a variety of performance tests, as well as biochemical, hematological, and electrocardiographic tests. Physical fitness and physical activity are interrelated concepts; some degree of physical fitness is inherited, yet increases in physical activity can increase physical fitness in an individual. Physical fitness and health and well-being are interrelated concepts as well; physical fitness can serve as a predictor for health conditions or mortality [248, 249], and health conditions have been demonstrated to predict fitness level [250, 251].

Investigators have examined the role of physical fitness as a predictor for the risk of developing health conditions, such as cardiovascular disease [248, 252], injury [253], and diabetes [254, 255]. A growing body of research has explored physical fitness as a predictor for the risk of cancer mortality. The epidemiological data available for physical fitness and cancer mortality are derived from observational studies: primarily prospective cohort studies conducted in the United States; one study has been conducted in Japan. The majority of published data is on men, and the main parameter of fitness measured is cardiorespiratory fitness.

1.2.2 Body of Evidence

To date, eight publications have reported findings on the association between physical fitness and risk of cancer mortality [256, 257, 258, 259, 260, 261, 262, 263]. The primary data source for the publications is the Aerobics Center Longitudinal Study. The prospective cohort study began enrollment in 1970 and has followed patients who completed a comprehensive health examination at the Cooper Institute in Dallas, Texas. The study population is primarily white, well-educated, and middle-to-upper socioeconomic status individuals in the age range of 20–88 years. Participants had to have no personal history of myocardial infarction, stroke, or cancer at baseline study entry. The baseline fitness assessment measured cardiorespiratory fitness by maximal treadmill test using the Balke protocol. Participants walked at a speed of 88 m/min (3.3 mph) with periodic changes in the percent grade. After 25 min the grade remained constant and the speed increased by 5.4 m/min (0.2 mph) until the participant reached exhaustion or the test was stopped by the supervising physician for medical reasons. Total test duration was used to define physical fitness because test duration correlates highly with measured maximal oxygen uptake.

Within this cohort, investigators have completed analyses for all cancer mortality, breast and digestive cancer mortality, and all cancer mortality within men with prediabetes and diabetes. All three analyses on all cancer mortality and cardiorespiratory fitness in men have reported statistically significant trends in decreased risk with increased fitness level [256, 257, 258], average relative risk or hazard ratio of 0.39 when comparing the most to the least fit men. The test for trend and hazard ratio for all cancer mortality in women were not significant [257], nor was the trend for increased fitness and all cancer mortality significant in men with prediabetes or diabetes [263]. Investigators reported statistically significant tests for trend in decreased risk of breast and digestive cancer mortality with increased fitness level [259, 260], hazard ratios of 0.45 (95% CI, 0.22–0.95) and 0.51 (95% CI, 0.37–0.70), respectively.

One analysis using Aerobic Center Longitudinal Study data examined physical fitness and all cancer mortality through a measure of muscular strength. Between the years of 1980 and 1989, a subset of 10,265 men completed upper body and lower body one-repetition maximum tests at their baseline enrollment visit. A strength score was computed for each participant by combining standardized values of bench and leg press. Investigators reported a significant test for trend and nearly 40% reduced risk of all cancer mortality with increased level of muscular strength [261]. Adjustment for BMI, percent body fat, waist circumference, and cardiorespiratory fitness had little effect on the statistical significance of the association.

Cancer mortality and cardiorespiratory fitness has also been examined in Japan. Men working at the Tokyo Gas Company were followed from 1982 to 1988. Participants included 9,039 healthy men (no diagnosis of cancer, cardiovascular disease, diabetes mellitus, gastrointestinal disease, or tuberculosis) aged 19–59 years who underwent annual health examinations. Participants completed a cycle ergometer test, in which maximal oxygen uptake was estimated based on the work rate obtained on the last 1 min and the heart rate obtained on the last 10 s of the test. After adjusting for age, BMI, systolic blood pressure, alcohol habit, and smoking habit, investigators reported a significant test for trend in decreased relative risk of all cancer mortality and increased cardiorespiratory fitness level [262], RR = 0.41 (95% CI, 0.23–0.74).

1.2.3 Conclusions

Research findings demonstrate that physical fitness is a measurable concept that can be used to assess or predict health conditions and outcomes. There is a growing body of research examining the relation of physical fitness and risk of cancer mortality. Evidence suggests that increased levels of physical fitness decrease the risk of cancer mortality by more than 50% in men. Evidence as to the association in women is limited, and additional research is needed in this area. Further, analyses should extend beyond all cancer mortality and examine specific cancer sites in order to determine whether the impact of physical fitness varies by type of cancer. Finally, there is a lack in understanding as to the association between physical fitness and risk of developing cancer. Researchers should evaluate whether existing cohorts contain the appropriate data to answer such questions or if physical fitness measures can be incorporated in ongoing follow-up to assess the exposure of interest.

References

1. Jemal A, Siegel R, Ward E et al (2009) Cancer statistics, 2009. CA Cancer J Clin 59:225–249
2. International Agency for Research on Cancer (2002) Weight control and physical activity, vol. 6. IARC Handbooks of Cancer Prevention. IARC Press, Lyon, France
3. Czene K, Lichtenstein P, Hemminki K (2002) Environmental and heritable causes of cancer among 9.6 million individuals in the Swedish Family-Cancer Database. Int J Cancer 99: 260–266
4. Friedenreich CM (2001) Physical activity and cancer prevention: from observational to intervention research. Cancer Epidemiol Biomarkers Prev 10:287–301
5. World Cancer Research Fund (1997) Food, nutrition, and the prevention of cancer: a global perspective. American Institute for Cancer Research, Washington, DC
6. Washburn RA, Montoye HJ (1986) The assessment of physical activity by questionnaire. Am J Epidemiol 123:563–576
7. Coughlin SS (1990) Recall bias in epidemiologic studies. J Clin Epidemiol 43:87–91
8. Rothman K (1986) Modern epidemiology. Little Brown and Company, Boston, MA
9. Dorgan JF, Brown C, Barrett M et al (1994) Physical activity and risk of breast cancer in the Framingham Heart Study. Am J Epidemiol 139:662–669
10. Bardia A, Hartmann LC, Vachon CM et al (2006) Recreational physical activity and risk of postmenopausal breast cancer based on hormone receptor status. Arch Intern Med 166: 2478–2483
11. Breslow RA, Ballard-Barbash R, Munoz K et al (2001) Long-term recreational physical activity and breast cancer in the National Health and Nutrition Examination Survey I epidemiologic follow-up study. Cancer Epidemiol Biomarkers Prev 10:805–808
12. Cerhan JR, Chiu BC, Wallace RB et al (1998) Physical activity, physical function, and the risk of breast cancer in a prospective study among elderly women. J Gerontol A Biol Sci Med Sci 53:M251–M256

13. Chang SC, Ziegler RG, Dunn B et al (2006) Association of energy intake and energy balance with postmenopausal breast cancer in the prostate, lung, colorectal, and ovarian cancer screening trial. Cancer Epidemiol Biomarkers Prev 15:334–341
14. Colditz GA, Feskanich D, Chen WY et al (2003) Physical activity and risk of breast cancer in premenopausal women. Br J Cancer 89:847–851
15. Dallal CM, Sullivan-Halley J, Ross RK et al (2007) Long-term recreational physical activity and risk of invasive and in situ breast cancer: the California teachers study. Arch Intern Med 167:408–415
16. Dirx MJ, Voorrips LE, Goldbohm RA et al (2001) Baseline recreational physical activity, history of sports participation, and postmenopausal breast carcinoma risk in the Netherlands Cohort Study. Cancer 92:1638–1649
17. Fraser GE, Shavlik D (1997) Risk factors, lifetime risk, and age at onset of breast cancer. Ann Epidemiol 7:375–382
18. Howard RA, Leitzmann MF, Linet MS et al (2009) Physical activity and breast cancer risk among pre- and postmenopausal women in the U.S. Radiologic Technologists cohort. Cancer Causes Control 20:323–333
19. Lahmann PH, Friedenreich C, Schuit AJ et al (2007) Physical activity and breast cancer risk: the European Prospective Investigation into Cancer and Nutrition. Cancer Epidemiol Biomarkers Prev 16:36–42
20. Lee IM, Rexrode KM, Cook NR et al (2001) Physical activity and breast cancer risk: the Women's Health Study (United States). Cancer Causes Control 12:137–145
21. Leitzmann MF, Moore SC, Peters TM et al (2008) Prospective study of physical activity and risk of postmenopausal breast cancer. Breast Cancer Res 10:R92
22. Luoto R, Latikka P, Pukkala E et al (2000) The effect of physical activity on breast cancer risk: a cohort study of 30,548 women. Eur J Epidemiol 16:973–980
23. Margolis KL, Mucci L, Braaten T et al (2005) Physical activity in different periods of life and the risk of breast cancer: the Norwegian-Swedish Women's Lifestyle and Health cohort study. Cancer Epidemiol Biomarkers Prev 14:27–32
24. Maruti SS, Willett WC, Feskanich D et al (2008) A prospective study of age-specific physical activity and premenopausal breast cancer. J Natl Cancer Inst 100:728–737
25. McTiernan A, Kooperberg C, White E et al (2003) Recreational physical activity and the risk of breast cancer in postmenopausal women: the Women's Health Initiative Cohort Study. JAMA 290:1331–1336
26. Mertens AJ, Sweeney C, Shahar E et al (2006) Physical activity and breast cancer incidence in middle-aged women: a prospective cohort study. Breast Cancer Res Treat 97:209–214
27. Moore DB, Folsom AR, Mink PJ et al (2000) Physical activity and incidence of postmenopausal breast cancer. Epidemiology 11:292–296
28. Moradi T, Adami HO, Ekbom A et al (2002) Physical activity and risk for breast cancer a prospective cohort study among Swedish twins. Int J Cancer 100:76–81
29. Patel AV, Callel EE, Bernstein L et al (2003) Recreational physical activity and risk of postmenopausal breast cancer in a large cohort of US women. Cancer Causes Control 14:519–529
30. Peters TM, Schatzkin A, Gierach GL et al (2009) Physical activity and postmenopausal breast cancer risk in the NIH-AARP diet and health study. Cancer Epidemiol Biomarkers Prev 18:289–296
31. Rintala P, Pukkala E, Laara E et al (2003) Physical activity and breast cancer risk among female physical education and language teachers: a 34-year follow-up. Int J Cancer 107: 268–270
32. Rockhill B, Willett WC, Hunter DJ et al (1999) A prospective study of recreational physical activity and breast cancer risk. Arch Intern Med 159:2290–2296
33. Schnohr P, Gronbaek M, Petersen L et al (2005) Physical activity in leisure-time and risk of cancer: 14-year follow-up of 28,000 Danish men and women. Scand J Public Health 33: 244–249

34. Sesso HD, Paffenbarger RS Jr., Lee IM (1998) Physical activity and breast cancer risk in the College Alumni Health Study (United States). Cancer Causes Control 9:433–439
35. Silvera SA, Jain M, Howe GR et al (2006) Energy balance and breast cancer risk: a prospective cohort study. Breast Cancer Res Treat 97:97–106
36. Suzuki S, Kojima M, Tokudome S et al (2008) Effect of physical activity on breast cancer risk: findings of the Japan collaborative cohort study. Cancer Epidemiol Biomarkers Prev 17:3396–3401
37. Tehard B, Friedenreich CM, Oppert JM et al (2006) Effect of physical activity on women at increased risk of breast cancer: results from the E3N cohort study. Cancer Epidemiol Biomarkers Prev 15:57–64
38. Thune I, Brenn T, Lund E et al (1997) Physical activity and the risk of breast cancer. N Engl J Med 336:1269–1275
39. Wyshak G, Frisch RE (2000) Breast cancer among former college athletes compared to non-athletes: a 15-year follow-up. Br J Cancer 82:726–730
40. Adams SA, Matthews CE, Hebert JR et al (2006) Association of physical activity with hormone receptor status: the Shanghai Breast Cancer Study. Cancer Epidemiol Biomarkers Prev 15:1170–1178
41. Adams-Campbell LL, Rosenberg L, Rao RS et al (2001) Strenuous physical activity and breast cancer risk in African-American women. J Natl Med Assoc 93:267–275
42. Bernstein L, Henderson BE, Hanisch R et al (1994) Physical exercise and reduced risk of breast cancer in young women. J Natl Cancer Inst 86:1403–1408
43. Bernstein L, Patel AV, Ursin G et al (2005) Lifetime recreational exercise activity and breast cancer risk among black women and white women. J Natl Cancer Inst 97: 1671–1679
44. Carpenter CL, Ross RK, Paganini-Hill A et al (2003) Effect of family history, obesity and exercise on breast cancer risk among postmenopausal women. Int J Cancer 106: 96–102
45. Chen CL, White E, Malone KE et al (1997) Leisure-time physical activity in relation to breast cancer among young women (Washington, United States). Cancer Causes Control 8:77–84
46. Coogan PF, Newcomb PA, Clapp RW et al (1997) Physical activity in usual occupation and risk of breast cancer (United States). Cancer Causes Control 8:626–631
47. Dorn J, Vena J, Brasure J et al (2003) Lifetime physical activity and breast cancer risk in pre- and postmenopausal women. Med Sci Sports Exerc 35:278–285
48. Friedenreich CM, Rohan TE (1995) Physical activity and risk of breast cancer. Eur J Cancer Prev 4:145–151
49. Friedenreich CM, Bryant HE, Courneya KS (2001) Case-control study of lifetime physical activity and breast cancer risk. Am J Epidemiol 154:336–347
50. Friedenreich CM, Courneya KS, Bryant HE (2001) Influence of physical activity in different age and life periods on the risk of breast cancer. Epidemiology 12:604–612
51. Friedenreich CM, Courneya KS, Bryant HE (2001) Relation between intensity of physical activity and breast cancer risk reduction. Med Sci Sports Exerc 33:1538–1545
52. Gammon MD, Schoenberg JB, Britton JA et al (1998) Recreational physical activity and breast cancer risk among women under age 45 years. Am J Epidemiol 147:273–280
53. Gilliland FD, Li YF, Baumgartner K et al (2001) Physical activity and breast cancer risk in hispanic and non-hispanic white women. Am J Epidemiol 154:442–450
54. Hirose K, Hamajima N, Takezaki T et al (2003) Physical exercise reduces risk of breast cancer in Japanese women. Cancer Sci 94:193–199
55. Hu YH, Nagata C, Shimizu H et al (1997) Association of body mass index, physical activity, and reproductive histories with breast cancer: a case-control study in Gifu, Japan. Breast Cancer Res Treat 43:65–72
56. John EM, Horn-Ross PL, Koo J (2003) Lifetime physical activity and breast cancer risk in a multiethnic population: the San Francisco Bay area breast cancer study. Cancer Epidemiol Biomarkers Prev 12:1143–1152

57. Kruk J (2007) Association of lifestyle and other risk factors with breast cancer according to menopausal status: a case-control study in the Region of Western Pomerania (Poland). Asian Pac J Cancer Prev 8:513–524
58. Kruk J (2007) Lifetime physical activity and the risk of breast cancer: a case-control study. Cancer Detect Prev 31:18–28
59. Kruk J (2007) Self-reported childhood physical activity and breast cancer in adulthood. Asian Pac J Cancer Prev 8:63–68
60. Kruk J (2009) Intensity of lifetime physical activity and breast cancer risk among Polish women. J Sports Sci 27:437–445
61. Kumar NB, Riccardi D, Cantor A et al (2005) A case-control study evaluating the association of purposeful physical activity, body fat distribution, and steroid hormones on premenopausal breast cancer risk. Breast J 11:266–272
62. Lee IM, Cook NR, Rexrode KM et al (2001) Lifetime physical activity and risk of breast cancer. Br J Cancer 85:962–965
63. Levi F, Pasche C, Lucchini F et al (1999) Occupational and leisure time physical activity and the risk of breast cancer. Eur J Cancer 35:775–778
64. Magnusson CM, Roddam AW, Pike MC et al (2005) Body fatness and physical activity at young ages and the risk of breast cancer in premenopausal women. Br J Cancer 93:817–824
65. Malin A, Matthews CE, Shu XO et al (2005) Energy balance and breast cancer risk. Cancer Epidemiol Biomarkers Prev 14:1496–1501
66. Marcus PM, Newman B, Moorman PG et al (1999) Physical activity at age 12 and adult breast cancer risk (United States). Cancer Causes Control 10:293–302
67. Matthews CE, Shu XO, Jin F et al (2001) Lifetime physical activity and breast cancer risk in the Shanghai Breast Cancer Study. Br J Cancer 84:994–1001
68. McTiernan A, Stanford JL, Weiss NS et al (1996) Occurrence of breast cancer in relation to recreational exercise in women age 50–64 years. Epidemiology 7:598–604
69. Mezzetti M, La Vecchia C, Decarli A et al (1998) Population attributable risk for breast cancer: diet, nutrition, and physical exercise. J Natl Cancer Inst 90:389–394
70. Mittendorf R, Longnecker MP, Newcomb PA et al (1995) Strenuous physical activity in young adulthood and risk of breast cancer (United States). Cancer Causes Control 6:347–353
71. Moradi T, Nyren O, Zack M et al (2000) Breast cancer risk and lifetime leisure-time and occupational physical activity (Sweden). Cancer Causes Control 11:523–531
72. Patel AV, Press MF, Meeske K et al (2003) Lifetime recreational exercise activity and risk of breast carcinoma in situ. Cancer 98:2161–2169
73. Peplonska B, Lissowska J, Hartman TJ et al (2008) Adulthood lifetime physical activity and breast cancer. Epidemiology 19:226–236
74. Schmidt ME, Steindorf K, Mutschelknauss E et al (2008) Physical activity and postmenopausal breast cancer: effect modification by breast cancer subtypes and effective periods in life. Cancer Epidemiol Biomarkers Prev 17:3402–3410
75. Shin A, Matthews CE, Shu XO et al (2009) Joint effects of body size, energy intake, and physical activity on breast cancer risk. Breast Cancer Res Treat 113:153–161
76. Shoff SM, Newcomb PA, Trentham-Dietz A et al (2000) Early-life physical activity and postmenopausal breast cancer: effect of body size and weight change. Cancer Epidemiol Biomarkers Prev 9:591–595
77. Slattery ML, Edwards S, Murtaugh MA et al (2007) Physical activity and breast cancer risk among women in the southwestern United States. Ann Epidemiol 17:342–353
78. Sprague BL, Trentham-Dietz A, Newcomb PA et al (2007) Lifetime recreational and occupational physical activity and risk of in situ and invasive breast cancer. Cancer Epidemiol Biomarkers Prev 16:236–243
79. Sprague BL, Trentham-Dietz A, Egan KM et al (2008) Proportion of invasive breast cancer attributable to risk factors modifiable after menopause. Am J Epidemiol 168:404–411
80. Steindorf K, Schmidt M, Kropp S et al (2003) Case-control study of physical activity and breast cancer risk among premenopausal women in Germany. Am J Epidemiol 157:121–130

81. Taioli E, Barone J, Wynder EL (1995) A case-control study on breast cancer and body mass. The American Health Foundation – Division of Epidemiology. Eur J Cancer 31A:723–728
82. Ueji M, Ueno E, Osei-Hyiaman D et al (1998) Physical activity and the risk of breast cancer: a case-control study of Japanese women. J Epidemiol 8:116–122
83. Verloop J, Rookus MA, van der Kooy K et al (2000) Physical activity and breast cancer risk in women aged 20-54 years. J Natl Cancer Inst 92:128–135
84. Yang D, Bernstein L, Wu AH (2003) Physical activity and breast cancer risk among Asian-American women in Los Angeles: a case-control study. Cancer 97:2565–2575
85. Monninkhof EM, Elias SG, Vlems FA et al (2007) Physical activity and breast cancer: a systematic review. Epidemiology 18:137–157
86. Brinton LA, Richesson DA, Gierach GL et al (2008) Prospective evaluation of risk factors for male breast cancer. J Natl Cancer Inst 100:1477–1481
87. Hsing AW, McLaughlin JK, Cocco P et al (1998) Risk factors for male breast cancer (United States). Cancer Causes Control 9:269–275
88. Johnson KC, Pan S, Mao Y (2002) Risk factors for male breast cancer in Canada, 1994–1998. Eur J Cancer Prev 11:253–263
89. Carpenter CL, Ross RK, Paganini-Hill A et al (1999) Lifetime exercise activity and breast cancer risk among post-menopausal women. Br J Cancer 80:1852–1858
90. Enger SM, Bernstein L (2004) Exercise activity, body size and premenopausal breast cancer survival. Br J Cancer 90:2138–2141
91. Albanes D, Blair A, Taylor PR (1989) Physical activity and risk of cancer in the NHANES I population. Am J Public Health 79:744–750
92. Andersson SO, Baron J, Wolk A et al (1995) Early life risk factors for prostate cancer: a population-based case-control study in Sweden. Cancer Epidemiol Biomarkers Prev 4: 187–192
93. Bairati I, Larouche R, Meyer F et al (2000) Lifetime occupational physical activity and incidental prostate cancer (Canada). Cancer Causes Control 11:759–764
94. Brownson RC, Chang JC, Davis JR et al (1991) Physical activity on the job and cancer in Missouri. Am J Public Health 81:639–642
95. Cerhan JR, Torner JC, Lynch CF et al (1997) Association of smoking, body mass, and physical activity with risk of prostate cancer in the Iowa 65+ Rural Health Study (United States). Cancer Causes Control 8:229–238
96. Clarke G, Whittemore AS (2000) Prostate cancer risk in relation to anthropometry and physical activity: the National Health and Nutrition Examination Survey I Epidemiological Follow-Up Study. Cancer Epidemiol Biomarkers Prev 9:875–881
97. Darlington GA, Kreiger N, Lightfoot N et al (2007) Prostate cancer risk and diet, recreational physical activity and cigarette smoking. Chronic Dis Can 27:145–153
98. Dosemeci M, Hayes RB, Vetter R et al (1993) Occupational physical activity, socioeconomic status, and risks of 15 cancer sites in Turkey. Cancer Causes Control 4:313–321
99. Friedenreich CM, McGregor SE, Courneya KS et al (2004) Case-control study of lifetime total physical activity and prostate cancer risk. Am J Epidemiol 159:740–749
100. Gallus S, Foschi R, Talamini R et al (2007) Risk factors for prostate cancer in men aged less than 60 years: a case-control study from Italy. Urology 70:1121–1126
101. Giovannucci EL, Liu Y, Leitzmann MF et al (2005) A prospective study of physical activity and incident and fatal prostate cancer. Arch Intern Med 165:1005–1010
102. Giovannucci E, Liu Y, Platz EA et al (2007) Risk factors for prostate cancer incidence and progression in the health professionals follow-up study. Int J Cancer 121:1571–1578
103. Hartman TJ, Albanes D, Rautalahti M et al (1998) Physical activity and prostate cancer in the Alpha-Tocopherol, Beta-Carotene (ATBC) Cancer Prevention Study (Finland). Cancer Causes Control 9:11–18
104. Hsing AW, McLaughlin JK, Zheng W et al (1994) Occupation, physical activity, and risk of prostate cancer in Shanghai, People's Republic of China. Cancer Causes Control 5: 136–140

105. Ilic M, Vlajinac H, Marinkovic J (1996) Case-control study of risk factors for prostate cancer. Br J Cancer 74:1682–1686
106. Inoue M, Yamamoto S, Kurahashi N et al (2008) Daily total physical activity level and total cancer risk in men and women: results from a large-scale population-based cohort study in Japan. Am J Epidemiol 168:391–403
107. Jian L, Shen ZJ, Lee AH et al (2005) Moderate physical activity and prostate cancer risk: a case-control study in China. Eur J Epidemiol 20:155–160
108. Krishnadasan A, Kennedy N, Zhao Y et al (2008) Nested case-control study of occupational physical activity and prostate cancer among workers using a job exposure matrix. Cancer Causes Control 19:107–114
109. Lacey JV Jr, Deng J, Dosemeci M et al (2001) Prostate cancer, benign prostatic hyperplasia and physical activity in Shanghai, China. Int J Epidemiol 30:341–349
110. Lagiou A, Samoli E, Georgila C et al (2008) Occupational physical activity in relation with prostate cancer and benign prostatic hyperplasia. Eur J Cancer Prev 17:336–339
111. Le Marchand L, Kolonel LN, Yoshizawa CN (1991) Lifetime occupational physical activity and prostate cancer risk. Am J Epidemiol 133:103–111
112. Lee IM, Paffenbarger RS Jr, Hsieh CC (1992) Physical activity and risk of prostatic cancer among college alumni. Am J Epidemiol 135:169–179
113. Lee IM, Paffenbarger RS Jr (1994) Physical activity and its relation to cancer risk: a prospective study of college alumni. Med Sci Sports Exerc 26:831–837
114. Lee IM, Sesso HD, Paffenbarger RS Jr (2001) A prospective cohort study of physical activity and body size in relation to prostate cancer risk (United States). Cancer Causes Control 12:187–193
115. Littman AJ, Kristal AR, White E (2006) Recreational physical activity and prostate cancer risk (United States). Cancer Causes Control 17:831–841
116. Liu S, Lee IM, Linson P et al (2000) A prospective study of physical activity and risk of prostate cancer in US physicians. Int J Epidemiol 29:29–35
117. Lund Nilsen TI, Johnsen R, Vatten LJ (2000) Socio-economic and lifestyle factors associated with the risk of prostate cancer. Br J Cancer 82:1358–1363
118. Moore SC, Peters TM, Ahn J et al (2008) Physical activity in relation to total, advanced, and fatal prostate cancer. Cancer Epidemiol Biomarkers Prev 17:2458–2466
119. Nilsen TI, Romundstad PR, Vatten LJ (2006) Recreational physical activity and risk of prostate cancer: a prospective population-based study in Norway (the HUNT study). Int J Cancer 119:2943–2947
120. Norman A, Moradi T, Gridley G et al (2002) Occupational physical activity and risk for prostate cancer in a nationwide cohort study in Sweden. Br J Cancer 86:70–75
121. Oliveria SA, Kohl HW 3rd, Trichopoulos D et al (1996) The association between cardiorespiratory fitness and prostate cancer. Med Sci Sports Exerc 28:97–104
122. Paffenbarger RS Jr, Hyde RT, Wing AL (1987) Physical activity and incidence of cancer in diverse populations: a preliminary report. Am J Clin Nutr 45:312–317
123. Paffenbarger RS Jr, Lee IM, Wing AL (1992) The influence of physical activity on the incidence of site-specific cancers in college alumni. Adv Exp Med Biol 322:7–15
124. Patel AV, Rodriguez C, Jacobs EJ et al (2005) Recreational physical activity and risk of prostate cancer in a large cohort of U.S. men. Cancer Epidemiol Biomarkers Prev 14: 275–279
125. Pierotti B, Altieri A, Talamini R et al (2005) Lifetime physical activity and prostate cancer risk. Int J Cancer 114:639–642
126. Platz EA, Leitzmann MF, Michaud DS et al (2003) Interrelation of energy intake, body size, and physical activity with prostate cancer in a large prospective cohort study. Cancer Res 63:8542–8548
127. Polednak AP (1976) College athletics, body size, and cancer mortality. Cancer 38:382–387
128. Pukkala E, Kaprio J, Koskenvuo M et al (2000) Cancer incidence among Finnish world class male athletes. Int J Sports Med 21:216–220

129. Putnam SD, Cerhan JR, Parker AS et al (2000) Lifestyle and anthropometric risk factors for prostate cancer in a cohort of Iowa men. Ann Epidemiol 10:361–369
130. Sass-Kortsak AM, Purdham JT, Kreiger N et al (2007) Occupational risk factors for prostate cancer. Am J Ind Med 50:568–576
131. Severson RK, Nomura AM, Grove JS et al (1989) A prospective analysis of physical activity and cancer. Am J Epidemiol 130:522–529
132. Steenland K, Nowlin S, Palu S (1995) Cancer incidence in the National Health and Nutrition Survey I. Follow-up data: diabetes, cholesterol, pulse and physical activity. Cancer Epidemiol Biomarkers Prev 4:807–811
133. Strom SS, Yamamura Y, Flores-Sandoval FN et al (2008) Prostate cancer in Mexican-Americans: identification of risk factors. Prostate 68:563–570
134. Sung JF, Lin RS, Pu YS et al (1999) Risk factors for prostate carcinoma in Taiwan: a case-control study in a Chinese population. Cancer 86:484–491
135. Thune I, Lund E (1994) Physical activity and the risk of prostate and testicular cancer: a cohort study of 53,000 Norwegian men. Cancer Causes Control 5:549–556
136. Vena JE, Graham S, Zielezny M et al (1987) Occupational exercise and risk of cancer. Am J Clin Nutr 45:318–327
137. Villeneuve PJ, Johnson KC, Kreiger N et al (1999) Risk factors for prostate cancer: results from the Canadian National Enhanced Cancer Surveillance System. The Canadian Cancer Registries Epidemiology Research Group. Cancer Causes Control 10:355–367
138. Wannamethee SG, Shaper AG, Walker M (2001) Physical activity and risk of cancer in middle-aged men. Br J Cancer 85:1311–1316
139. West DW, Slattery ML, Robison LM et al (1991) Adult dietary intake and prostate cancer risk in Utah: a case-control study with special emphasis on aggressive tumors. Cancer Causes Control 2:85–94
140. Whittemore AS, Paffenbarger RS Jr, Anderson K et al (1985) Early precursors of site-specific cancers in college men and women. J Natl Cancer Inst 74:43–51
141. Whittemore AS, Kolonel LN, Wu AH et al (1995) Prostate cancer in relation to diet, physical activity, and body size in blacks, whites, and Asians in the United States and Canada. J Natl Cancer Inst 87:652–661
142. Wiklund F, Lageros YT, Chang E et al (2008) Lifetime total physical activity and prostate cancer risk: a population-based case-control study in Sweden. Eur J Epidemiol 23:739–746
143. Yu H, Harris RE, Wynder EL (1988) Case-control study of prostate cancer and socioeconomic factors. Prostate 13:317–325
144. Yun YH, Lim MK, Won YJ et al (2008) Dietary preference, physical activity, and cancer risk in men: national health insurance corporation study. BMC Cancer 8:366
145. Zeegers MP, Dirx MJ, van den Brandt PA (2005) Physical activity and the risk of prostate cancer in the Netherlands cohort study, results after 9.3 years of follow-up. Cancer Epidemiol Biomarkers Prev 14:1490–1495
146. Bonovas S, Filioussi K, Tsantes A (2004) Diabetes mellitus and risk of prostate cancer: a meta-analysis. Diabetologia 47:1071–1078
147. Calton BA, Chang SC, Wright ME et al (2007) History of diabetes mellitus and subsequent prostate cancer risk in the NIH-AARP Diet and Health Study. Cancer Causes Control 18: 493–503
148. Leitzmann MF, Ahn J, Albanes D et al (2008) Diabetes mellitus and prostate cancer risk in the prostate, lung, colorectal, and ovarian cancer screening trial. Cancer Causes Control 19:1267–1276
149. Bostick RM, Potter JD, Kushi LH et al (1994) Sugar, meat, and fat intake, and non-dietary risk factors for colon cancer incidence in Iowa women (United States. Cancer Causes Control 5:38–52
150. Calton BA, Lacey JV Jr, Schatzkin A et al (2006) Physical activity and the risk of colon cancer among women: a prospective cohort study (United States). Int J Cancer 119: 385–391

151. Chao A, Connell CJ, Jacobs EJ et al (2004) Amount, type, and timing of recreational physical activity in relation to colon and rectal cancer in older adults: the Cancer Prevention Study II Nutrition Cohort. Cancer Epidemiol Biomarkers Prev 13:2187–2195
152. Colbert LH, Hartman TJ, Malila N et al (2001) Physical activity in relation to cancer of the colon and rectum in a cohort of male smokers. Cancer Epidemiol Biomarkers Prev 10: 265–268
153. Fraser G, Pearce N (1993) Occupational physical activity and risk of cancer of the colon and rectum in New Zealand males. Cancer Causes Control 4:45–50
154. Friedenreich C, Norat T, Steindorf K et al (2006) Physical activity and risk of colon and rectal cancers: the European prospective investigation into cancer and nutrition. Cancer Epidemiol Biomarkers Prev 15:2398–2407
155. Garabrant DH, Peters JM, Mack TM et al (1984) Job activity and colon cancer risk. Am J Epidemiol 119:1005–1014
156. Gerhardsson M, Norell SE, Kiviranta H et al (1986) Sedentary jobs and colon cancer. Am J Epidemiol 123:775–780
157. Gerhardsson M, Floderus B, Norell SE (1988) Physical activity and colon cancer risk. Int J Epidemiol 17:743–746
158. Giovannucci E, Ascherio A, Rimm EB et al (1995) Physical activity, obesity, and risk for colon cancer and adenoma in men. Ann Intern Med 122:327–334
159. Howard RA, Freedman DM, Park Y et al (2008) Physical activity, sedentary behavior, and the risk of colon and rectal cancer in the NIH-AARP Diet and Health Study. Cancer Causes Control 19:939–953
160. Johnsen NF, Christensen J, Thomsen BL et al (2006) Physical activity and risk of colon cancer in a cohort of Danish middle-aged men and women. Eur J Epidemiol 21:877–884
161. Larsson SC, Rutegard J, Bergkvist L et al (2006) Physical activity, obesity, and risk of colon and rectal cancer in a cohort of Swedish men. Eur J Cancer 42:2590–2597
162. Lee IM, Paffenbarger RS Jr, Hsieh C (1991) Physical activity and risk of developing colorectal cancer among college alumni. J Natl Cancer Inst 83:1324–1329
163. Lee IM, Manson JE, Ajani U et al (1997) Physical activity and risk of colon cancer: the Physicians' Health Study (United States). Cancer Causes Control 8:568–574
164. Lee KJ, Inoue M, Otani T et al (2007) Physical activity and risk of colorectal cancer in Japanese men and women: the Japan Public Health Center-based prospective study. Cancer Causes Control 18:199–209
165. Lynge E, Thygesen L (1988) Use of surveillance systems for occupational cancer: data from the Danish National system. Int J Epidemiol 17:493–500
166. Mai PL, Sullivan-Halley J, Ursin G et al (2007) Physical activity and colon cancer risk among women in the California Teachers Study. Cancer Epidemiol Biomarkers Prev 16: 517–525
167. Martinez ME, Giovannucci E, Spiegelman D et al (1997) Leisure-time physical activity, body size, and colon cancer in women. Nurses' Health Study Research Group. J Natl Cancer Inst 89:948–955
168. Moradi T, Gridley G, Bjork J et al (2008) Occupational physical activity and risk for cancer of the colon and rectum in Sweden among men and women by anatomic subsite. Eur J Cancer Prev 17:201–208
169. Nilsen TI, Romundstad PR, Petersen H et al (2008) Recreational physical activity and cancer risk in subsites of the colon (the Nord-Trondelag Health Study). Cancer Epidemiol Biomarkers Prev 17:183–188
170. Takahashi H, Kuriyama S, Tsubono Y et al (2007) Time spent walking and risk of colorectal cancer in Japan: the Miyagi Cohort study. Eur J Cancer Prev 16:403–408
171. Thune I, Lund E (1996) Physical activity and risk of colorectal cancer in men and women. Br J Cancer 73:1134–1140
172. Wei EK, Giovannucci E, Wu K et al (2004) Comparison of risk factors for colon and rectal cancer. Int J Cancer 108:433–442

173. Wolin KY, Lee IM, Colditz GA et al (2007) Leisure-time physical activity patterns and risk of colon cancer in women. Int J Cancer 121:2776–2781
174. Brownson RC, Zahm SH, Chang JC et al (1989) Occupational risk of colon cancer. An analysis by anatomic subsite. Am J Epidemiol 130:675–687
175. Fredriksson M, Bengtsson NO, Hardell L et al (1989) Colon cancer, physical activity, and occupational exposures. A case-control study. Cancer 63:1838–1842
176. Vena JE, Graham S, Zielezny M et al (1985) Lifetime occupational exercise and colon cancer. Am J Epidemiol 122:357–365
177. Gerhardsson de Verdier M, Steineck G, Hagman U et al (1990) Physical activity and colon cancer: a case-referent study in Stockholm. Int J Cancer 46:985–989
178. Arbman G, Axelson O, Fredriksson M et al (1993) Do occupational factors influence the risk of colon and rectal cancer in different ways? Cancer 72:2543–2549
179. Fernandez E, Gallus S, La Vecchia C et al (2004) Family history and environmental risk factors for colon cancer. Cancer Epidemiol Biomarkers Prev 13:658–661
180. Hou L, Ji BT, Blair A et al (2004) Commuting physical activity and risk of colon cancer in Shanghai, China. Am J Epidemiol 160:860–867
181. Isomura K, Kono S, Moore MA et al (2006) Physical activity and colorectal cancer: the Fukuoka Colorectal Cancer Study. Cancer Sci 97:1099–1104
182. Juarranz M, Calle-Puron ME, Gonzalez-Navarro A et al (2002) Physical exercise, use of Plantago ovata and aspirin, and reduced risk of colon cancer. Eur J Cancer Prev 11:465–472
183. Kato I, Tominaga S, Ikari A (1990) A case-control study of male colorectal cancer in Aichi Prefecture, Japan: with special reference to occupational activity level, drinking habits and family history. Jpn J Cancer Res 81:115–121
184. Kotake K, Koyama Y, Nasu J et al (1995) Relation of family history of cancer and environmental factors to the risk of colorectal cancer: a case-control study. Jpn J Clin Oncol 25:195–202
185. La Vecchia C, Gallus S, Talamini R et al (1999) Interaction between selected environmental factors and familial propensity for colon cancer. Eur J Cancer Prev 8:147–150
186. Levi F, Pasche C, Lucchini F et al (1999) Occupational and leisure-time physical activity and the risk of colorectal cancer. Eur J Cancer Prev 8:487–493
187. Marcus PM, Newcomb PA, Storer BE (1994) Early adulthood physical activity and colon cancer risk among Wisconsin women. Cancer Epidemiol Biomarkers Prev 3:641–644
188. Slattery ML, Abd-Elghany N, Kerber R et al (1990) Physical activity and colon cancer: a comparison of various indicators of physical activity to evaluate the association. Epidemiology 1:481–485
189. Slattery ML, Edwards SL, Ma KN et al (1997) Physical activity and colon cancer: a public health perspective. Ann Epidemiol 7:137–145
190. Slattery ML, Potter J, Caan B et al (1997) Energy balance and colon cancer–beyond physical activity. Cancer Res 57:75–80
191. Slattery ML, Potter JD (2002) Physical activity and colon cancer. Confounding or interaction? Med Sci Sports Exerc 34:913–919
192. Slattery ML, Edwards S, Curtin K et al (2003) Physical activity and colorectal cancer. Am J Epidemiol 158:214–224
193. Tang R, Wang JY, Lo SK et al (1999) Physical activity, water intake and risk of colorectal cancer in Taiwan: a hospital-based case-control study. Int J Cancer 82:484–489
194. Tavani A, Braga C, La Vecchia C et al (1999) Physical activity and risk of cancers of the colon and rectum: an Italian case-control study. Br J Cancer 79:1912–1916
195. Vetter R, Dosemeci M, Blair A et al (1992) Occupational physical activity and colon cancer risk in Turkey. Eur J Epidemiol 8:845–850
196. Vineis P, Ciccone G, Magnino A (1993) Asbestos exposure, physical activity and colon cancer: a case-control study. Tumori 79:301–303
197. White E, Jacobs EJ, Daling JR (1996) Physical activity in relation to colon cancer in middle-aged men and women. Am J Epidemiol 144:42–50

198. Whittemore AS, Wu-Williams AH, Lee M et al (1990) Diet, physical activity, and colorectal cancer among Chinese in North America and China. J Natl Cancer Inst 82:915–926
199. Yeh CC, Hsieh LL, Tang R et al (2003) Risk factors for colorectal cancer in Taiwan: a hospital-based case-control study. J Formos Med Assoc 102:305–312
200. Zhang Y, Cantor KP, Dosemeci M et al (2006) Occupational and leisure-time physical activity and risk of colon cancer by subsite. J Occup Environ Med 48:236–243
201. Wolin KY, Yan Y, Colditz GA et al (2009) Physical activity and colon cancer prevention: a meta-analysis. Br J Cancer 100:611–616
202. Mao Y, Pan S, Wen SW et al (2003) Physical inactivity, energy intake, obesity and the risk of rectal cancer in Canada. Int J Cancer 105:831–837
203. Lee IM, Oguma Y (2006) Physical activity. In: Schottenfeld D and Fraumeni JF (eds) Cancer epidemiology and prevention. Oxford University Press, New York, NY
204. Alfano CM, Klesges RC, Murray DM et al (2004) Physical activity in relation to all-site and lung cancer incidence and mortality in current and former smokers. Cancer Epidemiol Biomarkers Prev 13:2233–2241
205. Bak H, Christensen J, Thomsen BL et al (2005) Physical activity and risk for lung cancer in a Danish cohort. Int J Cancer 116:439–444
206. Colbert LH, Hartman TJ, Tangrea JA et al (2002) Physical activity and lung cancer risk in male smokers. Int J Cancer 98:770–773
207. Kubik A, Zatloukal P, Tomasek L et al (2004) Lung cancer risk among nonsmoking women in relation to diet and physical activity. Neoplasma 51:136–143
208. Kubik AK, Zatloukal P, Tomasek L et al (2004) Dietary habits and lung cancer risk among non-smoking women. Eur J Cancer Prev 13:471–480
209. Kubik A, Zatloukal P, Tomasek L et al (2007) Interactions between smoking and other exposures associated with lung cancer risk in women: diet and physical activity. Neoplasma 54:83–88
210. Kubik A, Zatloukal P, Tomasek L et al (2008) A case-control study of lifestyle and lung cancer associations by histological types. Neoplasma 55:192–199
211. Lee IM, Sesso HD, Paffenbarger RS Jr (1999) Physical activity and risk of lung cancer. Int J Epidemiol 28:620–625
212. Leitzmann MF, Koebnick C, Abnet CC et al (2009) Prospective study of physical activity and lung cancer by histologic type in current, former, and never smokers. Am J Epidemiol 169:542–553
213. Mao Y, Pan S, Wen SW et al (2003) Physical activity and the risk of lung cancer in Canada. Am J Epidemiol 158:564–575
214. Sinner P, Folsom AR, Harnack L et al (2006) The association of physical activity with lung cancer incidence in a cohort of older women: the Iowa Women's Health Study. Cancer Epidemiol Biomarkers Prev 15:2359–2363
215. Sprague BL, Trentham-Dietz A, Klein BE et al (2008) Physical activity, white blood cell count, and lung cancer risk in a prospective cohort study. Cancer Epidemiol Biomarkers Prev 17:2714–2722
216. Steindorf K, Friedenreich C, Linseisen J et al (2006) Physical activity and lung cancer risk in the European Prospective Investigation into Cancer and Nutrition Cohort. Int J Cancer 119:2389–2397
217. Thune I, Lund E (1997) The influence of physical activity on lung-cancer risk: A prospective study of 81,516 men and women. Int J Cancer 70:57–62
218. Colbert LH, Lacey JV Jr, Schairer C et al (2003) Physical activity and risk of endometrial cancer in a prospective cohort study (United States). Cancer Causes Control 14:559–567
219. Friberg E, Mantzoros CS, Wolk A (2006) Physical activity and risk of endometrial cancer: a population-based prospective cohort study. Cancer Epidemiol Biomarkers Prev 15: 2136–2140

220. Friedenreich C, Cust A, Lahmann PH et al (2007) Physical activity and risk of endometrial cancer: the European prospective investigation into cancer and nutrition. Int J Cancer 121:347–355
221. Furberg AS, Thune I (2003) Metabolic abnormalities (hypertension, hyperglycemia and overweight), lifestyle (high energy intake and physical inactivity) and endometrial cancer risk in a Norwegian cohort. Int J Cancer 104:669–676
222. Gierach GL, Chang SC, Brinton LA et al (2009) Physical activity, sedentary behavior, and endometrial cancer risk in the NIH-AARP Diet and Health Study. Int J Cancer 124: 2139–2147
223. Goodman MT, Hankin JH, Wilkens LR et al (1997) Diet, body size, physical activity, and the risk of endometrial cancer. Cancer Res 57:5077–5085
224. Hirose K, Tajima K, Hamajima N et al (1996) Subsite (cervix/endometrium)-specific risk and protective factors in uterus cancer. Jpn J Cancer Res 87:1001–1009
225. Kalandidi A, Tzonou A, Lipworth L et al (1996) A case-control study of endometrial cancer in relation to reproductive, somatometric, and life-style variables. Oncology 53: 354–359
226. Littman AJ, Voigt LF, Beresford SA et al (2001) Recreational physical activity and endometrial cancer risk. Am J Epidemiol 154:924–933
227. Matthews CE, Xu WH, Zheng W et al (2005) Physical activity and risk of endometrial cancer: a report from the Shanghai endometrial cancer study. Cancer Epidemiol Biomarkers Prev 14:779–785
228. Moradi T, Nyren O, Bergstrom R et al (1998) Risk for endometrial cancer in relation to occupational physical activity: a nationwide cohort study in Sweden. Int J Cancer 76: 665–670
229. Moradi T, Weiderpass E, Signorello LB et al (2000) Physical activity and postmenopausal endometrial cancer risk (Sweden). Cancer Causes Control 11: 829–837
230. Olson SH, Vena JE, Dorn JP et al (1997) Exercise, occupational activity, and risk of endometrial cancer. Ann Epidemiol 7:46–53
231. Patel AV, Feigelson HS, Talbot JT et al (2008) The role of body weight in the relationship between physical activity and endometrial cancer: results from a large cohort of US women. Int J Cancer 123:1877–1882
232. Salazar-Martinez E, Lazcano-Ponce EC, Lira-Lira GG et al (2000) Case-control study of diabetes, obesity, physical activity and risk of endometrial cancer among Mexican women. Cancer Causes Control 11:707–711
233. Schouten LJ, Goldbohm RA, van den Brandt PA (2004) Anthropometry, physical activity, and endometrial cancer risk: results from the Netherlands Cohort Study. J Natl Cancer Inst 96:1635–1638
234. Terry P, Baron JA, Weiderpass E et al (1999) Lifestyle and endometrial cancer risk: a cohort study from the Swedish Twin Registry. Int J Cancer 82:38–42
235. Olsen CM, Green AC, Whiteman DC et al (2007) Obesity and the risk of epithelial ovarian cancer: a systematic review and meta-analysis. Eur J Cancer 43:690–709
236. Lahmann PH, Friedenreich C, Schulz M et al (2009) Physical activity and ovarian cancer risk: the European Prospective Investigation into Cancer and Nutrition. Cancer Epidemiol Biomarkers Prev 18:351–354
237. Chiaffarino F, Parazzini F, Bosetti C et al (2007) Risk factors for ovarian cancer histotypes. Eur J Cancer 43:1208–1213
238. Bao Y, Michaud DS (2008) Physical activity and pancreatic cancer risk: a systematic review. Cancer Epidemiol Biomarkers Prev 17:2671–2682
239. Jiao L, Mitrou PN, Reedy J et al (2009) A combined healthy lifestyle score and risk of pancreatic cancer in a large cohort study. Arch Intern Med 169:764–770

240. Stevens RJ, Roddam AW, Spencer EA et al (2009) Factors associated with incident and fatal pancreatic cancer in a cohort of middle-aged women. Int J Cancer 124: 2400–2405
241. Eberle CA, Bracci PM, Holly EA (2005) Anthropometric factors and pancreatic cancer in a population-based case-control study in the San Francisco Bay area. Cancer Causes Control 16:1235–1244
242. Hanley AJ, Johnson KC, Villeneuve PJ et al (2001) Physical activity, anthropometric factors and risk of pancreatic cancer: results from the Canadian enhanced cancer surveillance system. Int J Cancer 94:140–147
243. Lee IM, Sesso HD, Oguma Y et al (2003) Physical activity, body weight, and pancreatic cancer mortality. Br J Cancer 88:679–683
244. Michaud DS, Giovannucci E, Willett WC et al (2001) Physical activity, obesity, height, and the risk of pancreatic cancer. JAMA 286:921–929
245. Patel AV, Rodriguez C, Bernstein L, et al (2005) Obesity, recreational physical activity, and risk of pancreatic cancer in a large U.S. Cohort. Cancer Epidemiol Biomarkers Prev 14: 459–466
246. Sinner PJ, Schmitz KH, Anderson KE et al (2005) Lack of association of physical activity and obesity with incident pancreatic cancer in elderly women. Cancer Epidemiol Biomarkers Prev 14:1571–1573
247. Berrington de Gonzalez A, Spencer EA, Bueno-de-Mesquita HB et al (2006) Anthropometry, physical activity, and the risk of pancreatic cancer in the European prospective investigation into cancer and nutrition. Cancer Epidemiol Biomarkers Prev 15: 879–885
248. Ekelund LG, Haskell WL, Johnson JL et al (1988) Physical fitness as a predictor of cardiovascular mortality in asymptomatic North American men. The Lipid Research Clinics Mortality Follow-up Study. N Engl J Med 319:1379–1384
249. Sandvik L, Erikssen J, Thaulow E et al (1993) Physical fitness as a predictor of mortality among healthy, middle-aged Norwegian men. N Engl J Med 328:533–537
250. Huang C, Ross PD, Wasnich RD (1996) Vertebral fracture and other predictors of physical impairment and health care utilization. Arch Intern Med 156:2469–2475
251. Stafford M, Hemingway H, Marmot M (1998) Current obesity, steady weight change and weight fluctuation as predictors of physical functioning in middle aged office workers: the Whitehall II Study. Int J Obes Relat Metab Disord 22:23–31
252. Hasselstrom H, Hansen SE, Froberg K et al (2002) Physical fitness and physical activity during adolescence as predictors of cardiovascular disease risk in young adulthood. Danish Youth and Sports Study. An eight-year follow-up study. Int J Sports Med 23(Suppl 1): S27–S31
253. Peate WF, Bates G, Lunda K et al (2007) Core strength: a new model for injury prediction and prevention. J Occup Med Toxicol 2:3
254. Katzmarzyk PT, Craig CL, Gauvin L (2007) Adiposity, physical fitness and incident diabetes: the physical activity longitudinal study. Diabetologia 50:538–544
255. Lee DC, Sui X, Church TS et al (2009) Associations of cardiorespiratory fitness and obesity with risks of impaired fasting glucose and type 2 diabetes in men. Diabetes Care 32: 257–262
256. Farrell SW, Cortese GM, LaMonte MJ et al (2007) Cardiorespiratory fitness, different measures of adiposity, and cancer mortality in men. Obesity 15:3140–3149
257. Kampert JB, Blair SN, Barlow CE et al (1996) Physical activity, physical fitness, and all-cause and cancer mortality: a prospective study of men and women. Ann Epidemiol 6: 452–457
258. Lee CD, Blair SN (2002) Cardiorespiratory fitness and smoking-related and total cancer mortality in men. Med Sci Sports Exerc 34:735–739
259. Peel JB, Sui X, Adams SA et al (2009) A prospective study of cardiorespiratory fitness and breast cancer mortality. Med Sci Sports Exerc 41:742–748

260. Peel JB, Sui X, Matthews CE et al (2009) Cardiorespiratory fitness and digestive cancer mortality: findings from the aerobics center longitudinal study. Cancer Epidemiol Biomarkers Prev 18:1111–1117
261. Ruiz JR, Sui X, Lobelo F et al (2009) Muscular strength and adiposity as predictors of adulthood cancer mortality in men. Cancer Epidemiol Biomarkers Prev 18: 1468–1476
262. Sawada SS, Muto T, Tanaka H et al (2003) Cardiorespiratory fitness and cancer mortality in Japanese men: a prospective study. Med Sci Sports Exerc 35:1546–1550
263. Thompson AM, Church TS, Janssen I et al (2008) Cardiorespiratory fitness as a predictor of cancer mortality among men with pre-diabetes and diabetes. Diabetes Care 31:764–769

Chapter 4
Energetics and Cancer: Exploring a Road Less Traveled

Henry J. Thompson, Weiqin Jiang, and Zongjian Zhu

Abstract As the number of individuals who are overweight or obese continues to increase in a worldwide epidemic of positive energy imbalance, identification of the mechanisms that account for the effects of energetics on the development of cancer becomes increasingly important. In this brief review, attention is directed to the contributions of extracellular mediators and intracellular energy-sensing mechanisms to the regulation of the carcinogenic process. The signaling pathways regulated by intracellular energy sensors are integrally linked to pathways that communicate to the intracellular milieu, information about effects of the host's energy status on the extracellular environment. Thus, the effects of energetics on cancer are likely to be accounted for by interactions among systemic factors, manifest in plasma concentrations of hormones, growth factors, and various cytokines including those arising from adipose and skeletal muscle tissues, and direct and indirect effects of energetic status on intracellular energy messengers and the proteins that detect changes in their concentrations. Collectively, the pathways regulated by energy status exert effects on cell survival/proliferation, cell death (apoptosis, autophagy, necrosis), tissue blood supply (vasculogenesis and angiogenesis), and resistance to metabolic stress, processes that are misregulated during the development of cancer.

1 Introduction

As the prevalence of overweight and obesity has increased worldwide at epidemic rates, the impact of the dysregulation of energy balance that results in the occurrence of excessive body weight relative to height on a number of chronic diseases

---

H.J. Thompson (✉)
Cancer Prevention Laboratory, Colorado State University, Fort Collins, CO 80523, USA
e-mail: henry.thompson@colostate.edu; thomph@lamar.colostate.edu

This work was supported by United States Public Health Services Grant U54-CA116847 from the National Cancer Institute.

A. McTiernan (ed.), *Physical Activity, Dietary Calorie Restriction, and Cancer*,
Energy Balance and Cancer 3, DOI 10.1007/978-1-4419-7551-5_4,

including cancer has been receiving increasing attention and the literature related to the cancer sites that are affected has been reviewed [1, 2]. Many questions have begun to emerge about the factors that account for the differences in susceptibility to cancer at various organ sites in individuals whose body weight relative to their height ranges from being underweight to morbidly obese. The resolution of these questions will undoubtedly benefit from a deeper understanding of mechanisms that underlie energetics and cancer. This chapter was designed to go beyond the most commonly discussed mechanisms relative to energetics and cancer [3], and thus to journey on a road less traveled. For the remainder of this chapter, examples are drawn from experience in working with women at risk for breast cancer and from rodent models for mammary carcinogenesis since breast cancer research has been the focus of our work for many years. It is anticipated that much of what is learned relative to the association between energetics and breast cancer will have relevance to cancer at other organ sites and in some cases to other chronic disease processes, e.g., type-2 diabetes and cardiovascular disease as discussed in [4].

2 Body Mass Index and Energy Balance

The journey down the path to this particular less traveled road began with the following consideration. Body weight relative to an individual's height (body mass index, BMI) provides an accepted index by which to categorize the prevalence of individuals who are underweight, normal weight, overweight, obese, or morbidly obese in adult populations around the world [1]. While individuals can vary markedly in their BMI at various stages of their lives, it is clear that in a cross section of a population at any given time, there is a full range of BMIs for individuals of any particular height. Let us argue that many individuals of the same height in each BMI category, e.g., between 15 and 40, will be in weight equilibrium, i.e., they will be neither gaining nor losing weight at a particular point in time. As shown in Table 4.1, at any particular level of physical activity and age (several are shown), the amount of energy required to maintain body weight for the same individual whose BMI is 15, 20, 25, 30, 35, or 40 can differ by as much as 35%. Our quest has been to understand experimentally how this single fact of energetics in relationship to weight maintenance over a wide range of BMIs translates into varying susceptibility to the development of cancer. We refer to the paradigm described in Table 4.1 as an energetics continuum, and argue that it illustrates how individuals could vary in their plane of energy nutrition depending on their body weight. We further argue that all tissues are exposed to energetic differences based on the plane of energy nutrition of the host, and that the challenge is to determine how both systemic and local responses to differing energetics planes of nutrition are integrated within cells in both tissue-specific and cell-type-specific manners such that the probability for transformed clones of cells residing within those tissues to progress to clinically detectable cancer is either inhibited or enhanced. These concepts are illustrated in Fig. 4.1.

Table 4.1 Energy requirements for an individual with the same height but different body weights ranging from underweight to morbidly obese

Height inches	Weight lbs	BMI[a]	Age	RMR[b] kcal/d	TEE[c] Sedentary kcal/d	TEE Moderately active kcal/d	TEE Vigorously active kcal/d
64	86	15	35	1,165	1,398	1,806	2,010
64	115	20	35	1,292	1,550	2,002	2,228
64	145	25	35	1,422	1,706	2,204	2,453
64	175	30	35	1,553	1,863	2,406	2,678
64	205	35	35	1,683	2,020	2,609	2,903
64	235	40	35	1,814	2,176	2,811	3,128
64	86	15	50	1,095	1,314	1,697	1,889
64	115	20	50	1,221	1,465	1,893	2,106
64	145	25	50	1,352	1,622	2,095	2,331
64	175	30	50	1,482	1,778	2,297	2,557
64	205	35	50	1,613	1,935	2,499	2,782
64	235	40	50	1,743	2,092	2,702	3,007

[a]Body mass index, BMI: Weight in lbs/Height in inches × 703
[b]Resting metabolic rate, RMR: For women = 655 + (4.35 × weight in pounds) + (4.7 × height in inches) – (4.7 × age in years)
[c]Total daily energy expenditure, TEE for a sedentary activity (RMR × 1.2); moderate activity (RMR × 1.55), and vigorous activity (RMR × 1.725) in kcal/d

3 Mechanistic Overview

Arguably, it can be stated that the preponderance of mechanistic work on energetics and cancer has focused on the impact of different energetic states on circulating levels of growth factors and hormones, prominent among which are insulin, insulin-like growth factor-1 (IGF-1), and hormones such as cortisol, estrogen, and progesterone [3]. Related to this has been the recognition of adipose tissue as an endocrine organ and the identification of cytokines secreted within adipose tissue, referred to as adipokines, for which there is accumulating but controversial evidence of their ability to affect processes misregulated during carcinogenesis [5–7]. Moreover, it has recently been reported that skeletal muscle, depending on the nature of the physical activity to which it is subjected, is also capable of synthesizing cytokines, referred to as myokines, some of which are released into circulation [8]. Since skeletal muscle generally constitutes a dominant proportion of body weight in individuals with a normal BMI, and the amount of muscle and its synthetic activity are impacted in normal weight versus overweight/obese individuals who generally are physically inactive, it will be surprising if changes in the biosynthetic activity of muscle versus adipose tissue in the production and release into circulation of their respective cytokines is not a topic given increasing attention relative to energetics and cancer. However, that is not the road less traveled which is explored in this chapter. Rather, the focus of this review is on how the overall energetics of the organism is actually reflected in the concentration of various energy-related substrates within the cell, which are referred to as energy messengers, and the proteins that detect changes in

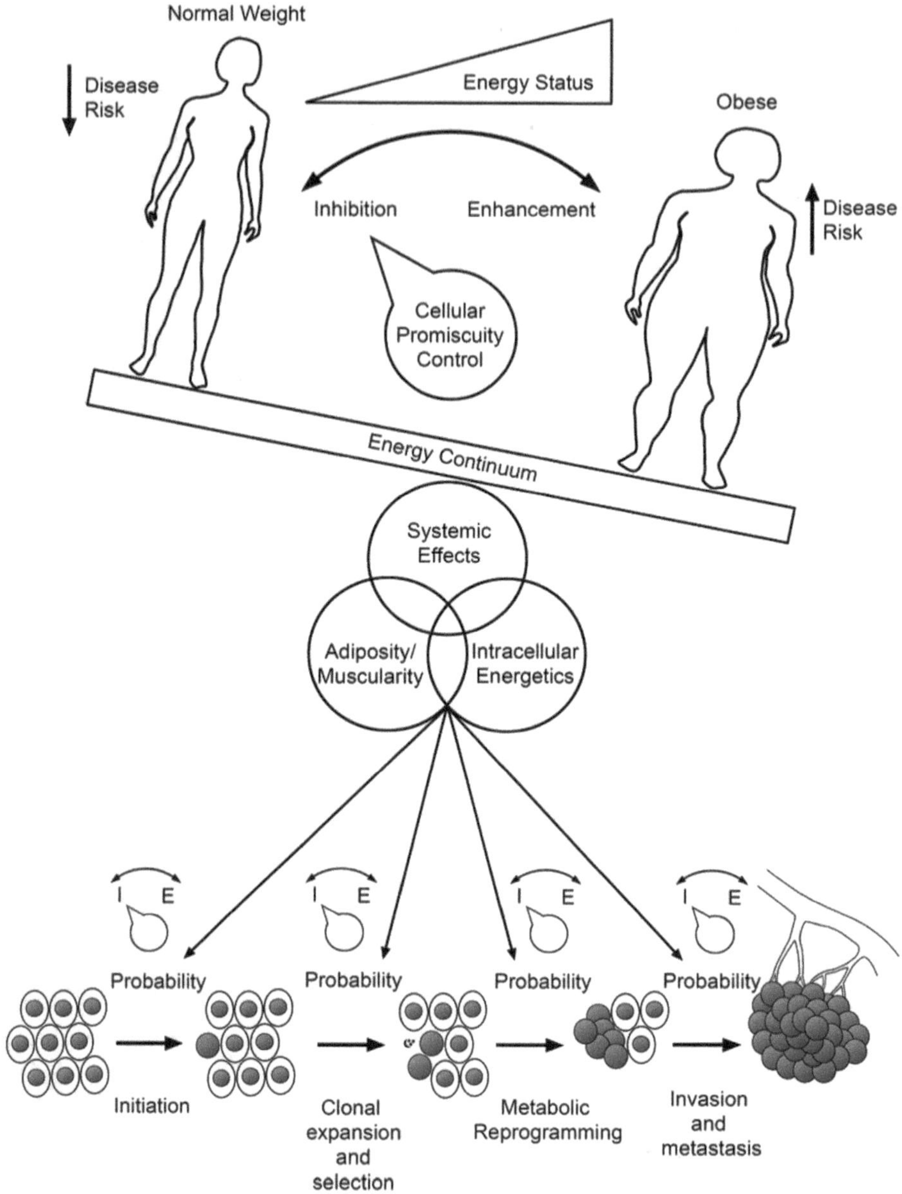

Fig. 4.1 Individuals with lower body weight for a particular height have a lower risk for a number of chronic diseases including cancer. Differences in cancer risk are due to combinatorial effects of energy balance on systemic factors, secretory products of adipose tissue and skeletal muscle, and energy-sensing mechanisms within the cell. These combined effects influence the probability of progression through multiple steps in the carcinogenic process, with low-energy status being associated with inhibition and high-energy status being associated with enhancement

their concentration, which are referred to as energy sensors [9, 10]. The function of the intracellular energy sensing network is not viewed as being independent of systemic effects mediated by circulating factors, but rather as being integrated with their activities as emphasized in Fig. 4.1.

There has been a natural tendency for mechanistic studies of excessive weight gain, and specifically obesity, to focus heavily on neuroendocrine-mediated effects of imbalances of energy homeostasis on appetite and growth and on contributions of adipose tissue per se to disease pathogenesis [11–13]. This focus is clearly important and has provided many insights about mechanisms of energy balance regulation and disease pathogenesis. Nonetheless, it is also important to recognize that all tissues within the body are exposed to the same energetic milieu that results in well-studied neuroendocrine responses. Thus, while a perception may exist that neuroendocrine-mediated effects, and the many systemic changes they induce, function to keep the energy status of most cells within the body invariant, the reality is that cells can survive not only with markedly different intracellular concentrations of free fatty acids, glycogen, and reducing equivalents ($NAD^+/NADH$, $NADP^+/NADPH$) but also with different concentrations of high-energy phosphate compounds [14]. However, it is also clear that cells have evolved multiple mechanisms through which they sense these intracellular energy substrates and regulate metabolism in order to provide sufficient sources of energy to avoid cell death and promote survival ([9, 10]). It also is clear that different energy sensors play dominant roles in a tissue-specific and cell-type-specific manner. Understanding the coordinated flow of information through metabolic, energetic, and cell signaling pathways as impacted by energy status of the host and the development of cancer is necessary to provide insight about the differential effects of overweight and obesity on tumor development at various organ sites.

4 Intracellular Energy Sensing

Recognized cellular energy messengers and their sensors are shown in Fig. 4.2. They include [1]: AMP and glycogen, which are sensed by AMP-activated protein kinase [15–17, 2]; ATP, which is sensed by soluble guanylyl cyclase [18, 3]; $NAD^+/NADH$, which are sensed by sirtuins [19–21]; and [4] free fatty acids and other lipid metabolites, which are sensed by peroxisome proliferator-activated receptors (PPARs, α, β/δ, and γ) [22–24]. Not surprisingly, these energy messenger–sensor pairings can be shown to have tight linkages with cell cycle regulatory machinery, various cell death mechanisms, mechanisms associated with blood vessel formation and maintenance, and adaptive mechanisms that protect cells against metabolic stresses as illustrated in Fig. 4.3. However, the number of cell signaling pathways modulated by each energy messenger–energy sensor pair is large and influenced in a tissue- and cell-type-specific manner; this precludes a comprehensive discussion of each energy messenger–energy sensing pair in this short review. Therefore, we will first briefly discuss each major class of energy sensor shown in Fig. 4.2 and then focus on one

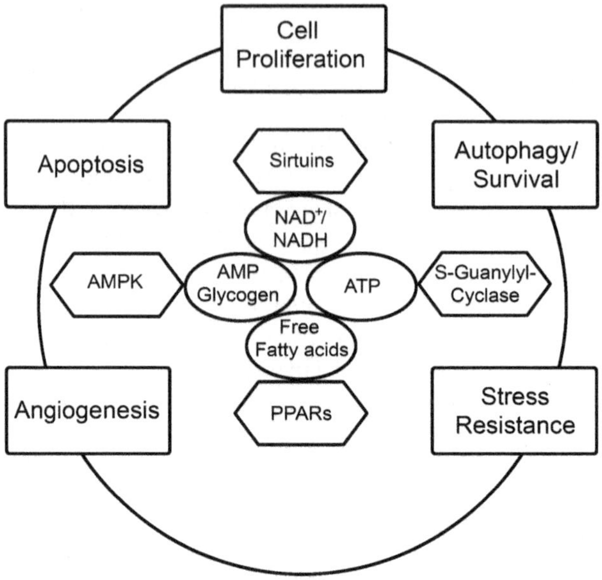

Fig. 4.2 Recognized cellular energy messengers (*ovals*) and their sensors (*hexagons*) include: AMP and glycogen, which are sensed by AMP-activated protein kinase (AMPK); ATP, which is sensed by soluble guanylyl cyclase (sGC); NAD^+/NADH, which are sensed by sirtuins; and free fatty acids and other lipid metabolites, which are sensed by peroxisome proliferator-activated receptors (PPARs, α, β/δ, and γ). These energy messenger–sensor pairings can be shown to have tight linkages with cell cycle regulatory machinery, various cell death mechanisms, mechanisms associated with blood vessel formation and maintenance, and adaptive mechanisms that protect cells against metabolic stresses

messenger–sensor pair (AMP-AMPK) and one of the metabolic hubs with which this pair communicates, i.e., the mammalian target of rapamycin (mTOR). This focus was chosen not only because mTOR activity has direct relevance to cancer but also because mTOR integrates signals from the extracellular environment, via the IGF-1R receptor, with intracellular energy status via AMPK as well as signals mediated via adipokines that also can regulate the activity of AMPK.

5 Guanylyl Cyclase

Soluble guanylyl cyclase (sGC) is an intracellular receptor for nitric oxide (NO) that is regulated by the concentration of ATP within the cell [25]. Thus sGC couples the energy charge of the cell measured as ATP with the functions of NO that include regulation of the supply of energy by improving the delivery of substrates and oxygen to tissues, regulating the intracellular delivery of metabolic substrates, selection of substrates that support metabolism, oxidation of metabolic substrates, generation of ATP by improving metabolic efficiency, and biogenesis of mitochondria (reviewed in [25]). sGC activity and NO production have been reported to be induced by

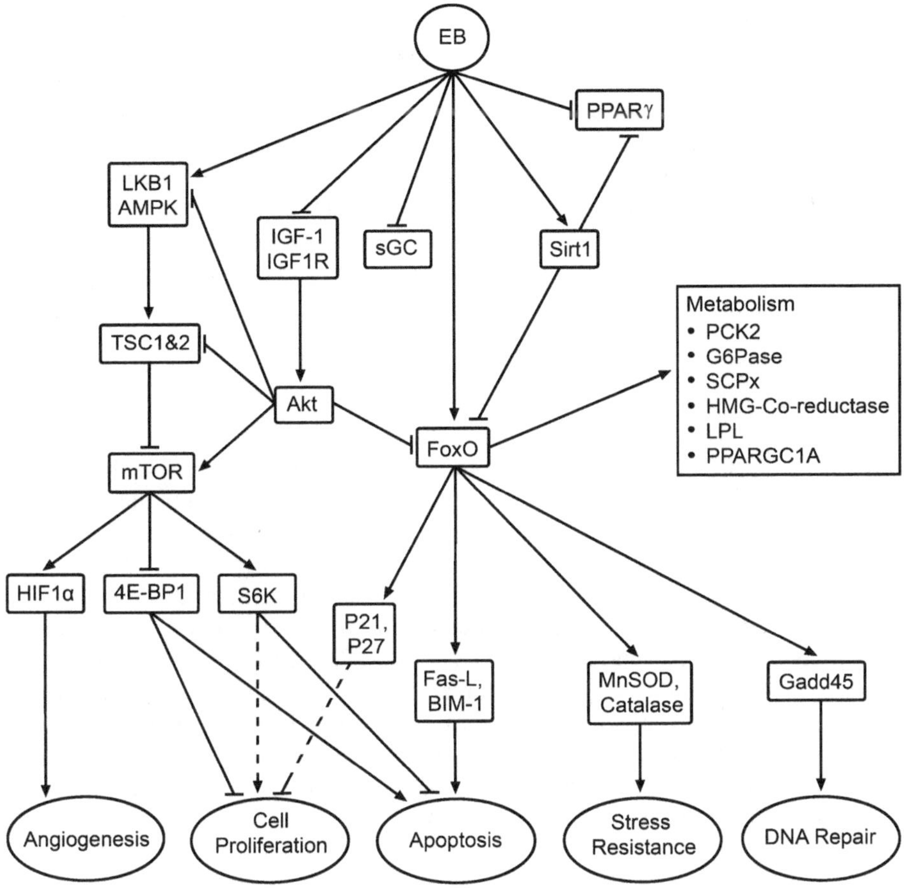

Fig. 4.3 This diagram illustrates the effects of energy sensor activity, cell signaling, and the cellular processes misregulated during carcinogenesis when energy status (EB, energy balance) is protective against the development of cancer. Note that energy sensors are components of a network of signaling that can downregulate cellular processes which are misregulated during the development of cancer

diet-induced obesity [26]. NO effects are tissue- and cell-type-specific [27], and the activities of enzymes that catalyze NO synthesis have been implicated in tumor growth and metastasis [28].

6 Sirtuins

The Sir family of proteins (sirtuins) are a group of nicotinamide (NAD^+)-dependent deacetylases/ADP-ribosyltransferases initially discovered in yeast that are conserved in diverse organisms including humans [29]. There are seven homologs of the yeast *Sir2* gene (SIR 1-7) that localize to the nucleus, cytoplasm, or mitochondria, and which utilize various substrates and exhibit a broad spectrum of functions [30]. It has been demonstrated that SIRT1 is one mediator of the effects of calorie restriction on longevity. Many proteins are deacetylated by SIRT1, and the deacetylated proteins either lose their effect on apoptotic cell death, e.g., p53, or have enhanced activity, e.g., FoxO, resulting in effects on cell survival and longevity. Evidence of tissue-specific and cell-type-specific effects of sirtuins has been reported, and recent findings indicate that SIRT1 may be a critical regulator of carcinogenesis although whether it serves the role of an oncogene or as a tumor suppressor remains controversial [31]. The activity of SIRT1 has recently been reported to be modulated by AMPK [32].

7 PPARs

Peroxisome proliferator-activated receptors (PPARα, -β/δ, and -γ), members of the ligand-activated nuclear receptor superfamily, are the key transcriptional regulators in fatty acid metabolism and are involved in energy homeostasis [14]. The various members of this gene family act in a tissue- and cell-type-specific manner. For example, PPARγ is expressed in adipose tissue where it regulates diverse functions such as the development of fat cells and their capacity to store lipids [33]. However, in a variety of malignant and nonmalignant tissues, PPARγ and its ligands have been reported to inhibit cell cycle progression at the G1/S checkpoint and cell proliferation by arresting the cells in G0/G1 phase, as well as inducing apoptosis [34]. A specific role of PPARγ as an energy sensor has been reported via its co-activator, peroxisome proliferator-activated receptor γ coactivator-1-α (PGC-1α); the activity of PGC-1α is modulated by sirtuins and AMPK [10].

8 AMP-Activated Protein Kinase

AMPK serves as a metabolic checkpoint, downregulating cell growth and cell division in the absence of an adequate supply of biosynthetic and energy substrates [15]. In this respect, AMPK has been likened in its function to p53 that serves as a guardian of genome integrity. AMPK has been shown to be an exquisitely sensitive detector of small changes in the intracellular ratio of AMP to ATP, and some investigators have even proposed that AMPK plays a central role in homeostatic regulation of whole body energy metabolism [16]. We have reported that reduced energy intake or increased energy expenditure via physical activity result in AMPK activation [35]. This suggests that these interventions, which are the primary affectors of overall energy balance are either altering substrate availability (the fuel mixture presented to tissues throughout the body) or that activation is being induced via alterations in the ratio of intracellular AMP to ATP. It is becoming clear that additional factors control the activation of AMPK, including various cytokines [17].

9 Extracellular Inputs

9.1 Insulin-Like Growth Factor-1 (IGF-1)

The insulin-like growth factor (IGF) signaling system plays a critical role in the growth and development of many tissues and regulates overall growth ([36] and references therein). The IGF system has also been implicated in various pathophysiological conditions, and is thought to play a particularly prominent role in tumorigenesis. The IGF system comprised the IGF ligands (IGF-I and IGF-II); cell-surface receptors that mediate the biological effects of the IGFs, including the IGF-I receptor (IGF-IR), the IGF-II receptor (IGF-IIR); and the insulin receptor (IR), as well as a family of IGF-binding proteins (IGFBPs). IGFBPs affect the half-lives and bioavailability of the IGFs in the circulation, in extracellular fluids, and may exert IGF-independent effects under certain conditions. Most, if not all, of the effects of IGF-I result from its activation of the IGF-IR and lead to activation of the mitogen-activated protein kinase (MAP kinase) and PI3 kinase cascades. The ultimate targets of the MAP kinase and PI3 kinase cascades include members of mTOR network and forkhead transcription factor families. Regulation of transcription factors provides a mechanism by which IGF action at the cell surface can elicit changes in gene expression that eventually mediate the proliferative, differentiating, and apoptotic effects of IGF-1. We have found that the level of plasma IGF-1 are reduced by either decreased levels of energy intake or increased levels of energy expenditure as physical activity [37].

9.2 Protein Kinase B (Akt)

Interventions that favor lower body weights have been reported to decrease circulating levels of IGF-1[35, 37–39]. Lower levels of IGF-1 would be expected to downregulate signaling via the pathway of which IGF-1 receptor, phosphoinositide kinase-3 (PI3K), and Akt are components. Of these proteins, activated Akt, a serine/threonine kinase, is the critical affecter molecule. Akt is activated by its phosphorylation on Ser473. Phospho-Akt serves important roles in cell proliferation, cell survival, and new blood vessel formation that are associated with tumor development [40]. While it is clear that reduced levels of activated Akt are likely to affect proliferation, apoptosis, and angiogenesis by mechanisms independent of mTOR (reviewed in [41]), the finding that either reduced energy intake or increased energy expenditure via physical activity induced both AMPK activation and downregulation of growth factor signaling via Akt points to mTOR as a downstream target mediating the effects of overall energy equilibrium. Thus, mTOR may represent a molecular target that is regulated by the hosts energy balance to modulate the probability that transformed clones of cells will progress to cancer.

10 Network Integration: Mammalian Target of Rapamycin

mTOR is an intracellular protein that plays a key role in integrating the information received from the extracellular environment via the binding of growth factors and hormones with their cognate receptor tyrosine kinases (e.g., IGF-1: IGF1-R) with signals from metabolic checkpoints within the cell in a manner that affects cell growth, cell division, and cell survival or death [15]. mTOR is an evolutionarily conserved serine–threonine kinase that is a key regulator of protein translation and synthesis. mTOR is centrally involved in cell growth, i.e., increase in cell size and cell mass; and these processes are tightly coupled to cell division (reviewed in [42]). The regulation of mTOR is multifaceted and still being investigated. It has two biochemically and functionally distinct complexes, mTOR complex 1 (TORC1) and mTOR complex 2 (TORC2) [43]. TORC1 comprised mTOR, regulatory associated protein of mTOR (Raptor), and G protein beta subunit-like (Gβ1/also known as mLST8) and its activity is nutrient/energy-sensitive, whereas TORC2 comprised mTOR, rapamycin-insensitive companion of mTOR (Rictor), stress-activated-protein-kinase-interacting protein 1 (SIN1) and Gβ1) and plays a role in regulating the signaling pathway of which Akt is a component. A primary locus for control of mTOR is via the tuberous sclerosis protein complex (TSC), specifically TSC2, which is phosphorylated on different sites by either activated AMPK (Thr1227 and Ser1345 residues that correspond to Thr1271 and Ser1387, respectively, in human TSC2) or activated Akt (Thr1462 and Ser939 residues). A second locus for control of mTOR via AMPK and Akt is via the phosphorylation of TORC1 complex components raptor and PRAD, respectively [15]. mTOR mediates its effects on downstream targets via site-specific phosphorylation. Relative to its effects on cell growth and cell division, two principal targets of mTOR are 70-kDa ribosomal protein S6 kinase (p70S6K) and 4E binding protein 1 (4E-BP1). Activated mTOR phosphorylates p70S6K and this leads to increased ribosomal biogenesis ([44, 45]). 4E-BP1 is a repressor of translation initiation [46–48]. Activated mTOR phosphorylates 4E-BP1, which inactivates the protein. When it is hypophosphorylated, 4E-BP1 binds to and inhibits the rate-limiting translation initiation factor eIF4E (eukaryotic translation initiation factor 4E). Upon phosphorylation, eIF4E is released from 4E-BP1, allowing eIF4E to assemble with other translation initiation factors to initiate cap-dependent translation [48]. We have reported that reduced energy intake or increased energy expenditure via physical activity decreases the levels of both phosphorylated S6K and 4E-BP1[35, 38, 49].

11 Conclusions

It is clear that no one factor can be expected to explain the differential effects of energy status on the development of cancer in various organ sites. In this short review, a framework has been presented for considering how energetic, metabolic, and cell signaling pathways can exert integrated effects on the carcinogenic process. One of the key proteins through which these effects are likely to be mediated is mTOR. Regulation of mTOR activity illustrates a coordinated function within the cell that integrates inputs from the external environment with those transduced via intracellular sensors of energy status, specifically AMPK, sirtuins, PPARs, and sGC, the activities of which are functionally linked. We suggest that a broad view of cell signaling is needed to fully appreciate how energy status impacts carcinogenesis. Thus rather than thinking of a pathway, of which mTOR is a component, we view it as one of several "control hubs" at the center of a signaling network that regulates cell function and cell fate. It is notable that various components of this network are implicated as being defective in the majority of human cancers, that a number of tumor suppressor genes are components of the network, and that at least some of the misregulated proteins in the pathway play direct roles in intracellular energy metabolism mediated by the extracellular excessive energy. Identification of the differential activities of these network components in tissue-specific and cell-type-specific contexts is likely to reveal how both systemic and local responses to various planes of energy nutrition are integrated and affect the probability that transformed clones of cells residing within a specific organ site will progress to clinically detectable cancer.

Acknowledgments The authors thank Mary Playdon and John N. McGinley for their technical assistance in the preparation of this chapter.

References

1. IARC (2002) Weight control and physical activity, vol. 6. IARC Press, Lyon, pp 1–355. IARC Handbook of Cancer Prevention
2. Physical Activity Guidelines Advisory Committee (2008) Physical activity guidelines advisory committee report, 2008. US Department of Health and Human Services, Washington DC
3. Gunter MJ, Leitzmann MF (2006) Obesity and colorectal cancer: epidemiology, mechanisms and candidate genes. J Nutr Biochem 17:145–156
4. Marshall S (2006) Role of insulin, adipocyte hormones, and nutrient-sensing pathways in regulating fuel metabolism and energy homeostasis: a nutritional perspective of diabetes, obesity, and cancer. Sci STKE vol. 2006(346):re7, DOI: 10.1126/stke.3462006re7
5. Fenton JI, Birmingham JM, Hursting SD, Hord NG (2008) Adiponectin blocks multiple signaling cascades associated with leptin-induced cell proliferation in Apc Min/+ colon epithelial cells. Int J Cancer 122:2437–2445
6. Hursting SD, Nunez NP, Varticovski L, Vinson C (2007) The obesity-cancer link: lessons learned from a fatless mouse. Cancer Res 67:2391–2393
7. Hursting SD, Lashinger LM, Wheatley KW et al (2008) Reducing the weight of cancer: mechanistic targets for breaking the obesity-carcinogenesis link. Best Pract Res Clin Endocrinol Metab 22:659–669
8. Pedersen BK, Akerstrom TCA, Nielsen AR, Fischer CP (2007) Role of myokines in exercise and metabolism. J Appl Physiol 103:1093–1098
9. Freyssenet D (2007) Energy sensing and regulation of gene expression in skeletal muscle. J Appl Physiol 102:529–540
10. Canto C, Auwerx J (2009) PGC-1alpha, SIRT1 and AMPK, an energy sensing network that controls energy expenditure. Curr Opin Lipidol 20:98–105
11. Chaptini L, Peikin S (2008) Neuroendocrine regulation of food intake. Curr Opin Gastroenterol Mar;24(2):223–229

12. Castaneda TR, Jurgens H, Wiedmer P et al (2005) Obesity and the neuroendocrine control of energy homeostasis: the role of spontaneous locomotor activity. J Nutr 135:1314–1319
13. Kojima M, Kangawa K (2005) Ghrelin: Structure and Function. Physiol Rev 85:495–522
14. Auwerx J (1999) PPARgamma, the ultimate thrifty gene. Diabetologia 42:1033–1049
15. Gwinn DM, Shackelford DB, Egan DF et al (2008) AMPK phosphorylation of raptor mediates a metabolic checkpoint. Mol Cell 30:214–226
16. Hardie DG (2004) The AMP-activated protein kinase pathway–new players upstream and downstream. J Cell Sci 117:5479–5487
17. Kahn BB, Alquier T, Carling D, Hardie DG (2005) AMP-activated protein kinase: ancient energy gauge provides clues to modern understanding of metabolism. Cell Metab 1:15–25
18. Potter LR (2005) Domain analysis of human transmembrane guanylyl cyclase receptors: implications for regulation. Front Biosci 10:1205–1220
19. Milner J (2009) Cellular regulation of SIRT1. Curr Pharm Des 15:39–44
20. Imai S (2009) The NAD World: a new systemic regulatory network for metabolism and aging–Sirt1, systemic NAD biosynthesis, and their importance. Cell Biochem Biophys 53:65–74
21. Kim EJ, Um SJ (2008) SIRT1: roles in aging and cancer. BMB Rep 41:751–756
22. Dupont J, Froment P, Rame C, Pierre P, Coyral-Castel S, Chabrolle C (2008) Role of the fatty acids in ovarian functions: involvement of peroxisome proliferator-activated receptors (PPAR) and adipokines. Gynecol Obstet Fertil 36:1230–1238
23. Guri AJ, Hontecillas R, Bassaganya-Riera J (2006) Peroxisome proliferator-activated receptors: bridging metabolic syndrome with molecular nutrition. Clin Nutr 25:871–885
24. Bensinger SJ, Tontonoz P (2008) Integration of metabolism and inflammation by lipid-activated nuclear receptors. Nature 454:470–477
25. Ruiz-Stewart I, Tiyyagura SR, Lin JE et al (2004) Guanylyl cyclase is an ATP sensor coupling nitric oxide signaling to cell metabolism. Proc Natl Acad Sci USA 101:37–42
26. Jebelovszki E, Kiraly C, Erdei N et al (2008) High-fat diet-induced obesity leads to increased NO sensitivity of rat coronary arterioles: role of soluble guanylate cyclase activation. Am J Physiol Heart Circ Physiol 294:H2558–H2564
27. Engeli S, Janke J, Gorzelniak K et al (2004) Regulation of the nitric oxide system in human adipose tissue. J Lipid Res 45:1640–1648
28. Jadeski LC, Chakraborty C, Lala PK (2003) Nitric oxide-mediated promotion of mammary tumour cell migration requires sequential activation of nitric oxide synthase, guanylate cyclase and mitogen-activated protein kinase. Int J Cancer 106:496–504
29. Yang T, Fu M, Pestell R, Sauve AA (2006) SIRT1 and endocrine signaling. Trends Endocrinol Metab 17:186–191
30. Haigis MC, Guarente LP (2006) Mammalian sirtuins–emerging roles in physiology, aging, and calorie restriction. Genes Dev 20:2913–2921
31. Metoyer CF, Pruitt K (2008) The role of sirtuin proteins in obesity. Pathophysiology 15:103–108
32. Canto C, Gerhart-Hines Z, Feige JN et al (2009) AMPK regulates energy expenditure by modulating NAD+ metabolism and SIRT1 activity. Nature 458:1056–1060
33. Medina-Gomez G, Gray S, Vidal-Puig A (2007) Adipogenesis and lipotoxicity: role of peroxisome proliferator-activated receptor gamma (PPARgamma) and PPARgammacoactivator-1 (PGC1. Public Health Nutr 10:1132–1137
34. Sertznig P, Seifert M, Tilgen W, Reichrath J (2007) Present concepts and future outlook: function of peroxisome proliferator-activated receptors (PPARs) for pathogenesis, progression, and therapy of cancer. J Cell Physiol 212:1–12
35. Zhu Z, Jiang W, Sells JL, Neil ES, McGinley JN, Thompson HJ (2008) Effect of nonmotorized wheel running on mammary carcinogenesis: circulating biomarkers, cellular processes, and molecular mechanisms in rats. Cancer Epidemiol Biomarkers Prev 17:1920–1929
36. LeRoith D, Roberts CT Jr (2003) The insulin-like growth factor system and cancer. Cancer Lett 195:127–137

37. Zhu Z, Jiang W, McGinley JN, Thompson HJ (2009) Energetics and mammary carcinogenesis: effects of moderate-intensity running and energy intake on cellular processes and molecular mechanisms in rats. J Appl Physiol 106:911–918
38. Jiang W, Zhu Z, Thompson HJ (2009) Effects of physical activity and restricted energy intake on chemically induced mammary carcinogenesis. Cancer Prev Res (Phila PA) 2:338–344
39. Zhu Z, Jiang W, McGinley J, Wolfe P, Thompson HJ (2005) Effects of dietary energy repletion and IGF-1 infusion on the inhibition of mammary carcinogenesis by dietary energy restriction. Mol Carcinog 42:170–176
40. Hursting SD, Lavigne JA, Berrigan D, Perkins SN, Barrett JC (2003) Calorie restriction, aging, and cancer prevention: mechanisms of action and applicability to humans. Annu Rev Med 54:131–152
41. Younes H, Leleu X, Hatjiharissi E et al (2007) Targeting the phosphatidylinositol 3-kinase pathway in multiple myeloma. Clin Cancer Res 13:3771–3775
42. Motoshima H, Goldstein BJ, Igata M, Araki E (2006) AMPK and cell proliferation–AMPK as a therapeutic target for atherosclerosis and cancer. J Physiol 574:63–71
43. Sabatini DM (2006) mTOR and cancer: insights into a complex relationship. Nat Rev Cancer 6:729–734
44. Lee CC, Huang CC, Wu MY, Hsu KS (2005) Insulin stimulates postsynaptic density-95 protein translation via the phosphoinositide 3-kinase-Akt-mammalian target of rapamycin signaling pathway. J Biol Chem 280:18543–18550
45. Martin KA, Rzucidlo EM, Merenick BL et al (2004) The mTOR/p70 S6K1 pathway regulates vascular smooth muscle cell differentiation. Am J Physiol Cell Physiol 286:C507–C517
46. Gingras AC, Raught B, Sonenberg N (2001) Regulation of translation initiation by FRAP/mTOR. Genes Dev 15:807–826
47. Martin KA, Blenis J (2002) Coordinate regulation of translation by the PI 3-kinase and mTOR pathways. Adv Cancer Res 86:1–39
48. Sonenberg N, Gingras AC (1998) The mRNA 5' cap-binding protein eIF4E and control of cell growth. Curr Opin Cell Biol 10:268–275
49. Jiang W, Zhu Z, Thompson HJ (2008) Dietary energy restriction modulates the activity of AMP-activated protein kinase, Akt, and mammalian target of rapamycin in mammary carcinomas, mammary gland, and liver. Cancer Res 68:5492–5499

Chapter 5
Calorie Restriction, Exercise, and Colon Cancer Prevention: A Mechanistic Perspective

Connie J. Rogers, Lisa H. Colbert, Susan N. Perkins, and Stephen D. Hursting

Abstract The prevalence of obesity, an established epidemiologic risk factor for many cancers (including colon cancer), has risen steadily for the past several decades in the US. Particularly alarming are the increasing rates of obesity among children, portending continuing increases in the rates of obesity and obesity-related colon cancers for many years to come. Unfortunately, the mechanisms underlying the association between obesity and colon cancer are not well understood. In particular, the effects and mechanistic targets of interventions that modulate energy balance, such as reduced calorie diets and physical activity, on the colon carcinogenesis process have not been well characterized. The purpose of this chapter is to provide a strong foundation for future mechanism-based research in this area, with a focus on key physiologic processes and pathways underlying the colon cancer preventive effects of energy balance modulation. Clearly, no single pathway accounts for all of the effects of energy balance modulation on colon cancer, and components of the insulin/IGF-1/Akt and mTOR pathways, adipokine pathways, inflammatory pathways, and the sirtuin pathway have emerged as potential energy-responsive targets. Future studies that exploit the emerging mechanistic information to target energy balance-responsive pathways through combinations of lifestyle (particularly diet and physical activity) as well as pharmacologic approaches, will facilitate the translation of this research into effective colon cancer prevention and control strategies in humans.

1 Introduction

Colon cancer is the third most common noncutaneous cancer and cause of cancer death in both men and women in the United States [1]. The American Cancer Society estimates that in 2009 over 100,000 new cases of colon cancer will be diagnosed and that nearly 50,000 deaths from colorectal cancer will occur [1]. The

S.D. Hursting (✉)
Department of Nutritional Sciences, University of Texas, Austin, TX, USA
e-mail: shursting@mail.utexas.edu

A. McTiernan (ed.), *Physical Activity, Dietary Calorie Restriction, and Cancer*, Energy Balance and Cancer 3, DOI 10.1007/978-1-4419-7551-5_5,

recent estimates of colon cancer incidence and mortality are disturbing, given that lifestyle factors such as physical activity and nutritional interventions such as calorie restriction can play a significant role in colon cancer prevention. Furthermore, there is mounting evidence that obesity can significantly increase colon cancer risk and mortality [2, 3]. With more than two thirds of adults in the United States overweight or obese, the colon cancer death rate may in fact increase in the coming years (despite significant progress in screening and therapy) if active preventative strategies are not implemented. Therefore, gaining a better understanding of the biological mechanisms that contribute to colon cancer risk reduction observed with changes in energy balance (either via increasing energy expenditure through physical activity or reducing energy intake through calorie restriction) may lead to effective intervention strategies for colon cancer prevention, particularly in the face of the growing obesity epidemic.

2 Overview of Physical Activity and Colon Cancer Prevention

Numerous reviews have been published that summarize the epidemiological evidence linking physical activity and colon cancer prevention in humans [3–7]. In brief, there is an approximate 30% risk reduction in active men and women compared to their inactive peers [4, 6, 7]. One randomized clinical trial has been completed in humans, which explored possible mechanisms underlying the cancer-preventive effects of exercise. In this study, markers of inflammation were not changed following a 12-month exercise intervention [8, 9]; however, colonic crypt proliferation [10] and apoptosis [11] were altered by the exercise intervention.

There are few preclinical studies examining the effects of exercise on colon carcinogenesis. Studies to date have used either chemically induced tumors in rats or transgenic mice, specifically the Apc^{min} mouse, which carries a germline mutation in the *Apc* gene and develops intestinal tumors spontaneously [12–15]. Many of the studies have identified some form of protective effect of either voluntary running wheel or treadmill exercise on tumor incidence or number [12–15]. A few recent studies have begun to focus on possible biological mechanisms that might explain the effect of exercise on cancer prevention, including cellular proliferation and apoptosis, markers of inflammation, and gene expression studies [14, 15].

3 Overview of Calorie Restriction and Colon Cancer Prevention

In contrast to the large number of epidemiological studies demonstrating an association between increased levels of physical activity and reduced risk of colon cancer (see Chapter 3), the vast majority of studies using calorie restriction (CR) have been done in preclinical models. Over the past 30 years CR has emerged as the most potent, broadly acting dietary intervention for preventing carcinogenesis in rodent models of cancer [16]. CR is often described as "undernutrition without malnutrition," and CR experiments typically involve 10–40% reduction in calories relative to controls, coupled with adequate nutrition and a controlled physical environment [16]. CR regimens administered throughout life are generally more protective than adult-onset CR [16]. However, CR, both early and adult onset, prevents adult-onset obesity, significantly extends lifespan, and suppresses tumorigenesis, prompting many investigators to suggest that obesity prevention may be a key underlying factor in the anticancer effects of CR [16]. In terms of preclinical models relevant to colon cancer, we previously found a 57% lower polyp number in Apc^{min} mice on 40% CR vs. ad libitum fed control animals [17].

Most of these aforementioned studies have involved rodent models of chemically induced or oncogene-driven cancer. However, a recent report demonstrated extended lifespan and delayed spontaneous cancer development in response to CR in rhesus monkeys [18]. A 30% CR regimen reduced the incidence of cancer, cardiovascular disease, and brain atrophy, and 80% of the CR monkeys were still alive compared to 50% of the controls at the time of the report. These data suggest that CR provides benefits in nonhuman primates similar to those that have been repeatedly demonstrated in rodents. In humans, several observational studies further support the notion that CR has beneficial effects on longevity and cancer risk [16]. For example, inhabitants of Okinawa, Japan, who until recently consumed significantly fewer calories than residents of the main Japanese islands, have lower death rates from cancer and other chronic diseases than inhabitants of the Japanese mainland [19]. Furthermore, patients with early-onset anorexia nervosa (and hence periods of energy restriction) or other forms of CR during the premenopausal years have reduced risk of breast cancer later in life [20, 21]. While these observational studies suggest a beneficial effect of CR on cancer risk in humans, more well-controlled clinical studies are needed to support this hypothesis.

To this end, several National Institute of Aging (NIA)-funded clinical trials are underway to test the effects of CR in humans. The outcomes of these trials are biomarkers of age-related disease processes, including cancer, to compare and contrast the responses to CR in humans to the well-characterized effects of CR in rodents. Although each of these long-term trials is in the early stages, preliminary reports of biomarker responses in one of these studies (termed the CALERIE Study, conducted at the Pennington Biomedical Research Center) indicate that many of the same metabolic and endocrine changes observed in rodents and monkeys may also occur in humans in response to CR [22, 23].

These are important and encouraging findings that suggest the mechanisms characterized in animal model studies, and their translation into intervention targets and strategies will have relevance to the prevention and treatment of cancer (particularly those related to obesity) in humans. While no studies have directly examined the effect of CR on colon cancer risk in humans, it seems likely that some of the biological mediators that confer cancer risk reduction, in general, would also be relevant to colon cancer prevention.

4 Rationale for Exercise and Calorie Restriction Interventions in Humans

Translation of the beneficial effects of exercise or CR to human chronic disease prevention is especially critical, considering the staggering obesity trends in the Western world [24] and the relationship between obesity and colon cancer [25, 26]. Given these trends, the development of intervention strategies that either prevent obesity or disrupt the mechanistic link underlying obesity and colon cancer will become increasingly critical in the coming years. A first step toward developing intervention strategies is to have an understanding of the mechanisms underlying the beneficial effects of exercise and CR on cancer risk. While exploration of the mechanisms responsible for the observed effects of exercise or CR on colon cancer risk has begun, they are not completely understood. In addition, despite exercise and CR having similar beneficial effects on cancer prevention, with both interventions potentially resulting in a physiological condition of negative energy balance, the mechanisms that have been examined in response to these two intervention strategies have not been systematically explored in the same manner (i.e., very few studies have directly compared exercise and CR mechanistically) or to the same extent (e.g., DNA repair mechanisms have been evaluated following exercise, but not CR). Therefore, the objective of this review is to summarize our current knowledge of the biological mechanisms underlying the anticancer effects of both exercise and CR, and to compare and contrast the similarities and differences in these mechanisms among the two intervention strategies.

The mechanisms commonly cited as potential mediators of the beneficial effect of exercise on cancer prevention include enhanced antioxidant defense mechanisms; alterations in proliferation and apoptosis; changes in the growth factor milieu (e.g., changes in insulin, insulin-like growth factor (IGF)-1, and IGF-binding proteins); a reduction in chronic inflammation; enhanced antitumor immunity; and reduced tumor angiogenesis, some of which could be acting through similar pathways [15, 27, 28]. There are also cancer site-specific mechanisms that have been proposed, such as decreased colonic transit time in relation to colon cancer; however, there is little evidence that transit time in the colon influences cancer risk [29, 30]. A caveat to this review is that the effects of regular, moderate exercise training will be considered rather than the effects of an acute bout of exercise or exhaustive exercise, as the effects of regular, chronic physical activity on basal levels of any of the mediators discussed may be more relevant to the carcinogenic process. In contrast to exercise, the mechanisms often discussed as mediators of the anticancer effect of CR have been more focused on hormonal factors, such as the growth factors, insulin and IGF-1; glucocorticoids; and several adipose-derived factors, such as leptin and adiponectin, which are associated with inflammation and energy metabolism. Evidence regarding an association between CR and sirtuins, the family of proteins implicated in aging, is also beginning to emerge.

5 Biological Mechanisms: Exercise and Colon Cancer Prevention

5.1 Enhanced DNA Repair and Antioxidant Defenses

Reactive oxygen species (ROS) play an important role in a variety of normal processes within the body, including intracellular signaling, the immune response against pathogens, and vascular permeability. However, the accumulation of ROS as by-products of normal energy metabolism, in response to inflammatory conditions, or due to ROS-generating environmental exposures has been associated with the pathogenesis of cancer in rodents and humans [31, 32]. Experimental studies have shown that ROS contribute to tumor development by damaging critical cellular macromolecules, such as DNA, proteins, and lipids, and by acting as cell-signaling molecules, as nitric oxide does [31, 32]. The removal of ROS is dependent on scavenger and antioxidant systems. Antioxidant processes include the enzymes superoxide dismutase (SOD), glutathione peroxidase (GPX), and catalase (CAT); additionally, vitamin C, vitamin E, and β-carotene have been shown to be important in reducing free radical damage [33].

The idea that endogenous sources of these ROS may play a bigger role in colon carcinogenesis than exogenous sources (e.g., environmental carcinogens) is particularly relevant to exercise research, because an acute bout of exercise results in increased metabolism and a greater production of ROS [34–37]. At the same time, regular physical activity has been shown to be effective in reducing the risk of several types of cancer, suggesting that there may be physiological adaptations that occur in response to chronic exercise which prevent oxidative DNA damage. Moreover, chronic exercise training has been shown to be an important stimulus to upregulation of antioxidant enzymes [38], as well as nonenzymatic repair systems that work to prevent and/or repair the damage induced by ROS [35, 39–42].

ROS can attack many cellular structures, including lipids, proteins, and DNA; however, with respect to cancer, the effects of ROS on DNA are thought to be most important [43–45]. The most common oxidative modification of DNA involves the C-8 hydroxylation of guanine, which can be estimated by the measurement of 8-hydroxydeoxyguanosine (8-OH-dG) levels. Thus, the formation of 8-OH-dG as a result of oxidative DNA damage has been proposed to be a key biomarker relevant to carcinogenesis [46] and has been examined in response to exercise. Several studies have shown that 8-OH-dG levels are significantly lower in leukocyte DNA in physically active compared to sedentary men at baseline [47, 48] and in skeletal muscle of exercising rats [39]. In contrast, one recent study showed that moderate and strenuous exercise training did not alter 8-OH-dG levels in the liver of rats [49]. Taken together, these data suggest that chronic exercise may reduce oxidative damage, as measured by the formation of 8-OH-dG, but that these exercise-induced changes may be tissue-specific.

Exercise studies to date have largely focused on tissues relevant to exercise (e.g., skeletal muscle, heart) and not necessarily on target tissues like the colon. For example, a number of studies in both animal models and in humans have shown that chronic exercise increases gene expression [50] and/or protein levels [51, 52] of the antioxidant enzymes SOD and GPX in skeletal muscle. However, one study examined antioxidant defense mechanisms in cancer-relevant tissues following a 10-week treadmill training program in rats, and found that both SOD and CAT were upregulated with exercise in the lung and that UDP-glucuronosyl transferase was upregulated in both liver and lung [53]. Also, Nakatani and colleagues found that 10 weeks of swimming increased SOD activity in the diaphragm and kidney of rats treated with a renal carcinogen, Fe-nitrilotriacetic acid [52]. Additionally, the Phase II enzyme DT-diaphorase, a quinone reductase predominantly found in the liver, has also been shown to function as an antioxidant [54]. The activity of DT-diaphorase is elevated following 9 weeks of swimming in both young and middle-aged rats [39]. These data suggest that antioxidant enzymes may be upregulated in a variety of tissues in response to chronic exercise training. However, further studies are needed to explore specific antioxidant defense mechanisms in colonic epithelial cells.

In addition to the enzymatic antioxidant defense systems, DNA repair enzymes are upregulated with chronic exercise [39, 40, 42, 48, 51]. Mammalian cells have multiple repair enzymes to thwart the mutagenic effect of oxidative damage via 8-OH-dG and other mutagenic derivatives created by ROS. Human MutT homolog (hMTH1), one of several 8-OH-dG repair enzymes, prevents the incorporation of 8-OH-dG into DNA by hydrolyzing 8-OH-dGTP into 8-OH-dGMP [55, 56]. hMTH1 mRNA levels are significantly higher in physically active as compared to sedentary men [48]. Additionally, in both animal and human studies, exercise increases the activity of another 8-OH-dG repair enzyme, 8-oxoG DNA glycosylase (hOGG1) [51]. Furthermore, several studies have shown that chronic exercise increases the activity of the proteosome complex [39], which is thought to be important in the degradation of proteins that have been modified by oxidative stress [57]. In sum, these data suggest that chronic exercise may reduce oxidative damage by increasing a variety of DNA repair systems, as well as improve protein repair systems within the cell. Alteration of DNA and protein repair mechanisms by exercise may be a particularly important cancer prevention mechanism, given the potential exposure of epithelial cells in the colon to mutagens.

5.2 Alterations in Cellular Proliferation and Apoptosis

During tumor development clonal expansion of initiated cells occurs, resulting in preferential growth of the transformed cells. Tumor-promoting agents are not mutagenic, but rather alter the expression of genes whose products are associated with proliferation, apoptosis, and tissue remodeling. It has also become clear in recent years that proliferation and apoptosis are equally important in cell number homeostasis, and that the growth advantage manifested by initiated cells during tumor promotion is usually the net effect of increased proliferation and decreased apoptosis. Thus, both cell proliferation and apoptosis have emerged as critical targets for cancer prevention [58].

Recent studies in both animal models and humans have demonstrated an exercise effect on indices of cell proliferation and apoptosis. In rats, swim training significantly reduced cellular proliferation in the colonic mucosa, as measured by labeling of proliferative cellular nuclear antigen (PCNA) [59]. Furthermore, treadmill running reduced both the induction of aberrant crypt foci in carcinogen-induced colon cancer and the total number aberrant crypts [60]. In contrast to these two studies in rats, which suggest a reduction in colonic proliferation following exercise, treadmill running in Apc^{min} mice not only significantly reduced polyp number and size but also decreased the number of apoptotic cells (measured both by TUNEL staining and Bax protein expression) in adenomatous polyps [14]. These findings are counterintuitive and are likely complicated by the fact that apoptotic genes are upregulated in the polyps of Apc^{min} mice due to the mutation in the *Apc* gene. Results from the latter study suggest that Apc^{min} mice may not be the most appropriate model in which to study the effects of exercise on colonic cell proliferation and/or apoptosis, given the confounding associated with the presence of the Apc mutation.

In humans, one study examined the effect of a 12-month moderate-to-vigorous aerobic exercise intervention on markers of proliferation and apoptosis in the colonic crypts [10, 11]. McTiernan and colleagues demonstrated that in men, but not women, the exercise intervention altered colonic crypt height and reduced several measures of colonic crypt proliferation. Furthermore, a significant dose–response of exercise on proliferation was present, with a trend toward decreasing proliferation with increasing minutes of exercise per week [10]. This 12-month exercise intervention also significantly increased the expression of Bax protein (a proapoptotic marker) in the bottom of the colonic crypts of men, but in women decreased Bax expression in the middle of the crypt and increased the ratio of Bcl-2 (an antiapoptic marker) to Bax in the top of the crypt [11]. These results suggest that proliferation and apoptosis may be altered by exercise but that the effects seem to be greater in men than women. Additional preclinical and clinical studies are needed to further elucidate the effect of exercise on proliferation and apoptosis in colonic epithelial cells and to determine the underlying cause of the reported gender effect.

5.3 Altered Growth Factor Milieu

Insulin, particularly under conditions of chronic hyperinsulinemia and insulin resistance, increases the risk of colon cancer [61, 62]. Hyperinsulinemia and insulin resistance are common consequences of obesity. Higher cancer incidence and mortality are also reported in patients with type 2 diabetes or impaired glucose tolerance [63–65], further supporting the relationship between insulin dysregulation and tumor formation. Insulin can have a direct effect through insulin receptors on preneoplastic cells to stimulate proliferation and inhibit apoptosis [62]. Insulin can also have indirect effects on tumor development via IGF-1. High circulating levels of insulin promote the hepatic synthesis of IGF-1 and decrease the production of IGF-binding protein (IGFBP)-1, thus increasing the biologic activity of IGF-1 [62]. IGF-1, like insulin, can act as a growth factor to promote cancer cell proliferation and survival and decrease apoptosis. Additionally, insulin can enhance tumor development by regulating the synthesis and activity of reproductive hormones and altering the hepatic synthesis of steroid hormone-binding globulin, the main carrier of estrogen and testosterone [61].

Exercise is extremely effective in enhancing insulin sensitivity. An acute aerobic exercise bout can increase insulin sensitivity and improve glucose uptake in skeletal muscle for up to 12 h after a training session [66]. Chronic aerobic exercise training results in sustained improvements in insulin sensitivity over a longer period of time and can remedy insulin dysregulation in diabetes and conditions of impaired glucose tolerance [67, 68]. Finally, resistance training alone or combined with aerobic exercise can improve insulin sensitivity [69, 70]. Insulin sensitivity is linked closely to changes in body composition, with increasing adiposity correlated with decreasing insulin sensitivity. Despite this well-documented relationship, exercise-induced changes in insulin sensitivity can occur independently of changes in body weight or adiposity, suggesting that an uncoupling of weight and insulin sensitivity occurs when exercise is included in the equation. Thus, exercise-induced changes in insulin sensitivity may contribute to reduced cancer risk by reducing the direct and indirect effects of excess insulin on target tissues such as the colon.

Within the past several years, IGF-1 and its related binding proteins have received considerable attention as potential mediators of the protective effects of physical activity on cancer incidence. This interest has developed to some extent from the fact that CR works in part through IGF-1 (discussed in detail in the next section), and exercise and CR both can result in a state of negative energy balance. Although there is convincing evidence that IGF-1 is relevant to carcinogenesis [16, 61, 71], the data supporting the link between physical activity and IGF-1 are inconsistent. A recent review examining the relationship between IGF-1 and exercise in humans showed no consistency among published studies with increasing activity levels [72].

Data from animal studies on exercise and IGF-1 are much more limited. In one study, rats were run on a treadmill with and without added weight for five weeks in order to examine the effect on various bone growth factors. Exercise had no effect compared to control on circulating IGF-1 measured at the end of the training period [73]. In another study using female Apc^{min} mice, no change in serum IGF-1 was reported after 9 weeks of treadmill running [12]; however, IGFBP-3 levels were significantly elevated in the exercising mice in this study. In contrast, we showed that negative energy balance induced by voluntary wheel running for 10 weeks in male Apc^{min} mice resulted in significantly higher IGF-1 levels despite a significant (22%) reduction in polyp number [15]. We also recently demonstrated that neither treadmill nor voluntary wheel running in p53-deficient:MMTV-Wnt-1 transgenic mice altered IGF-1 levels [74]. Collectively, these experiments suggest that exercise training does not appear to consistently alter circulating levels of IGF-1, and thus IGF-1 may not be an important mediator in the cancer prevention effect of exercise.

5.4 Alterations in Chronic Inflammation

The association between chronic inflammation and cancer is well established [75], as is the link between obesity and inflammation [76]. In general, acute inflammation is a process that is beneficial to the host by providing protection from invading pathogens and initiating wound healing. This protection is mediated by a complex interplay between chemokines and cytokines that induce migration of immune cells (e.g., neutrophils, monocytes) to the site of tissue damage. The pro-inflammatory cytokines tumor necrosis factor-alpha (TNF-α) and interleukin 1-beta (IL-1β) are produced locally at the site of infection by macrophages and stimulate the release of IL-6, which has been shown to have both pro-inflammatory and anti-inflammatory effects [77]. An important effect of TNF-α, IL-1β, and IL-6 is the initiation of the acute phase response to a pathogenic or other challenge. This involves a shift in the proteins secreted by the liver into the blood, including C-reactive protein (CRP). Following initiation of the acute phase response and subsequent clearance of the infection, the production of IL-1β and TNF-α is dampened by the production and release of IL-1 receptor antagonist (IL-1ra) and soluble TNF-α receptor (sTNF-R), respectively, which block signal transduction via these receptors [78]. Additionally, IL-10, an anti-inflammatory cytokine that works by deactivating macrophages, is produced by T lymphocytes and is important in controlling the inflammatory response [79, 80].

Chronic, low-grade systemic inflammation, as occurs with obesity, has been described as a condition in which there is a two-to-threefold increase in the circulating levels of TNF-α, IL-1β, IL-6, IL-1ra, sTNF-R, and CRP. The origin of the cytokine cascade is typically not due to the presence of a foreign pathogen; however, the initial stimuli and the cause of this elevation in cytokines seen in chronic systemic inflammation are not completely understood. Several reports have demonstrated that macrophages reside in the adipose tissue of obese animals and humans, and these macrophages produce inflammatory cytokines, including TNF-α, IL-6, CRP, resistin, and MCP-1 [81–83]. In addition, the type of macrophage present in adipose tissue may also affect the extent and degree of the inflammatory response. Adipose tissue macrophages are recruited in response to the adipocyte enlargement that occurs due to excessive nutrient intake [84]. Activated macrophages can polarize into either a classic pro-inflammatory M1 phenotype or an immunosuppressive M2 phenotype depending on the cytokine and chemokine environment. In the context of obesity, adipose tissue is associated with an increase in M1 and a decrease in M2 macrophages; however, these phenotypes exhibit a high degree of plasticity and are reversible with environmental changes within the adipose tissue [85, 86].

In addition to cytokine release, inflammation is characterized by the release of arachidonic acid and its metabolism to eicosanoids [87]. Eicosanoids, which include the prostaglandins and hydroperoxy forms of arachidonic acid, are involved in many immune-mediated processes. Prostaglandin synthesis is regulated by cyclooxygenase (COX) gene expression. Two separate gene products, COX-1 and -2, have similar cyclooxygenase and peroxidase activities but are differentially regulated [87, 88]. Expression of COX-2 is upregulated in colonic polyps [89] and tumors

[90]. Nonsteroidal anti-inflammatory drugs (NSAIDs), which exert their anti-inflammatory effects by reducing prostaglandin production and by inhibiting COX-2 activity, have been shown to significantly decrease incidence of colon cancer in humans [91] and animal models [92]. These findings highlight the importance of this inflammatory pathway in colon carcinogenesis.

To date, numerous cross-sectional epidemiologic studies have shown an association between physical activity and alterations in systemic inflammation [93–101]. One mechanism by which physical activity could reduce cancer risk is via a reduction in chronic inflammation. As described previously, the cascade of cytokines that occurs sequentially following an acute infection begins with the release of TNF-α, IL-1β, and IL-6, followed by IL-1ra, sTNF-R, and IL-10. In contrast, the cytokine response to exercise [102–104] does not involve an increase in the pro-inflammatory cytokines TNF-α and IL-1β but rather is initiated by IL-6, followed by an increase in the anti-inflammatory mediators IL-1rα, sTNF-R, and IL-10 [105, 106]. In fact, Starkie and colleagues have shown that an acute bout of exercise prevents a rise in TNF-α following administration of a low dose of endotoxin in healthy volunteers [107], demonstrating a significant anti-inflammatory effect of exercise.

In support of this hypothesis, many human cross-sectional studies demonstrate an inverse relationship between regular physical activity and inflammatory markers, including CRP, TNF-α, and IL-6 [95–97, 100, 108–118]. However, human intervention studies have shown an effect of exercise on CRP in some [94, 119, 120], but not all studies [121–123]. Less work has been done with IL-6 in humans, but these results are conflicting as well [124]. Inflammatory cytokines have many physiological, metabolic, and immunological roles and can be produced by a myriad of tissues [102, 103]. The relationship between exercise and inflammatory mediators is complex. Additional studies are needed to determine (a) the dose, duration, and frequency of exercise needed to achieve an anti-inflammatory effect, if one exists; and (b) the timing of blood collection with respect to the exercise bout to adequately capture maximal cytokine levels.

Results from animal studies, although limited, demonstrate an anti-inflammatory role of exercise via multiple pathways. For example, exercise normalized the elevated levels of TNF-α in sTNF-R knock-out mice [125]. Treadmill exercise decreased the number of macrophages in polyps from Apc^{min} mice that may, in turn, contribute to a reduction in inflammatory cytokines [14] and also resulted in a lower circulating level of IL-6 [13]. COX-2 expression in polyps, however, was not changed with treadmill running in this same mouse model [14]. In contrast, swimming exercise reduced the number of COX-2-positive cells in rat colonocytes [59], and voluntary exercise decreased prostaglandin E_2 levels in serum and polyps from Apc^{min} mice [12]. These data suggest that several inflammatory pathways may be altered by exercise, but additional studies are needed to confirm these results.

5.5 Enhanced Antitumor Immunity

Many investigators have studied changes in immune function as a potential mechanism mediating the effect of exercise on cancer outcomes. Most of these have examined a variety of immunological functions following exercise, but few have focused on those components of the immune system that are most likely mediating antitumor immunity. For example, most studies have examined innate immune functions, specifically macrophage and natural killer (NK) cell cytotoxicity of tumor cells; however, only a few studies have examined adaptive immune responses that may be important in antitumor immunity (e.g., cytolytic T cell function) or interactions between innate and adaptive immunity that are essential in generating an in vivo antitumor response.

Several studies have examined exercise effects on immune function in the context of implanted tumors. In one study, moderate exercise training reduced the growth of the tumor, and, in this case, the survival of the rats [126]. Lymphocyte proliferative responses in the spleen were also increased in the trained rats in this study. We have demonstrated that exercise training in mice reduced the growth of implanted tumors concurrently with an enhancement of antigen-specific T cell function [127]. In other studies, tumor weights or volumes were unaffected by the various exercise regimens despite increases in various immune functions, such as splenocyte mitogen response and phagocytic activity of macrophages [128–130]. One study, which examined the growth and regression of allogeneic EL-4 lymphoma cells, found that repeated strenuous exercise delayed the time to peak tumor volume and resulted in a quicker regression of the tumor [130]. The heterogeneity of these results likely arises from the fact that different tumor types and training protocols were used in these studies.

Many studies have examined exercise effects on experimental tumor metastasis models in association with innate immune cell activity. Both an acute bout of exhaustive exercise and six days of hour-long bouts of higher-intensity exercise have been found to decrease the number of lung tumor foci following intravenous injection of B16 melanoma [131, 132]. In both studies, the same exercise was found to increase macrophage cytotoxicity against the same tumor in vitro. Additionally, studies with other models of exercise have found that both chronic and short-term repeated bouts of acute exercise can increase macrophage antitumoral cytotoxicity in vitro [128, 133, 134]. Collectively, these studies demonstrate a beneficial effect of many types of exercise on macrophage function, and, in the two cases examined, on experimental lung tumor metastasis.

NK cells and T lymphocytes are both important mediators of antitumor immunity [135–138]. The effect of exercise on NK cell function has been examined in both in vitro and in vivo experiments, as well as in a few studies in relation to tumor metastases. We and other investigators have identified a beneficial effect of exercise training on splenic NK cell cytotoxicity [139–141]. Chronic exercise enhanced in vivo and in vitro cytotoxic mechanisms of natural immunity in mice [139]. Additionally, tumor cell retention in the lungs following intravenous injection, considered by some to be a marker of NK cell activity, is reduced with exercise training [142]. The data in animals are promising. Exercise of many types and intensities appears to have beneficial effects on innate immunity, which may play a role in cancer prevention.

There have been considerably fewer studies examining the effect of exercise on T cell functions, either cytokine production or cytotoxicity of tumor cells. We have shown that moderate exercise enhances both mucosal T cell proliferation and cytokine production and enhances antigen-specific T cell-mediated immune responses after mucosal or systemic vaccination [140, 143]. This enhancement of mucosal immunity may provide selective protection from the growth and development of intestinal tumors. We have also demonstrated greater antigen-specific $CD8^+$ T cell proliferation and cytotoxicity, which may translate into greater antitumor activity (unpublished results). These results are exciting and suggest that regular exercise may in fact result in enhanced antitumor immune mechanisms.

5.6 Reduction in Angiogenesis

The process of angiogenesis is upregulated in skeletal and cardiac muscle following exercise training [144]. Additionally, an acute bout of exercise has been shown to decrease plasma vascular endothelial growth factor (VEGF) [145], increase circulating endostatin [145], and increase soluble VEGF receptor-1 [146] in healthy subjects, suggesting that exercise may decrease the amount of functionally available unbound plasma VEGF. However, only a few studies, to date, have measured markers of angiogenesis following exercise training in tumor-bearing animals. In one study, the growth and regression of allogeneic EL-4 lymphoma cells was compared in sedentary and exercising mice. This study found fewer inflammatory cells, as well as a decrease in blood vessel density within the tumors of exercising animals [130]. Furthermore, in a recent study, VEGF gene expression was lower in rat colonic mucosa following exercise training [147].

6 Biological Mechanisms: Calorie Restriction and Colon Cancer Prevention

6.1 Altered Growth Factor Milieu

CR (like exercise) improves insulin sensitivity and reduces fasting glucose, IGF-1, and insulin concentrations in rodents and monkeys [16, 18, 148–153]. The improvement in insulin sensitivity and the reduction in plasma glucose contribute significantly to the antiaging effects of CR [154]. However, accumulated evidence suggests that IGF-1 may be the major contributor to the anticancer effect of CR [16].

IGF-1, discussed previously in the context of exercise, is a mitogen so named because of its sequence homology to pro-insulin. IGF-1 plays a central role in regulating cell cycle progression from G1 to S phase by activating the phosphatidylinositol 3-kinase (PI3K)/Akt signal transduction pathway and modulating cyclin-dependent kinases [155–157]. IGF-1 can also significantly suppress apoptosis in a variety of cell types, and cells overexpressing IGF-1 receptor (IGF-1R) show decreased apoptosis [158]. IGF-1 is thus a major endocrine and paracrine regulator of tissue growth and metabolism. IGF-1's involvement in cancer was first suspected when in vitro studies consistently showed that supplementation of culture media with IGF-1 enhances the growth of a variety of cancer cell lines, including colon cancer cells [159–162]. There is also abundant epidemiologic evidence supporting the hypothesis that IGF-1 is involved in several types of human cancers, including colon cancer [163–168]. IGF-1 may be acting either directly on cells via its receptor, IGF-1R, or indirectly through interaction with other cancer-related molecules such as the insulin receptor (through heterodimerization) [156] or the p53 tumor suppressor [169, 170]. Levels of circulating IGF-1 are determined primarily by growth hormone-regulated hepatic synthesis, which is influenced by dietary intake of energy and protein [160]. To a lesser extent, IGF-1 synthesis can also occur in extrahepatic tissues, but this involves a complex integration of signals involving growth hormone, other hormones, and growth factors, as well as IGFBPs, which determine the local availability of IGF-1 and its systemic half-life [171].

There is increasing evidence that reduction in serum levels of IGF-1 mediates many of the antiproliferative, pro-apoptotic, and anticancer effects of CR through its role in an evolutionarily conserved regulatory pathway that is responsive to energy availability [16, 172]. In fact, restoration of IGF-1 levels in CR mice has been shown to abolish the antitumor effects of CR in multiple preclinical models [157, 173]. We have reported that the reduction in polyps in Apc^{min} mice in response to CR was associated with reduced IGF-1 levels [17]. We also showed that mice genetically deficient in circulating IGF-1 levels were resistant to azoxymethane-induced colon carcinogenesis [174] and chemically induced skin carcinogenesis [175]. Conversely, we have shown that diet-induced obesity can lead to insulin resistance, with increased IGF-1 and decreased IGFBP-1, all of which can result in enhanced IGF-1 signaling [176, 177].

Downstream targets of the IGF-1 and insulin receptors comprise a signaling network that regulates cellular growth and metabolism predominately through induction of the PI3K/Akt pathway, recently reviewed in [178, 179]. The importance of this signaling cascade in human cancers has recently been highlighted by the observation that it is one of the most commonly altered pathways in human epithelial tumors, including colon cancer [178, 180, 181]. Engagement of the PI3K/Akt pathway allows both intracellular and environmental cues, such as energy availability and growth factor supply, to affect cell growth, proliferation, survival, and metabolism.

Activation of receptor tyrosine kinases (RTKs) and/or the Ras proto-oncogene stimulates PI3K to produce the lipid second messenger, phosphatidyl-inositol-3,4,5-trisphosphate (PIP3). PIP3 recruits and anchors Akt to the cell membrane, where it can be further phosphorylated and activated [180, 182]. Akt is a cAMP-dependent, cGMP-dependent protein kinase C that, when constitutively active, is sufficient for cellular transformation by stimulating cell cycle progression, promoting cell survival, and inhibiting apoptosis [183, 184]. Frequently associated with the aberrant Akt signaling commonly seen in human cancers is an elevation in mammalian target of rapamycin (mTOR) signaling. mTOR is a highly conserved serine/threonine protein kinase that is activated by Akt and also inhibited by an opposing signal from AMP-activated kinase (AMPK). At the interface of the Akt and AMPK pathways, mTOR dictates translational control of new proteins in response to both growth factor signals and nutrient availability through phosphorylation of its downstream mediators, p70-S6 Kinase 1 and 4EBP-1 [185–191]. Ultimately, activation of mTOR results in cell growth, cell proliferation, and resistance to apoptosis.

Energy balance can influence both the Akt and the AMPK pathways of mTOR activation. For example, overweight and obese states are positively associated, as previously mentioned, with high serum levels of bioavailable IGF-1. We and others have found that obesity is associated with enhanced induction of the PI3K/Akt pathway [175, 192, 193,]. In contrast, CR reduces steady-state PI3K/Akt signaling as a result of decreased circulating levels of IGF-1 [175, 193]. Furthermore, genetic reduction of circulating IGF-1 mimics the effects of CR on tumor development and PI3K/Akt signaling [174, 177]. Additionally, the literature suggests that elevated cellular amino acid, glucose, and ATP concentrations, as are present under high-energy conditions, signal for mTOR activation [191, 192, 194]. Conversely, it has been shown that low glucose availability, high AMP/ATP ratios, and decreased amino acids, such as those attained during CR, can lead to growth arrest, apoptosis, and autophagy in colon and other tumor cells, through an AMPK-induced repression of mTOR [191, 192, 194].

6.2 Increased Glucocorticoids

Adrenal glucocorticoid hormones may also play a role in the anticancer effects of CR, especially at restriction levels above 30% CR, which markedly increase corticosterone levels in rodents [195–197]. Glucocorticoid hormones have long been known to inhibit tumor promotion [198]. In addition to the anti-inflammatory effects of corticosterone, it can induce p27 and thus influence cell cycle machinery [196]. Birt and colleagues have shown that the CR induction of corticosterone can inhibit protein kinase C and MAP kinase signaling, including reduced extracellular signal-regulated kinase (ERK)-1 and -2 signaling and AP-1:DNA binding [195]. We have also found that 40% CR can increase corticosterone more than threefold in APC^{min} mice, concomitant with the significant reduction in polyp number [17].

6.3 Alterations in Adipose-Derived Hormones

Leptin is a peptide hormone secreted from adipocytes, which is involved with appetite control and energy metabolism through its effects on the hypothalamus. In the nonobese state, rising leptin levels result in decreased appetite through a series of neuroendocrine changes. The obese state is associated with high circulating levels of leptin [199–202], suggesting that the obese may develop leptin resistance. This resistance appears to explain much of the inability of exogenous leptin administration to prevent weight gain and may result in a higher "set-point" for body weight [203]. The limited number of studies to date are suggestive of an association between circulating leptin levels and cancer risk, with the most consistent findings thus far for colon [204]. In vitro, leptin stimulates proliferation of multiple types of preneoplastic and neoplastic colon cells (but not "normal" cells, as reported by Fenton [162]), and in animal models it appears to promote angiogenesis and tumor invasion [205].

The primary physiologic role of leptin may be the regulation of energy homeostasis by providing a signal to the central nervous system regarding the size of fat stores, as circulating leptin levels correlate strongly with adipose tissue levels in animals and humans [206]. The canonical pathway that transduces leptin's signal from its receptor (OB-R) is the Janus kinase 2/signal transducer and activator of transcription 3 (JAK2/STAT3) pathway [207]. Leptin may also exert its metabolic effects, at least in part, by activating AMPK in muscle and liver, thus decreasing several anabolic pathways (including glucose-regulated transcription and fatty acid and triglyceride synthesis) and increasing several ATP-producing catabolic pathways [208]. In addition, there is emerging evidence of crosstalk between the JAK/STAT family of transcription factors, the insulin/IGF-1/Akt pathway, and the AMPK [209]. Furthermore, leptin plays a role in regulating the hypothalamus/pituitary/adrenal axis and thus influences IGF-1 synthesis [208]. Finally, leptin functions as an inflammatory cytokine and appears to influence immune function, possibly by triggering release of IL-6 and other obesity-related cytokines [162, 210]. Thus, although not well studied to date, leptin is certainly positioned as a central player in the energy balance and cancer association. Leptin levels were significantly reduced with CR in APC^{min} mice, consistent with their decreased fat mass [17].

Adiponectin is a peptide hormone produced by adipocytes and involved in the regulation of insulin sensitivity and carbohydrate and lipid metabolism. Plasma levels of adiponectin, in contrast with other adipokines, are decreased in response to several metabolic impairments, including type 2 diabetes, dyslipidemia, and extreme obesity. This obesity-related decrease can be partially reversed by weight loss, although these changes are relatively small unless there are drastic weight changes, such as occurs following severe CR or surgical intervention [211, 212]. The link between adiponectin and cancer risk is not well characterized, although several recent reviews show that the evidence is mounting for a possible relationship between low adiponectin levels and the risk of some types of cancer [213, 214, 215]. Recent findings also suggest that leptin and adiponectin may interact antagonistically to influence breast and colon carcinogenesis [216, 217].

6.4 Alterations in Chronic Inflammation

Obesity leads to a state of systemic chronic inflammation, as discussed previously. In contrast, CR exerts a potent anti-inflammatory effect [218, 219]. In animal studies, CR inhibits the dysregulation of TNF-α and IL-6 in aging mice [220]. Inflammatory responses to lipopolysaccharide (IL-1β, IL-6, and TNF-α) are significantly lower in CR animals [221]. Furthermore, the expression of several genes important in the TNF-α signaling pathway are downregulated by CR [222]. Adult-onset CR also exerts a powerful anti-inflammatory effect in nonhuman primates and humans. Adult-onset CR in rhesus monkeys reduces the production of IL-6 from peripheral blood mononuclear cells in response to oxidative stress [223]. In humans, a 1-year controlled trial involving 48 nonobese subjects who were placed on a 20% CR showed a significant reduction in CRP levels after the intervention [224]. Together, these data suggest CR consistently lowers markers of inflammation, which may contribute to the anticancer effects of CR.

6.5 Alterations in Sirtuins

Sirtuins are a family of proteins that have been implicated in the regulation of aging [225], transcription [226], endocrine signaling [227], stress-induced apoptosis [228], and most recently in metabolic changes associated with obesity (reviewed in [229]). Sirtuins were originally studied in the budding yeast *Saccharomyces cerevisiae* [230, 231] and nematode *Caenorhabditis elegans* [232], where CR was shown to increase lifespan as well as increase the levels and activity of the Sir2 protein. In mammals, levels of SIRT1, a mammalian homolog of Sir2, also rise during CR and promote long-term survival of cells [228]. SIRT1 is a NAD^+-dependent deacetylase that acts on Ku70, a protein that in turn sequesters the pro-apoptotic factor Bax from the mitochondria, thus inhibiting stress-induced apoptotic cell death [228]. Additionally, SIRT1 has been shown to repress peroxisome proliferator-activated receptor (PPAR)-γ by docking with its cofactors and thereby ultimately repressing PPAR-γ-responsive genes. This results in lipolysis in response to CR and SIRT1 upregulation [233]. Decreases in sirtuin levels during obesity, specifically SIRT1 levels, have been shown to regulate many other metabolic alterations linked to obesity. SIRT1 has been shown to play a role in regulation of adiponectin synthesis [234, 235], insulin secretion [236], plasma glucose levels and insulin sensitivity [237], and oxygen consumption and mitochondrial capacity [238, 239]. Another yeast Sir2 homolog, mammalian SIRT3, has been shown to be selectively downregulated at both the gene and the protein levels in a mouse model of type 2 diabetes, but not in a model of deficient insulin action without diabetes. In this study, muscle-specific insulin receptor-deficient (MIRKO) mice lacked muscle insulin receptors, but maintained normal levels of insulin, glucose, and insulin-regulated genes. The same MIRKO mice with streptozotocin (STZ)-induced diabetes, however, modeled the metabolic changes associated with type 2 diabetes, including downregulation of Sirt1 [240]. These findings further suggest that sirtuins may be involved in the control of important downstream transcriptional regulatory mechanisms involved in glucose metabolism.

While CR has long been shown to have a dramatic effect on lifespan and tumor suppression in almost every tumor type tested, the specific role of sirtuins in cancer development/progression has yet to be elucidated [241]. Studies have shown conflicting data as to whether SIRT1 can act as a tumor suppressor gene or an oncogene. SIRT1 is upregulated in several tumor types and can inhibit apoptosis and downregulate the expression of tumor suppressor genes to extend the longevity of epithelial cancer cells [242]. For example, SIRT1 is upregulated in tumors and cancer cells lacking the tumor suppressor gene, hypermethylated in cancer (HIC)1 [243], and upregulated in mouse and human prostate cancers [244]. In addition, deleted in breast cancer (DBC) 1-mediated repression of SIRT1 was shown to increase p53 function [245, 246]. In contrast, several studies suggest SIRT1 can act to suppress intestinal tumorigenesis [247, 248, 249].

7 Summary

This chapter considered the key physiologic processes and pathways underlying the colon cancer-preventive effects of increasing energy expenditure through physical activity or reducing energy intake through CR. Clearly, no single pathway accounts for all of the effects of energy balance modulation on colon cancer, and components of the insulin/IGF-1/Akt/mTOR pathway, adipokine pathways, inflammatory pathways, and the sirtuin pathway have emerged as potential energy-responsive targets. As with most chronic disease intervention strategies, combination approaches that target multiple pathways (and that maximize efficacy and minimize adverse effects) will likely be most successful for colon cancer prevention, particularly for offsetting the impact of obesity on colon carcinogenesis. Future studies that exploit the emerging mechanistic information to target energy balance-responsive pathways through combinations of lifestyle changes (particularly diet and physical activity), as well as pharmacologic approaches, will facilitate the translation of this research into effective colon cancer prevention and control strategies in humans.

References

1. American Cancer Society. (2009) Cancer facts and figures. American Cancer Society, Inc. No. 500809
2. Calle EE, Rodriguez C, Walker-Thurmond K et al (2003 Apr 24) Overweight, obesity, and mortality from cancer in a prospectively studied cohort of U.S. adults. N Engl J Med 348(17):1625–1638
3. World Cancer Research Fund/American Institute for Cancer Research (2007) Food, nutrition, physical activity and the prevention of cancer: a global perspective. AICR, Washington, DC
4. Physical Activity Guidelines Advisory Committee (2008) physical activity guidelines advisory committee report. U.S. Department of Health and Human Services, Washington, DC
5. Trojian TH, Mody K, Chain P (2007 Apr) Exercise and colon cancer: primary and secondary prevention. Curr Sports Med Rep 6(2):120–124
6. Samad AK, Taylor RS, Marshall T et al (2005 May) A meta-analysis of the association of physical activity with reduced risk of colorectal cancer. Colorectal Dis 7(3):204–213
7. Harriss DJ, Atkinson G, Batterham A et al (2009 Sep) Lifestyle factors and colorectal cancer risk (2): a systematic review and meta-analysis of associations with leisure-time physical activity. Colorectal Dis 11(7):689–701

8. Abrahamson PE, King IB, Ulrich CM et al (2007 Nov) No effect of exercise on colon mucosal prostaglandin concentrations: a 12-month randomized controlled trial. Cancer Epidemiol Biomarkers Prev 16(11):2351–2356
9. Campbell KL, Campbell PT, Ulrich CM et al (2008 Jul) No reduction in C-reactive protein following a 12-month randomized controlled trial of exercise in men and women. Cancer Epidemiol Biomarkers Prev 17(7):1714–1718
10. McTiernan A, Yasui Y, Sorensen B et al (2006 Sep) Effect of a 12-month exercise intervention on patterns of cellular proliferation in colonic crypts: a randomized controlled trial. Cancer Epidemiol Biomarkers Prev 15(9):1588–1597
11. Campbell KL, McTiernan A, Li SS et al (2007 Sep) Effect of a 12-month exercise intervention on the apoptotic regulating proteins Bax and Bcl-2 in colon crypts: a randomized controlled trial. Cancer Epidemiol Biomarkers Prev 16(9):1767–1774
12. Ju J, Nolan B, Cheh M et al (2008) Voluntary exercise inhibits intestinal tumorigenesis in Apc(Min/+) mice and azoxymethane/dextran sulfate sodium-treated mice. BMC Cancer 8:316
13. Mehl K, Davis J, Clements J, Berger F, Pena M, Carson J (2005) Decreased intestinal polyp multiplicity is related to exercise mode and gender in $APC^{Min/+}$ mice. J Appl Physiol 98:2219–2225
14. Baltgalvis KA, Berger FG, Pena MM et al (2008 Apr) Effect of exercise on biological pathways in ApcMin/+ mouse intestinal polyps. J Appl Physiol 104(4):1137–4315
15. Colbert LH, Mai V, Tooze JA et al (2006 Oct) Negative energy balance induced by voluntary wheel running inhibits polyp development in APCMin mice. Carcinogenesis 27(10):2103–2107
16. Hursting SD, Lavigne JA, Berrigan D et al (2003) Calorie restriction, aging, and cancer prevention: mechanisms of action and applicability to humans. Annu Rev Med 54:131–152
17. Mai V, Colbert LH, Berrigan D, Perkins S, Pfeiffer R, Lavigne J, Lanza E, Haines D, Schatzkin A,, Hursting S (2003) Calorie restriction and diet composition modulate spontaneous intestinal tumorigenesis in APC^{Min} mice through different mechanisms. Cancer Res 63:1752–1755
18. Colman RJ, Anderson RM, Johnson SC et al (2009 Jul 10) Caloric restriction delays disease onset and mortality in rhesus monkeys. Science 325(5937):201–204
19. Kagawa Y (1978 Jun) Impact of Westernization on the nutrition of Japanese: changes in physique, cancer, longevity and centenarians. Prev Med 7(2):205–217
20. Michels KB, Ekbom A (2004 Mar 10) Caloric restriction and incidence of breast cancer. JAMA 291(10):1226–1230
21. Howell A, Chapman M, Harvie M (2009) Energy restriction for breast cancer prevention. Recent results. Cancer Res 181:97–111
22. Heilbronn LK, de Jonge L, Frisard MI et al (2006 Apr 5) Effect of 6-month calorie restriction on biomarkers of longevity, metabolic adaptation, and oxidative stress in overweight individuals: a randomized controlled trial. JAMA 295(13):1539–1548
23. Redman LM, Heilbronn LK, Martin CK et al (2009) Metabolic and behavioral compensations in response to caloric restriction: implications for the maintenance of weight loss. PLoS One 4(2):e4377
24. Caballero B (2007) The global epidemic of obesity: an overview. Epidemiol Rev 29:1–5
25. Gunter MJ, Leitzmann MF (2006 Mar) Obesity and colorectal cancer: epidemiology, mechanisms and candidate genes. J Nutr Biochem 17(3):145–156
26. Harriss DJ, Atkinson G, George K et al (2009 Jul) Lifestyle factors and colorectal cancer risk (1): systematic review and meta-analysis of associations with body mass index. Colorectal Dis 11(6):547–563
27. Rogers CJ, Colbert LH, Berrigan D, Greiner JW, Perkins SN, Hursting SD (2008) Physical activity and cancer prevention: Pathways and targets for intervention. Sports Med 38(4): 221–257

28. Campbell KL, McTiernan A (2007 Jan) Exercise and biomarkers for cancer prevention studies. J Nutr 137(1 Suppl):161S–169S
29. MacLennan R, Jensen OM, Mosbech J et al (1978 Oct) Diet, transit time, stool weight, and colon cancer in two Scandinavian populations. Am J Clin Nutr 31(10 Suppl):S239–S242
30. Dukas L, Willett WC, Colditz GA et al (2000 May 15) Prospective study of bowel movement, laxative use, and risk of colorectal cancer among women. Am J Epidemiol 151(10):958–964
31. Perchellet JP, Perchellet EM, Gali HU et al (1995) In: Mukhtar H (ed) Oxidant stress and multistage carcinogenesis. CRC Press, Boca Raton, FL, pp 145–180
32. Trush MA, Kensler TW (1991) An overview of the relationship between oxidative stress and chemical carcinogenesis. Free Radic Biol Med 10:201–207
33. Valko M, Izakovic M, Mazur M et al (2004 Nov) Role of oxygen radicals in DNA damage and cancer incidence. Mol Cell Biochem 266(1–2):37–56
34. Davies KJ, Quintanilha AT, Brooks GA et al (1982 Aug 31) Free radicals and tissue damage produced by exercise. Biochem Biophys Res Commun 107(4):1198–1205
35. Ji LL (1999 Dec) Antioxidants and oxidative stress in exercise. Proc Soc Exp Biol Med 222(3):283–292
36. Marnett LJ (2000 Mar) Oxyradicals and DNA damage. Carcinogenesis 21(3):361–370
37. McArdle A, Dillmann WH, Mestril R et al (2004 Feb) Overexpression of HSP70 in mouse skeletal muscle protects against muscle damage and age-related muscle dysfunction. Faseb J 18(2):355–357
38. McArdle A, Jackson MJ (2000 Nov) Exercise, oxidative stress and ageing. J Anat 197(Pt 4):539–541
39. Radak Z, Kaneko T, Tahara S et al (1999 Jul) The effect of exercise training on oxidative damage of lipids, proteins, and DNA in rat skeletal muscle: evidence for beneficial outcomes. Free Radic Biol Med 27(1–2):69–74
40. Radak Z, Taylor AW, Ohno H et al (2001) Adaptation to exercise-induced oxidative stress: from muscle to brain. Exerc Immunol Rev 7:90–107
41. Fehrenbach E, Northoff H (2001) Free radicals, exercise, apoptosis, and heat shock proteins. Exerc Immunol Rev 7:66–89
42. Wittwer M, Billeter R, Hoppeler H et al (2004 Feb) Regulatory gene expression in skeletal muscle of highly endurance-trained humans. Acta Physiol Scand 180(2):217–227
43. Ames BN, Gold LS, Willett WC (1995 Jun 6) The causes and prevention of cancer. Proc Natl Acad Sci USA 92(12):5258–5265
44. Clayson DB, Mehta R, Iverson F (1994 Feb) International commission for protection against environmental mutagens and carcinogens. Oxidative DNA damage–the effects of certain genotoxic and operationally non-genotoxic carcinogens. Mutat Res 317(1):25–42
45. Feig DI, Reid TM, Loeb LA (1994 Apr 1) Reactive oxygen species in tumorigenesis. Cancer Res 54(7 Suppl):1890s–1894s
46. Kasai H, Nishimura S (1984 Feb 24) Hydroxylation of deoxyguanosine at the C-8 position by ascorbic acid and other reducing agents. Nucleic Acids Res 12(4):2137–2145
47. Asami S, Hirano T, Yamaguchi R et al (1998 Dec) Reduction of 8-hydroxyguanine in human leukocyte DNA by physical exercise. Free Radic Res 29(6):581–584
48. Sato Y, Nanri H, Ohta M et al (2003 May 30) Increase of human MTH1 and decrease of 8-hydroxydeoxyguanosine in leukocyte DNA by acute and chronic exercise in healthy male subjects. Biochem Biophys Res Commun 305(2):333–338
49. Ogonovszky H, Sasvari M, Dosek A et al (2005 Apr) The effects of moderate, strenuous, and overtraining on oxidative stress markers and DNA repair in rat liver. Can J Appl Physiol 30(2):186–195
50. Ennezat PV, Malendowicz SL, Testa M et al (2001 Jul) Physical training in patients with chronic heart failure enhances the expression of genes encoding antioxidative enzymes. J Am Coll Cardiol 38(1):194–198

51. Radak Z, Naito H, Kaneko T et al (2002 Nov) Exercise training decreases DNA damage and increases DNA repair and resistance against oxidative stress of proteins in aged rat skeletal muscle. Pflugers Arch 445(2):273–278
52. Nakatani K, Komatsu M, Kato T et al (2005 Sep) Habitual exercise induced resistance to oxidative stress. Free Radic Res 39(9):905–911
53. Duncan K, Harris S, Ardies CM (1997 Jun 24) Running exercise may reduce risk for lung and liver cancer by inducing activity of antioxidant and phase II enzymes. Cancer Lett 116(2):151–158
54. Beyer RE, Segura-Aguilar J, Di Bernardo S et al (1996 Mar 19) The role of DT-diaphorase in the maintenance of the reduced antioxidant form of coenzyme Q in membrane systems. Proc Natl Acad Sci USA 93(6):2528–2532
55. Sakumi K, Furuichi M, Tsuzuki T et al (1993 Nov 5) Cloning and expression of cDNA for a human enzyme that hydrolyzes 8-oxo-dGTP, a mutagenic substrate for DNA synthesis. J Biol Chem 268(31):23524–23530
56. Kang JJ, Yokoi TJ, Holland MJ (1995 Dec 1) Binding sites for abundant nuclear factors modulate RNA polymerase I-dependent enhancer function in Saccharomyces cerevisiae. J Biol Chem 270(48):28723–28732
57. Goto S, Takahashi R, Kumiyama AA et al (2001 Apr) Implications of protein degradation in aging. Ann N Y Acad Sci 928:54–64
58. Thompson HJ, Strange R, Schedin PJ (1992 Nov–Dec) Apoptosis in the genesis and prevention of cancer. Cancer Epidemiol Biomarkers Prev 1(7):597–602
59. Demarzo MM, Martins LV, Fernandes CR et al (2008 Apr) Exercise reduces inflammation and cell proliferation in rat colon carcinogenesis. Med Sci Sports Exerc 40(4):618–621
60. Fuku N, Ochiai M, Terada S et al (2007 Jan) Effect of running training on DMH-induced aberrant crypt foci in rat colon. Med Sci Sports Exerc 39(1):70–74
61. Kaaks R, Lukanova A (2001 Feb) Energy balance and cancer: the role of insulin and insulin-like growth factor-I. Proc Nutr Soc 60(1):91–106
62. Calle EE, Kaaks R (2004 Aug) Overweight obesity and cancer: epidemiological evidence and proposed mechanisms. Nat Rev Cancer 4(8):579–591
63. Hu FB, Manson JE, Liu S et al (1999 Mar 17) Prospective study of adult onset diabetes mellitus (type 2) and risk of colorectal cancer in women. J Natl Cancer Inst 91(6):542–547
64. Saydah SH, Loria CM, Eberhardt MS et al (2003 Jun 15) Abnormal glucose tolerance and the risk of cancer death in the United States. Am J Epidemiol 157(12):1092–1100
65. Saydah SH, Platz EA, Rifai N et al (2003 May) Association of markers of insulin and glucose control with subsequent colorectal cancer risk. Cancer Epidemiol Biomarkers Prev 12(5):412–418
66. Wilmore J, Costill C (eds) Physiology of sport and exercise, 2005, Human Kinetics, Champaign, IL
67. Regensteiner JG, Mayer EJ, Shetterly SM et al (1991 Nov) Relationship between habitual physical activity and insulin levels among nondiabetic men and women. San Luis Valley Diabetes Study. Diabetes Care 14(11):1066–1074
68. Regensteiner JG, Shetterly SM, Mayer EJ et al (1995 Apr) Relationship between habitual physical activity and insulin area among individuals with impaired glucose tolerance. The San Luis Valley Diabetes Study. Diabetes Care 18(4):490–497
69. Ivy JL (1997 Nov) Role of exercise training in the prevention and treatment of insulin resistance and non-insulin-dependent diabetes mellitus. Sports Med 24(5):321–336
70. Poehlman ET, Dvorak RV, DeNino WF et al (2000 Jul) Effects of resistance training and endurance training on insulin sensitivity in nonobese, young women: a controlled randomized trial. J Clin Endocrinol Metab 85(7):2463–2468
71. Yu H, Rohan T (2000 Sep 20) Role of the insulin-like growth factor family in cancer development and progression. J Natl Cancer Inst 92(18):1472–1489
72. Orenstein M, Friedenreich C (2004) Review of physical activity and the IGF family. J Physical Act Aging 1:291–320

73. Bravenboer N, Engelbregt MJ, Visser NA et al (2001 Sep) The effect of exercise on systemic and bone concentrations of growth factors in rats. J Orthop Res 19(5):945–949
74. Colbert LH, Westerlind KC, Perkins SN et al (2009 Aug) Exercise effects on tumorigenesis in a p53-deficient mouse model of breast cancer. Med Sci Sports Exerc 41(8):1597–1605
75. Coussens LM, Werb Z (2002 Dec 19–26) Inflammation and cancer. Nature 420(6917): 860–867
76. Hotamisligil GS, Shargill NS, Spiegelman BM (1993 Jan 1) Adipose expression of tumor necrosis factor-alpha: direct role in obesity-linked insulin resistance. Science 259(5091): 87–91
77. Tilg H, Dinarello CA, Mier JW (1997 Sep) IL-6 and APPs: anti-inflammatory and immunosuppressive mediators. Immunol Today 18(9):428–432
78. Dinarello CA (2000 Sep 7) The role of the interleukin-1-receptor antagonist in blocking inflammation mediated by interleukin-1. N Engl J Med 343(10):732–734
79. Moore KW, O'Garra A, de Waal Malefyt R et al (1993) Interleukin-10. Annu Rev Immunol 11:165–190
80. Pretolani M (1999 Sep) Interleukin-10: an anti-inflammatory cytokine with therapeutic potential. Clin Exp Allergy 29(9):1164–1171
81. Weisberg SP, McCann D, Desai M et al (2003 Dec) Obesity is associated with macrophage accumulation in adipose tissue. J Clin Invest 112(12):1796–1808
82. Xu H, Barnes GT, Yang Q et al (2003 Dec) Chronic inflammation in fat plays a crucial role in the development of obesity-related insulin resistance. J Clin Invest 112(12): 1821–1830
83. Subramanian V, Ferrante AW Jr (2009) Obesity, inflammation, and macrophages. Nestle Nutr Workshop Ser Pediatr Program 63:151–159; Discussion 159–162, 259–268
84. Lumeng CN, Deyoung SM, Bodzin JL et al (2007 Jan) Increased inflammatory properties of adipose tissue macrophages recruited during diet-induced obesity. Diabetes 56(1):16–23
85. Mantovani A, Sozzani S, Locati M et al (2002 Nov) Macrophage polarization: tumor-associated macrophages as a paradigm for polarized M2 mononuclear phagocytes. Trends Immunol 23(11):549–555
86. Sica A, Larghi P, Mancino A et al (2008) Macrophage polarization in tumour progression. Semin Cancer Biol 18:349–355
87. Furstenberger G, Marks F (1985) In: Honn KV, Martin LJ (eds) Prostaglandinsepidermal hyperplasia and skin tumor promotion. Prostaglandins, leukotrienes and cancer. Marinus Nijhoff Publishers, Boston, MA, pp 28–50
88. Sigal E (1991 Feb) The molecular biology of mammalian arachidonic acid metabolism. Am J Physiol 260(2 Pt 1):L13–L28
89. McLean MH, Murray GI, Fyfe N et al (2008 Jun) COX-2 expression in sporadic colorectal adenomatous polyps is linked to adenoma characteristics. Histopathology 52(7):806–815
90. Wang D, Dubois RN (2009 Nov 30) The role of COX-2 in intestinal inflammation and colorectal cancer. Oncogene 2010; 29:781–788
91. Lanas A (2009 Aug) Nonsteroidal antiinflammatory drugs and cyclooxygenase inhibition in the gastrointestinal tract: a trip from peptic ulcer to colon cancer. Am J Med Sci 338(2): 96–106
92. Muller-Decker K, Furstenberger G (2007 Aug) The cyclooxygenase-2-mediated prostaglandin signaling is causally related to epithelial carcinogenesis. Mol Carcinog 46(8):705–710
93. Smith JK, Dykes R, Douglas JE et al (1999 May 12) Long-term exercise and atherogenic activity of blood mononuclear cells in persons at risk of developing ischemic heart disease. JAMA 281(18):1722–1727
94. Mattusch F, Dufaux B, Heine O et al (2000 Jan) Reduction of the plasma concentration of C-reactive protein following nine months of endurance training. Int J Sports Med 21(1):21–24

95. Taaffe DR, Harris TB, Ferrucci L et al (2000 Dec) Cross-sectional and prospective relationships of interleukin-6 and C-reactive protein with physical performance in elderly persons: MacArthur studies of successful aging. J Gerontol A Biol Sci Med Sci 55(12):M709–M715
96. Fallon KE, Fallon SK, Boston T (2001 Jun) The acute phase response and exercise: court and field sports. Br J Sports Med 35(3):170–173
97. Geffken DF, Cushman M, Burke GL et al (2001 Feb 1) Association between physical activity and markers of inflammation in a healthy elderly population. Am J Epidemiol 153(3): 242–250
98. Abramson JL, Vaccarino V (2002 Jun 10) Relationship between physical activity and inflammation among apparently healthy middle-aged and older US adults. Arch Intern Med 162(11):1286–1292
99. Wannamethee SG, Lowe GD, Whincup PH et al (2002 Apr 16) Physical activity and hemostatic and inflammatory variables in elderly men. Circulation 105(15):1785–1790
100. King DE, Carek P, Mainous AG 3rd et al (2003 Apr) Inflammatory markers and exercise: differences related to exercise type. Med Sci Sports Exerc 35(4):575–581
101. Fischer CP, Berntsen A, Perstrup LB et al (2006 Nov 1) Plasma levels of interleukin-6 and C-reactive protein are associated with physical inactivity independent of obesity. Scand J Med Sci Sports 2007; 17:580–587
102. Pedersen BK, Fischer CP (2007 May) Physiological roles of muscle-derived interleukin-6 in response to exercise. Curr Opin Clin Nutr Metab Care 10(3):265–271
103. Pedersen BK, Hoffman-Goetz L (2000 Jul) Exercise and the immune system: regulation, integration, and adaptation. Physiol Rev 80(3):1055–1081
104. Pedersen BK, Steensberg A, Schjerling P (2001 Oct 15) Muscle-derived interleukin-6: possible biological effects. J Physiol 536(Pt 2):329–337
105. Ostrowski K, Rohde T, Asp S et al (1999 Feb 15) Pro- and anti-inflammatory cytokine balance in strenuous exercise in humans. J Physiol 515(Pt 1):287–291
106. Ostrowski K, Schjerling P, Pedersen BK (2000 Dec) Physical activity and plasma interleukin-6 in humans–effect of intensity of exercise. Eur J Appl Physiol 83(6): 512–515
107. Starkie R, Ostrowski SR, Jauffred S et al (2003 May) Exercise and IL-6 infusion inhibit endotoxin-induced TNF-alpha production in humans. FASEB J 17(8):884–886
108. Rohde LE, Hennekens CH, Ridker PM (1999 Nov 1) Survey of C-reactive protein and cardiovascular risk factors in apparently healthy men. Am J Cardiol 84(9):1018–1022
109. Church TS, Barlow CE, Earnest CP et al (2002 Nov 1) Associations between cardiorespiratory fitness and C-reactive protein in men. Arterioscler Thromb Vasc Biol 22(11):1869–1876
110. Ford ES (2002 Sept) Does exercise reduce inflammation? Physical activity and C-reactive protein among U.S. adults. Epidemiology 13(5):561–568
111. Rothenbacher D, Hoffmeister A, Brenner H et al (2003 May 26) Physical activity, coronary heart disease, and inflammatory response. Arch Intern Med 163(10):1200–1205
112. LaMonte MJ, Durstine JL, Yanowitz FG et al (2002 Jul 23) Cardiorespiratory fitness and C-reactive protein among a tri-ethnic sample of women. Circulation 106(4):403–406
113. Pitsavos C, Panagiotakos DB, Chrysohoou C et al (2005 Apr) The associations between physical activity, inflammation, and coagulation markers, in people with metabolic syndrome: the ATTICA study. Eur J Cardiovasc Prev Rehabil 12(2):151–158
114. Reuben DB, Judd-Hamilton L, Harris TB et al (2003 Aug) The associations between physical activity and inflammatory markers in high-functioning older persons: Macarthur Studies of Successful Aging. J Am Geriatr Soc 51(8):1125–1130
115. Stauffer BL, Hoetzer GL, Smith DT et al (2004 Jan) Plasma C-reactive protein is not elevated in physically active postmenopausal women taking hormone replacement therapy. J Appl Physiol 96(1):143–148
116. Colbert LH, Visser M, Simonsick EM et al (2004 Jul) Physical activity, exercise, and inflammatory markers in older adults: findings from the Health, Aging and Body Composition Study. J Am Geriatr Soc 52(7):1098–1104

117. Pischon T, Hankinson SE, Hotamisligil GS et al (2003 Sep) Leisure-time physical activity and reduced plasma levels of obesity-related inflammatory markers. Obes Res 11(9): 1055–1064
118. Otani T, Iwasaki M, Sasazuki S et al (2006 Apr) Plasma C-reactive protein and risk of colorectal cancer in a nested case-control study: Japan Public Health Center-based prospective study. Cancer Epidemiol Biomarkers Prev 15(4):690–695
119. Esposito K, Pontillo A, Di Palo C et al (2003 Apr 9) Effect of weight loss and lifestyle changes on vascular inflammatory markers in obese women: a randomized trial. JAMA 289(14):1799–1804
120. Wegge JK, Roberts CK, Ngo TH et al (2004 Mar) Effect of diet and exercise intervention on inflammatory and adhesion molecules in postmenopausal women on hormone replacement therapy and at risk for coronary artery disease. Metabolism 53(3):377–381
121. Marcell TJ, McAuley KA, Traustadottir T et al (2005 Apr) Exercise training is not associated with improved levels of C-reactive protein or adiponectin. Metabolism 54(4):533–541
122. Nicklas BJ, Ambrosius W, Messier SP et al (2004 Apr) Diet-induced weight loss, exercise, and chronic inflammation in older, obese adults: a randomized controlled clinical trial. Am J Clin Nutr 79(4):544–551
123. Rauramaa R, Halonen P, Vaisanen SB et al (2004 Jun 15) Effects of aerobic physical exercise on inflammation and atherosclerosis in men: the DNASCO Study: a six-year randomized, controlled trial. Ann Intern Med 140(12):1007–1014
124. Wetmore CM, Ulrich CM (eds) (2004) Mechanisms associating physical activity with cancer incidence: exercise and immune function. CRC Taylor Francis, Boca Raton, FL
125. Keller C, Keller P, Giralt M et al (2004 Aug 13) Exercise normalises overexpression of TNF-alpha in knockout mice. Biochem Biophys Res Commun 321(1):179–182
126. Bacuau RF, Belmonte MA, Seelaender MC et al (2000 Dec) Effect of a moderate intensity exercise training protocol on the metabolism of macrophages and lymphocytes of tumour-bearing rats. Cell Biochem Funct 18(4):249–258
127. Rogers CJ, Hance KW, Zaharoff DA et al (2008) Exercise, alone and in combination with an anti-CEA vaccine, reduces pancreatic tumor cell growth and enhances survival in mice. Vaccine 26:5407–5415
128. Woods JA, Davis JM, Kohut ML et al (1994 Sep) Effects of exercise on the immune response to cancer. Med Sci Sports Exerc 26(9):1109–1115
129. Shewchuk LD, Baracos VE, Field CJ (1997 Jan) Dietary L-glutamine supplementation reduces the growth of the Morris Hepatoma 7777 in exercise-trained and sedentary rats. J Nutr 127(1):158–166
130. Zielinski MR, Muenchow M, Wallig MA et al (2004 Jun) Exercise delays allogeneic tumor growth and reduces intratumoral inflammation and vascularization. J Appl Physiol 96(6):2249–2256
131. Davis JM, Kohut ML, Colbert LH et al (1997 Nov) Exercise, alveolar macrophage function, and susceptibility to respiratory infection. J Appl Physiol 83(5):1461–1466
132. Murphy EA, Davis JM, Brown AS et al (2004 Sep) Effects of moderate exercise and oat beta-glucan on lung tumor metastases and macrophage antitumor cytotoxicity. J Appl Physiol 97(3):955–959
133. Woods JA, Davis JM, Mayer EP et al (1993 Aug) Exercise increases inflammatory macrophage antitumor cytotoxicity. J Appl Physiol 75(2):879–886
134. Lu Q, Ceddia MA, Price EA et al (1999 Feb) Chronic exercise increases macrophage-mediated tumor cytolysis in young and old mice. Am J Physiol 276(2 Pt 2): R482–R489
135. Barlozzari T, Leonhardt J, Wiltrout RH et al (1985 Apr) Direct evidence for the role of LGL in the inhibition of experimental tumor metastases. J Immunol 134(4):2783–2789
136. Cerwenka A, Baron JL, Lanier LL (2001 Sep 25) Ectopic expression of retinoic acid early inducible-1 gene (RAE-1) permits natural killer cell-mediated rejection of a MHC class I-bearing tumor in vivo. Proc Natl Acad Sci USA 98(20):11521–11526

137. Imai K, Matsuyama S, Miyake S et al (2000 Nov 25) Natural cytotoxic activity of peripheral-blood lymphocytes and cancer incidence: an 11-year follow-up study of a general population. Lancet 356(9244):1795–1799
138. Kaplan DH, Shankaran V, Dighe AS et al (1998 Jun 23) Demonstration of an interferon gamma-dependent tumor surveillance system in immunocompetent mice. Proc Natl Acad Sci USA 95(13):7556–7561
139. MacNeil B, Hoffman-Goetz L (1993 Jan) Chronic exercise enhances in vivo and in vitro cytotoxic mechanisms of natural immunity in mice. J Appl Physiol 74(1):388–395
140. Rogers CJ, Berrigan D, Zaharoff DA et al (2008 Jan) Energy restriction and exercise differentially enhance components of systemic and mucosal immunity in mice. J Nutr 138(1):115–122
141. Hoffman-Goetz L, May KM, Arumugam Y (1994 Nov–Dec) Exercise training and mouse mammary tumour metastasis. Anticancer Res 14(6B):2627–2631
142. MacNeil B, Hoffman-Goetz L (1993 Aug) Effect of exercise on natural cytotoxicity and pulmonary tumor metastases in mice. Med Sci Sports Exerc 25(8):922–928
143. Rogers CJ, Zaharoff DA, Hance KW et al (2008 Oct 3) Exercise enhances vaccine-induced antigen-specific T cell responses. Vaccine 26(42):5407–5415
144. Bloor CM (2005) Angiogenesis during exercise and training. Angiogenesis 8(3):263–271
145. Gu JW, Gadonski G, Wang J et al (2004 Jan) Exercise increases endostatin in circulation of healthy volunteers. BMC Physiol 16(4):2
146. Bailey AP, Shparago M, Gu JW (2006 Feb) Exercise increases soluble vascular endothelial growth factor receptor-1 (sFlt-1) in circulation of healthy volunteers. Med Sci Monit 12(2):CR45–CR50
147. Buehlmeyer K, Doering F, Daniel H et al (2008) Alteration of gene expression in rat colon mucosa after exercise. Ann Anat 190(1):71–80
148. Masoro EJ, McCarter RJ, Katz MS et al (1992 Nov) Dietary restriction alters characteristics of glucose fuel use. J Gerontol 47(6):B202–B208
149. Kemnitz JW, Roecker EB, Weindruch R et al (1994 Apr) Dietary restriction increases insulin sensitivity and lowers blood glucose in rhesus monkeys. Am J Physiol 266(4 Pt 1): E540–E547
150. Lane MA, Ball SS, Ingram DK et al (1995 May) Diet restriction in rhesus monkeys lowers fasting and glucose-stimulated glucoregulatory end points. Am J Physiol 268(5 Pt 1): E941–E948
151. Cefalu WT, Wagner JD, Wang ZQ et al (1997 Jan) A study of caloric restriction and cardiovascular aging in cynomolgus monkeys (*Macaca fascicularis*): a potential model for aging research. J Gerontol A Biol Sci Med Sci 52(1):B10–19
152. Barzilai N, Banerjee S, Hawkins M et al (1998 Apr 1) Caloric restriction reverses hepatic insulin resistance in aging rats by decreasing visceral fat. J Clin Invest 101(7): 1353–1361
153. Gresl TA, Colman RJ, Roecker EB et al (2001 Oct) Dietary restriction and glucose regulation in aging rhesus monkeys: a follow-up report at 8.5 yr. Am J Physiol Endocrinol Metab 281(4):E757–E765
154. Cerami A (1985 Sep) Hypothesis. Glucose as a mediator of aging. J Am Geriatr Soc 33(9):626–634
155. Baserga R (1994 Dec 16) Oncogenes and the strategy of growth factors. Cell 79(6):927–930
156. Sara VR, Hall K (1990 Jul) Insulin-like growth factors and their binding proteins. Physiol Rev 70(3):591–614
157. Dunn SE, Kari FW, French J et al (1997) Dietary restriction reduces insulin-like growth factor I levels, which modulates apoptosis, cell proliferation, and tumor progression in p53-deficient mice. Cancer Res 57:4667–4672
158. Resnicoff M, Abraham D, Yutanawiboonchai W et al (1995 Jun 1) The insulin-like growth factor I receptor protects tumor cells from apoptosis in vivo. Cancer Res 55(11): 2463–2469

159. Macaulay VM (1992 Mar) Insulin-like growth factors and cancer. Br J Cancer 65(3): 311–320
160. LeRoith D, Baserga R, Helman L et al (1995 Jan 1) Insulin-like growth factors and cancer. Ann Intern Med 122(1):54–59
161. Singh P, Dai B, Yallampalli U et al (1996 May) Proliferation and differentiation of a human colon cancer cell line (CaCo2) is associated with significant changes in the expression and secretion of insulin-like growth factor (IGF) IGF-II and IGF binding protein-4: role of IGF-II. Endocrinology 137(5):1764–1774
162. Fenton JI, Hord NG, Lavigne JA et al (2005 Jul) Leptin, insulin-like growth factor-1, and insulin-like growth factor-2 are mitogens in ApcMin/+ but not Apc+/+ colonic epithelial cell lines. Cancer Epidemiol Biomarkers Prev 14(7):1646–1652
163. Hankinson SE, Willett WC, Colditz GA et al (1998 May 9) Circulating concentrations of insulin-like growth factor-I and risk of breast cancer. Lancet 351(9113): 1393–1396
164. Chan JM, Stampfer MJ, Giovannucci E et al (1998 Jan 23) Plasma insulin-like growth factor-I and prostate cancer risk: a prospective study. Science 279(5350):563–566
165. Ma J, Pollak M, Giovannucci E, Chan J, Tao Y, Hennekens C, Stampfer M (1999) Prospective study of colorectal cancer risk in men and plasma levels of insulin-like growth factor (IGF-1) and IGF-Binding Protein-3. J Natl Cancer Inst 91:620–625
166. Yu H, Spitz MR, Mistry J et al (1999 Jan 20) Plasma levels of insulin-like growth factor-I and lung cancer risk: a case-control analysis. J Natl Cancer Inst 91(2):151–156
167. Giovannucci E, Pollak MN, Platz EA et al (2000 Apr) A prospective study of plasma insulin-like growth factor-1 and binding protein-3 and risk of colorectal neoplasia in women. Cancer Epidemiol Biomarkers Prev 9(4):345–349
168. Manousos O, Souglakos J, Bosetti C, Tzonou A, Chatzikdakis V, Trichopoulos D, Adami H-O, Mantzoros C (1999) IGF-1 and IGF-II in relation to colorectal cancer. Int J Cancer 83:15–17
169. Buckbinder L, Talbott R, Velasco-Miguel S et al (1995) Induction of the growth inhibitor IGF-binding protein 3 by p53. Nature 377:646–649
170. Takahashi K, Suzuki K (1993 Sep 30) Association of insulin-like growth-factor-I-induced DNA synthesis with phosphorylation and nuclear exclusion of p53 in human breast cancer MCF-7 cells. Int J Cancer 55(3):453–458
171. Butler AA, LeRoith D (2001 May) Minireview: tissue-specific versus generalized gene targeting of the igf1 and igf1r genes and their roles in insulin-like growth factor physiology. Endocrinology 142(5):1685–1688
172. Gems D, Partridge L (2001 Jun) Insulin/IGF signalling and ageing: seeing the bigger picture. Curr Opin Genet Dev 11(3):287–292
173. Hursting SD, Switzer BR, French JE et al (1993 Jun 15) The growth hormone: insulin-like growth factor 1 axis is a mediator of diet restriction-induced inhibition of mononuclear cell leukemia in Fischer rats. Cancer Res 53(12):2750–2757
174. Olivo-Marston S, Hursting SD, Lavigne J, Perkins SN, Marouf R, Yakar S, Haris CC (2009) Genetic reduction of insulin-like growth factor-1 inhibits azoxymethane-induced colon tumorigenesis in mice. Mol Carcinogenesis 2009, 48:1071–1076
175. Moore T, Carbajal S, Beltran L et al (2008 May 15) Reduced susceptibility to two-stage skin carcinogenesis in mice with low circulating insulin-like growth factor I levels. Cancer Res 68(10):3680–3688
176. Yakar S, Nunez NP, Pennisi P et al (2006 Dec) Increased tumor growth in mice with diet-induced obesity: impact of ovarian hormones. Endocrinology 147(12):5826–5834
177. Moore T, Beltran L, Carbajal S et al (2008) Dietary energy balance modulates signaling through the Akt/mammalian target of rapamycin pathways in multiple epithelial tissues. Cancer Prev Res 1:65–76
178. Pollak MN, Schernhammer ES, Hankinson SE (2004) Insulin-like growth factors and neoplasia. Nat Rev Cancer 4(7):505–518

179. Pollak M (2008 Dec) Insulin and insulin-like growth factor signalling in neoplasia. Nat Rev Cancer 8(12):915–928
180. Yuan TL, Cantley LC (2008 Sep 18) PI3K pathway alterations in cancer: variations on a theme. Oncogene 27(41):5497–5510
181. Engelman JA (2009 Aug) Targeting PI3K signalling in cancer: opportunities, challenges and limitations. Nat Rev Cancer 9(8):550–562
182. Franke TF (2008 Oct 27) PI3K/Akt: getting it right matters. Oncogene 27(50):6473–6488
183. Brazil DP, Yang ZZ, Hemmings BA (2004 May) Advances in protein kinase B signalling: AKTion on multiple fronts. Trends Biochem Sci 29(5):233–242
184. Guertin DA, Sabatini DM (2005 Aug) An expanding role for mTOR in cancer. Trends Mol Med 11(8):353–361
185. Shaw RJ, Bardeesy N, Manning BD et al (2004 Jul) The LKB1 tumor suppressor negatively regulates mTOR signaling. Cancer Cell 6(1):91–99
186. Corradetti MN, Inoki K, Bardeesy N et al (2004 Jul 1) Regulation of the TSC pathway by LKB1: evidence of a molecular link between tuberous sclerosis complex and Peutz-Jeghers syndrome. Genes Dev 18(13):1533–1538
187. Shaw RJ, Kosmatka M, Bardeesy N et al (2004 Mar 9) The tumor suppressor LKB1 kinase directly activates AMP-activated kinase and regulates apoptosis in response to energy stress. Proc Natl Acad Sci USA 101(10):3329–3335
188. Astrinidis A, Henske EP (2005 Nov 14) Tuberous sclerosis complex: linking growth and energy signaling pathways with human disease. Oncogene 24(50):7475–7481
189. Inoki K, Corradetti MN, Guan KL (2005 Jan) Dysregulation of the TSC-mTOR pathway in human disease. Nat Genet 37(1):19–24
190. Tee AR, Blenis J (2005 Feb) mTOR, translational control and human disease. Semin Cell Dev Biol 16(1):29–37
191. Memmott RM, Dennis PA (2009 May) Akt-dependent and -independent mechanisms of mTOR regulation in cancer. Cell Signal 21(5):656–664
192. Huang XF, Chen JZ (2009 Nov) Obesity, the PI3K/Akt signal pathway and colon cancer. Obes Rev 10(6):610–616
193. Jiang W, Zhu Z, Thompson HJ (2008) Dietary energy restriction modulates the activity of AMP-activated protein kinase, Akt, and mammalian target of rapamycin in mammary carcinomas, mammary gland, and liver. Cancer Res 68:5492–5499
194. Avruch J, Hara K, Lin Y et al (2006 Oct 16) Insulin and amino-acid regulation of mTOR signaling and kinase activity through the Rheb GTPase. Oncogene 25(48):6361–6372
195. Birt DF, Przybyszewski J, Wang W et al (2004 Feb 1) Identification of molecular targets for dietary energy restriction prevention of skin carcinogenesis: an idea cultivated by Edward Bresnick. J Cell Biochem 91(2):258–264
196. Jiang W, Zhu Z, Bhatia N et al (2002 Sep 15) Mechanisms of energy restriction: effects of corticosterone on cell growth, cell cycle machinery, and apoptosis. Cancer Res 62(18): 5280–5287
197. Pashko LL, Schwartz AG (1992 Oct) Reversal of food restriction-induced inhibition of mouse skin tumor promotion by adrenalectomy. Carcinogenesis 13(10):1925–1928
198. Boutwell RK (1964) Some biological aspects of skin carcinogenisis. Prog Exp Tumor Res 4:207–250
199. Woods SC, Seeley RJ, Porte D Jr et al (1998 May 29) Signals that regulate food intake and energy homeostasis. Science 280(5368):1378–1383
200. Zhang Y, Leibel R (1998) Molecular physiology of leptin and its receptor. Growth Genet Hormones 14:17–35
201. Lonnqvist F, Wennlund A, Arner P (1997 Apr) Relationship between circulating leptin and peripheral fat distribution in obese subjects. Int J Obes Relat Metab Disord 21(4):255–260
202. Montague CT, Prins JB, Sanders L et al (1997 Mar) Depot- and sex-specific differences in human leptin mRNA expression: implications for the control of regional fat distribution. Diabetes 46(3):342–347

203. Brennan AM, Mantzoros CS (2006 Jun) Drug Insight: the role of leptin in human physiology and pathophysiology–emerging clinical applications. Nat Clin Pract Endocrinol Metab 2(6):318–327
204. Stattin P, Lukanova A, Biessy C et al (2004 Mar) Obesity and colon cancer: does leptin provide a link?. Int J Cancer 109(1):149–152
205. Bouloumie A, Drexler HC, Lafontan M et al (1998 Nov 16) Leptin, the product of Ob gene, promotes angiogenesis. Circ Res 83(10):1059–1066
206. Ostlund RE Jr., Yang JW, Klein S et al (1996 Nov) Relation between plasma leptin concentration and body fat, gender, diet, age, and metabolic covariates. J Clin Endocrinol Metab 81(11):3909–3913
207. Villanueva EC, Myers MG Jr. (2008 Dec) Leptin receptor signaling and the regulation of mammalian physiology. Int J Obes (London) 32(Suppl 7):S8–S12
208. Rajala MW, Scherer PE (2003 Sep) Minireview: The adipocyte–at the crossroads of energy homeostasis, inflammation, and atherosclerosis. Endocrinology 144(9):3765–3773
209. Gonzalez RR, Cherfils S, Escobar M et al (2006 Sep 8) Leptin signaling promotes the growth of mammary tumors and increases the expression of vascular endothelial growth factor (VEGF) and its receptor type two (VEGF-R2. J Biol Chem 281(36):26320–26328
210. Loffreda S, Yang SQ, Lin HZ et al (1998 Jan) Leptin regulates proinflammatory immune responses. FASEB J 12(1):57–65
211. Ryan AS, Nicklas BJ, Berman DM et al (2003 Sep) Adiponectin levels do not change with moderate dietary induced weight loss and exercise in obese postmenopausal women. Int J Obes Relat Metab Disord 27(9):1066–1071
212. Diker D, Vishne T, Maayan R et al (2006 Aug) Impact of gastric banding on plasma adiponectin levels. Obes Surg 16(8):1057–1061
213. Kelesidis I, Kelesidis T, Mantzoros CS (2006) Adiponectin and cancer: a systematic review. Br J Cancer 94:1221–1225
214. Freedland SJ, Williams CD, Masko EM (2010) Adipoenctin and prostate cancer mortality: to be or not to be skinny?. Clin Chem 56:1–3
215. Barb D, Williams CJ, Neuwirth AK, Mantzoros CS (2007) Adiponectin in relation to malignancies: a review of existing basic research and clinical evidence. Am J CLin Nutr 86:s856–s866
216. Cleary MP, Ray A, Rogozina OP, Dogan S, Grossmann ME (2009) Targeting the adiponectin:leptin ration for postmenopausal breast cancer prevention. Front Biosci 1: 329–357
217. Fenton JI, Birmingham JM, Hursting SD, Hord NG (2008) Adiponectin blocks multiple signaling cascades associated with leptin-induced cell proliferation in Apc Min/+ colon epithelial cells. Int J Cancer 122:2437–2445
218. Fontana L, Klein S (2007 Mar 7) Aging adiposity, and calorie restriction. JAMA 297(9): 986–994
219. Fontana L (2009 Jan–Feb) Neuroendocrine factors in the regulation of inflammation: excessive adiposity and calorie restriction. Exp Gerontol 44(1–2):41–45
220. Spaulding CC, Walford RL, Effros RB (1997 Feb) Calorie restriction inhibits the age-related dysregulation of the cytokines TNF-alpha and IL-6 in C3B10RF1 mice. Mech Ageing Dev 93(1–3):87–94
221. Matsuzaki J, Kuwamura M, Yamaji R et al (2001 Aug) Inflammatory responses to lipopolysaccharide are suppressed in 40% energy-restricted mice. J Nutr 131(8): 2139–2144
222. Higami Y, Pugh TD, Page GP et al (2004 Feb) Adipose tissue energy metabolism: altered gene expression profile of mice subjected to long-term caloric restriction. FASEB J 18(2):415–417
223. Kim MJ, Aiken JM, Havighurst T et al (1997 Dec) Adult-onset energy restriction of rhesus monkeys attenuates oxidative stress-induced cytokine expression by peripheral blood mononuclear cells. J Nutr 127(12):2293–2301

224. Fontana L, Villareal DT, Weiss EP et al (2007 Jul) Calorie restriction or exercise: effects on coronary heart disease risk factors. A randomized, controlled trial. Am J Physiol Endocrinol Metab 293(1):E197–E202
225. Longo VD, Kennedy BK (2006 Jul 28) Sirtuins in aging and age-related disease. Cell 126(2):257–268
226. Anastasiou D, Krek W (2006 Dec) SIRT1: linking adaptive cellular responses to aging-associated changes in organismal physiology. Physiology (Bethesda) 21:404–410
227. Yang T, Fu M, Pestell R et al (2006 Jul) SIRT1 and endocrine signaling. Trends Endocrinol Metab 17(5):186–191
228. Cohen HY, Miller C, Bitterman KJ et al (2004 Jul 16) Calorie restriction promotes mammalian cell survival by inducing the SIRT1 deacetylase. Science 305(5682):390–392
229. Metoyer CF, Pruitt K (2008 Aug) The role of sirtuin proteins in obesity. Pathophysiology 15(2):103–108
230. Lin SJ, Defossez PA, Guarente L (2000 Sep 22) Requirement of NAD and SIR2 for life-span extension by calorie restriction in Saccharomyces cerevisiae. Science 289(5487): 2126–2128
231. Anderson RM, Bitterman KJ, Wood JG et al (2003 May 8) Nicotinamide and PNC1 govern lifespan extension by calorie restriction in Saccharomyces cerevisiae. Nature 423(6936):181–185
232. Tissenbaum HA, Guarente L (2001 Mar 8) Increased dosage of a sir-2 gene extends lifespan in Caenorhabditis elegans. Nature 410(6825):227–230
233. Picard F, Kurtev M, Chung N et al (2004 Jun 17) Sirt1 promotes fat mobilization in white adipocytes by repressing PPAR-gamma. Nature 429(6993):771–776
234. Qiang L, Wang H, Farmer SR (2007 Jul) Adiponectin secretion is regulated by SIRT1 and the endoplasmic reticulum oxidoreductase Ero1-L alpha. Mol Cell Biol 27(13):4698–4707
235. Qiao L, Shao J (2006) SIRT1 regulates adiponectin gene expression through Foxo1-C/enhancer-binding protein alpha transcriptional complex. J Biol Chem 281(52): 39915–39924
236. Bordone L, Cohen D, Robinson A et al (2007 Dec) SIRT1 transgenic mice show phenotypes resembling calorie restriction. Aging Cell 6(6):759–767
237. Ramsey KM, Mills KF, Satoh A et al (2008 Jan) Age-associated loss of Sirt1-mediated enhancement of glucose-stimulated insulin secretion in beta cell-specific Sirt1-overexpressing (BESTO) mice. Aging Cell 7(1):78–88
238. Nemoto S, Fergusson MM, Finkel T (2005 Apr 22) SIRT1 functionally interacts with the metabolic regulator and transcriptional coactivator PGC-1. J Biol Chem 280(16): 16456–16460
239. Nisoli E, Tonello C, Cardile A et al (2005 Oct 14) Calorie restriction promotes mitochondrial biogenesis by inducing the expression of eNOS. Science 310(5746):314–317
240. Yechoor VK, Patti ME, Ueki K et al (2004 Nov 23) Distinct pathways of insulin-regulated versus diabetes-regulated gene expression: an in vivo analysis in MIRKO mice. Proc Natl Acad Sci USA 101(47):16525–16530
241. Lim CS (2006) SIRT1: tumor promoter or tumor suppressor?. Med Hypotheses 67(2): 341–344
242. Ford J, Jiang M, Milner J (2005 Nov 15) Cancer-specific functions of SIRT1 enable human epithelial cancer cell growth and survival. Cancer Res 65(22):10457–10463
243. Chen WY, Wang DH, Yen RC et al (2005 Nov 4) Tumor suppressor HIC1 directly regulates SIRT1 to modulate p53-dependent DNA-damage responses. Cell 123(3):437–448
244. Huffman DM, Grizzle WE, Bamman MM et al (2007 Jul 15) SIRT1 is significantly elevated in mouse and human prostate cancer. Cancer Res 67(14):6612–6618
245. Kim JE, Chen J, Lou Z (2008 Jan 31) DBC1 is a negative regulator of SIRT1. Nature 451(7178):583–586
246. Zhao W, Kruse JP, Tang Y et al (2008 Jan 31) Negative regulation of the deacetylase SIRT1 by DBC1. Nature 451(7178):587–590

247. Firestein R, Blander G, Michan S et al (2008) The SIRT1 deacetylase suppresses intestinal tumorigenesis and colon cancer growth. PLoS One 3(4):e2020
248. Kabra N, Li Z, Chen L et al (2009) SIRT1 is an inhibitor of proliferation and tumor formation in colon cancer. J Biol Chem 284:18210–18217
249. Pruitt K, Zinn RL, Ohm JE (2006) Inhibition of SIRT1 reactivates silenced cancer genes without loss of promoter DNA hypermethylation. PLoS Genet 2:e40

Chapter 6
Mechanisms Linking Obesity to Cancer Risk

Ikuyo Imayama, Caitlin Mason, and Catherine Duggan

Abstract Increased body mass and adiposity are linked to increased risk of many cancers, including postmenopausal breast, endometrial, prostate, and colon cancer [1]. Obesity levels are reaching epidemic proportions: the World Health Organization (WHO) estimated that in 2005, 1.6 billion individuals worldwide aged 15 years and older are overweight, of whom 400 million are obese. Projected figures for 2015 are 2.3 billion adults will be overweight, and 700 million obese [2]. Estimates attribute 14% of US cancer deaths [3] and 25% of cancer incidence worldwide [4] to excess adiposity.

The mechanisms through which overweight and increased adiposity influence cancer risk are still to be fully elucidated. Obesity is commonly associated with hyperinsulinemia; insulin resistance; alterations in levels of adipokines, such as adiponectin; alterations of steroid hormonal profiles thought to favor cancer growth; and an upregulation of inflammatory pathways.

To date, these are the principal candidates for explaining the association between increased adiposity/obesity and cancer risk, and will be discussed in detail in this chapter. Other potential mechanistic pathways are discussed elsewhere [6].

1 Definition and Measurement of Obesity

There are a variety of methods available to measure body composition and adiposity. The emergence of dual energy X-ray absorptiometry (DXA) scans and imaging technologies such as computed tomography (CT) and magnetic resonance imaging (MRI) has led to increasingly sophisticated and accurate means of quantifying

C. Duggan (✉)
Division of Public Health Sciences, Fred Hutchinson Cancer Research Center, Seattle, WA 98109-1024, USA
e-mail: cduggan@fhcrc.org

Ikuyo Imayama and Caitlin Mason contributed equally to the writing of this chapter

A. McTiernan (ed.), *Physical Activity, Dietary Calorie Restriction, and Cancer*, Energy Balance and Cancer 3, DOI 10.1007/978-1-4419-7551-5_6,

adipose tissue [7]. DXA can differentiate fat mass, lean mass, and bone mass, and is used to estimate whole-body or regional (arms, trunk, legs) fat tissue [7, 8]. CT and MRI scans are unique in their ability to differentiate subcutaneous and visceral abdominal fat depots, which are typically estimated from a single cross-sectional image, commonly taken at the level of the L4-L5 vertebrae [9].

Despite the validity and reliability of these methods, their widespread applicability remains limited due to factors such as cost, availability, and radiation exposure [10, 11]. Consequently, simple, inexpensive, and noninvasive anthropometric measures (weight, height, body mass index, waist and hip circumferences, skinfold thickness) or bioelectrical impedance are more routinely used in clinical and population studies [10, 11].

By far the most common measure of adiposity used in studies of obesity and chronic disease is body mass index (BMI; kgm^2), a simple ratio of weight to height first proposed by the Belgian statistician, Quetelet, in the 1830s [12]. BMI is independent of height and provides a better estimation of adipose tissue than weight alone [13]. It also provides a single value that can be easily compared across studies and between populations. BMI is directly correlated with the risk of medical complications, and the sum of evidence from a large body of epidemiological studies generally shows a J-shaped or U-shaped relation between BMI and risk of mortality [14, 15, 16] and disease, including cancer [4, 17, 18]. Based on these observed associations, several leading health organizations, including the WHO [19] and the US National Institutes of Health (NIH) [20], advocate a simple BMI-based system for classifying adiposity in adult men and women such that individuals with a BMI $\geq$30 are considered obese and are at greater health risk than those classified as overweight (BMI 25–29.9) who in turn have a greater risk than those in the normal weight (BMI 18.5–24.9) category. Further subclassifications of obesity (Class I, II, and III) (Table 6.1) are also important, as individuals with more extreme obesity most frequently experience serious metabolic complications and suffer greater morbidity [20].

Although BMI has the advantage of being easy to measure, reliable, and closely correlated with adult body fat ($r = 0.7$–0.8) [21, 22], it is also subject to certain limitations, most notably its inability to account for inter-individuals differences in the relative proportions of body fat and lean tissue, and to capture relative body fat distribution [23]. As a central distribution of adipose tissue is most strongly correlated with metabolic complications [24, 25, 26], it is important to note that there exists a substantial degree of heterogeneity in this regard, within each BMI category [27].

As a result, waist circumference or the ratio of waist-to-hip circumference (WHR) are sometimes used alone or in combination with BMI to assess the risks of obesity that may be more closely associated with body fat distribution than to generalized adiposity, particularly the adverse consequences of visceral fat accumulation [28, 29]. Waist circumference values greater than 35 inches in women and 40 inches in men and/or a WHR above 0.8 in women and 0.9 in men have come to be generally accepted cut-points reflecting elevated risk [30, 31].

Table 6.1 Classification of obesity-related health risk based on BMI and waist circumferencea

		Waist circumference	
Category	Men ≤102 cm BMI (kg/m²)	Men >102 cm Women ≤88 cm	Women >88 cm
Underweight	<18.5		
Normal weight	18.5–24.9	Normal	Increased
Overweight (pre-obese)	25–29.9	Increased	High
Obese	≥30		
Class I	30–34.9	High	Very high
Class II	35–39.9	Very high	Very high
Class III	≥40	Extremely high	Extremely high

[a]Based on WHO and US National Institutes of Health guidelines

Assessment of Insulin Sensitivity and Resistance

Several direct and indirect methods are currently employed to assess insulin sensitivity and the degree of insulin resistance (decreased sensitivity or responsiveness to actions of insulin) in humans, and there is no single method that is appropriate in all settings [32]. The hyperinsulinemic euglycemic clamp and the insulin suppression test allow direct assessment of insulin-mediated glucose uptake under steady-state conditions; however, these methods are complex, costly, and labor-intensive [33]. Alternatively, a simple measure of fasting blood glucose is commonly used to detect insulin resistance in clinical settings. Fasting glucose levels of 100–125 mg/dL (5.6–6.9 mmol/L) are termed "impaired" [2] because they are above normal but not high enough to be considered overt diabetes, which requires repeated measures >126 mg/dL />7 mmol/L on two separate occasions [34]. In many cases, insulin resistance or overt diabetes detected by fasting glucose measures is confirmed with a more sophisticated indirect measure known as an oral glucose tolerance test (OGTT). This involves serial blood samples for determination of glucose and insulin concentrations taken at set time intervals (e.g. 0, 30, 60, 120 min) following a standard oral glucose load (e.g. 75 g) or standard meal administered following an overnight fast [33]. Type 2 diabetes may also be diagnosed with a test of glycated hemoglobin (HbA1c), which is used to assess the average plasma glucose concentration over prolonged periods of time and does not need to be conducted in a fasted state. Values exceeding 6.5% are considered indicative of a diabetic state [35].

Several surrogate indices of insulin sensitivity/resistance (e.g., QUICKI, HOMA) can also be derived from blood concentrations of glucose, insulin and/or C-peptide under fasting conditions. The Quantitative insulin sensitivity check index (QUICKI=1/[log(fasting insulin, μU/mL) + log(fasting glucose, mg/dL)]) [36] and the Homeostatic Model Assessment (HOMA= fasting insulin (mU/L) × fasting glucose (mmol/L)/22.5 [5]), which can be expressed as insulin resistance (HOMA-IR) where lower values are more favorable, or, as its reciprocal, insulin sensitivity (HOMA-IS), are two of the most widely used. Each has its own strengths and limitations [33], but both correlate well with estimates from the euglycemic clamp [5, 36, 37]. Surrogate indices have the benefit of being relatively inexpensive and more feasible in diverse settings compared to other methods of assessing insulin sensitivity. For these reasons, they are well suited to large samples and epidemiological studies. For practical purposes, insulin resistance is defined by the WHO as the highest quartile of HOMA-IR in nondiabetic subjects; however, the clinical utility of surrogate indices is limited by the lack of exact reference values [38].

The different approaches to the measurement and characterization of insulin resistance may be one contributing factor to the heterogeneity in reported associations between obesity, insulin resistance, and cancer. Subject fasting status, blood sample handling, and specific assay characteristics have the potential to influence biological markers of insulin sensitivity as well as related analytes involved in their downstream metabolic pathways [32]. Greater standardization and accuracy of methodology including available assays will likely help to reconcile some apparent discrepancies in current evidence.

2 The Epidemiology of Insulin Resistance, the Insulin-Like Growth Factor (IGF) System, Sex Steroid Hormones, Inflammation, and Cancer

2.1 Insulin/Hyperinsulinemia

Chronic positive energy balance leading to obesity is associated with several metabolic and endocrine perturbations, including the development of insulin resistance and the progression to type 2 diabetes in susceptible individuals [39]. In healthy metabolic functioning, insulin is secreted by pancreatic β-cells in response to a rise in blood glucose concentrations and signals in insulin-sensitive tissues, mainly muscle and fat, to absorb glucose, thereby maintaining normoglycemia. In the obese state, pro-inflammatory cytokines released by adipocytes disrupt normal insulin action, leading to a reduced responsiveness of target tissues to the physiological actions of insulin and a compensatory rise in insulin secretion from pancreatic β-cells in order to avert high blood glucose levels [39].

Although insulin concentrations correlate with increasing adiposity as measured by BMI in nondiabetic individuals [40], it is the accumulation of abdominal visceral fat and the release of proinflammatory cytokines from this fat depot that are particularly implicated in metabolic dysregulation and the development of insulin resistance [25, 41, 42, 43, 44, 45].

Considerable in vitro and in vivo evidence now provides support for the hypothesized etiologic role of insulin resistance in the pathogenesis of various cancers and as a plausible mechanistic link between obesity and carcinogenesis. Despite this growing body of evidence, the exact molecular mechanisms involved have yet to be fully elucidated. The mechanistic links are likely to be complex, given the numerous and interrelated biological pathways involved in body weight regulation and energy metabolism. The sections below are not comprehensive in this regard, but will briefly discuss some of the current epidemiological evidence with respect to insulin-related pathways that are dysregulated in obesity and postulated to affect cancer risk.

In humans, numerous epidemiological studies support a direct link between hyperinsuliemia and cancers of the breast [46, 47, 48, 49, 50, 51, 52, 53], endometrium [54, 55, 56], colon [54, 57, 58, 59, 60, 61], and pancreas [62], while less consistent evidence exists for prostate cancer [63, 64, 65] and cancers at other sites [66]. Hyperinsulinemia has also been related to poor prognosis and mortality from colorectal [67], breast [52, 68, 69], prostate [70], and pancreatic cancers [71], while an increased risk of less prevalent cancers including esophageal adenocarcinomas [72] and liver cancer [73] has been reported among individuals with the metabolic syndrome – a clustering of metabolic abnormalities characterized by central adiposity, insulin resistance, dyslipidemia, hypertension, and chronic low-grade inflammation [74, 75]. Likewise, type 2 diabetes, a disease typically preceded by extended periods of insulin resistance and increased insulin secretion, is associated with higher risk of numerous cancers including colorectal [76], endometrial [51, 77], breast [48, 51, 52, 78, 79], pancreatic [80], and those of the kidney, liver, and biliary tract [81, 82, 83]. Type 2 diabetes is also associated with higher cancer mortality [84].

The effect of insulin on breast cancer incidence has been widely examined in diverse cohorts. Most [46, 49, 85, 86, 87], but not all [88, 89], have reported a modest positive effect with results from case–control studies generally reporting larger effects than cohort studies [90]. However, interpretation of the collective findings is complicated by the substantial heterogeneity in study designs with regards to the method and timing of insulin measurement, inclusion of pre- and/or postmenopausal women, and adjustment for potential confounders including exogenous hormone use.

In a nested case–control study from the Women's Health Initiative cohort study, breast cancer incidence was 2.4-fold greater among women in the highest quartile compared to the lowest quartile of fasting insulin ($p_{\text{trend}} < 0.001$) [46]. In this study, insulin was a major factor in explaining the observed relationship between BMI and breast cancer risk. Its positive effects were also independent of endogenous estradiol concentrations, providing support for insulin's involvement in breast cancer etiology through a pathway distinct from circulating estrogens.

In a separate analysis of endometrial cancer risk in women from the same prospective cohort [91], women in the highest compared to lowest quartile of fasting insulin had an increased risk of endometrioid adenocarcinoma, the most prevalent histologic type of endometrial cancer (Hazard ratio $(HR)_{Q4\text{-}Q1}$: 2.79, 95%CI:1.39–5.60). This association was only apparent in women not using hormone therapy (HT); however, the risk estimate remained significant after adjustment for BMI and endogenous estradiol, suggesting the observed association was not solely attributable to these factors. A similar magnitude of association was observed between C-peptide and endometrial cancer in pre- and postmenopausal women not using HT in the European Prospective Investigation into Cancer and Nutrition (EPIC) study. During an average 5 years of follow-up, the relative risk (RR) comparing the highest to lowest quartile of insulin was 2.13 (95%CI:1.33–3.41, $p_{trend} = 0.001$) [92]. In this cohort, the effect of C-peptide was diminished, but remained statistically significant after adjustment for BMI, while adjusting for free estradiol further attenuated the association in postmenopausal women (RR:1.28, 95% CI:0.67–2.45, $p_{trend} = 0.42$).

Results from a recent meta-analysis of 10 prospective studies of colorectal cancer determined a summary relative risk of 1.35 (95% CI: 1.13–1.61), comparing extreme categories of insulin and/or C-peptide concentrations [90]. In this analysis, the pooled RR was greater in men than women, although the difference was not statistically significant. The available evidence from studies of incident colorectal cancer suggest that insulin has effects that are independent of the insulin-like growth factor (IGF) system (see the Section on IGF) [58, 59, 91]. For example, among men in the Physician's Health Study, adjusting for insulin-like growth factor-1 (IGF-1) and its primary binding protein, IGF binding protein-3 (IGFBP), did not materially change the observed positive association between plasma C-peptide levels and risk of colorectal cancer (RR: 2.7, 95% CI: 1.2–6.2, $p_{trend} = 0.047$) [59]. Likewise, a positive association for C-peptide, but not IGFBP-1 or -2, was observed in the EPIC study [58]. In the Women's Health Initiative Observational Study (WHI-OS), insulin significantly attenuated the association between waist circumference and colorectal cancer risk, while adjustment for free IGF-1 had no effect [91].

Fewer studies have examined the influence of insulin or C-peptide on the development of pancreatic cancer. Their results have shown a consistent positive association with high levels of insulin/C-peptide generally being associated with approximately twofold increased risk compared to low levels [71, 93, 94].

In contrast, studies of insulin and prostate cancer have yielded conflicting results. For example, in a case–control study of Finnish men, the odds of prostate cancer associated with being in the highest vs. lowest quartile of serum insulin were 2.55 (95%CI: 1.18–5.51, $p_{trend} = 0.02$) [63]. Several prospective cohort studies have shown either a weak or no association [95, 96, 97, 98], while one reported an apparent risk reduction for nonaggressive tumors [65]. Recently, an analysis of prostate cancer cases in the Physician's Health Study showed that high baseline C-peptide levels were associated with greater prostate cancer mortality, suggesting a possible association with aggressive, high-grade tumors [99].

Of special note with relevance to the association between hyperinsulinemia and cancer are findings that the use of the antidiabetic drug metformin is associated with reduced cancer incidence among diabetic patients [100, 101, 102, 103, 104]. In a recent record linkage study involving more than 12,000 type 2 diabetics [103], the use of metformin, which stimulates the uptake of glucose into muscle cells via the AMPK/mTOR/S6K1 axis [105], was associated with a cancer incidence of 7.3% compared to 11.6% in non-users of metformin. In addition to reducing circulating insulin levels, it is hypothesized that metformin may act directly on cancer cells as an AMPK-dependent growth inhibitor [106]. Metformin has also been shown to interact with chemotherapy agents to inhibit cellular transformation in mice [107], and to disrupt crosstalk between G protein-coupled receptor and insulin receptor signaling systems, leading to inhibited pancreatic cell growth in vitro [108]. Finally, diabetic breast cancer patients using metformin experience a higher rate of pathologic complete response to neoadjuvant chemotherapy than those using other diabetic treatments (OR=2.95; $p = 0.04$) [109]

2.2 IGF-1 and the IGF System

Similar in structure to insulin, IGF-1 is a hormone and growth factor that shares several downstream signaling pathways with insulin and also exhibits potent mitogenic properties [110, 111]. It is released mainly by the liver in response to growth hormone (GH), but small amounts are also produced locally in most tissue types, including adipose tissue [112]. IGF-1 is part of a complex molecular network that includes insulin-like growth factor-2 (IGF-2), IGF-1 and IGF-2 receptors (IGF-1R, IGF-2R), and at least six binding proteins (IGFBP 1-6) with high affinity for IGF binding [110, 111]. The vast majority (>95%) of circulating IGF-1 is bound to a binding protein, principally IGFBP-3 [111], and once bound is unable to transfer from the circulation to the target tissues. High levels of insulin associated with overweight/obesity downregulate the secretion of IGFBP-1 and -2, leading in turn to greater bioavailability of free (unbound) IGF-1 [113, 114]. Certain IGFBPs may also have biologic effects relevant to carcinogenesis, which are independent of their IGF-binding properties [115].

Like insulin, IGF-1 is postulated to play a role in cancer development on account of its proliferative and antiapoptotic effects via binding to the IGF-1 receptor (IGF-1R) and several downstream signaling pathways. However, unlike insulin, IGF-1 levels are not elevated in obese individuals, but peak in persons with BMI values 24–27 kg/m^2 [40]. It is postulated that obesity-related hyperinsulinemia inhibits production of IGFBPs and results in elevated levels of free IGF-1. In turn this exerts a negative feedback on GH secretion, thereby lowering IGF-1 levels [116, 117, 118].

Nevertheless, in site-specific meta-analyses comparing highest versus lowest categories, IGF-1 levels have been positively associated with colorectal cancer [119], prostate cancer [66, 119, 120, 121], and premenopausal, but not postmenopausal, breast cancer [66, 122, 123], though the evidence for breast cancer remains highly heterogeneous, precluding clear conclusions. Limited data are available with respect to IGF-1 and pancreatic cancer, but published reports suggest that low IGFBP-1 may confer excess risk [124, 125]. Similarly, IGF-1 and IGFBP-3 have been implicated in the development and prognosis of esophageal cancer [126, 127]; however, studies to date have been limited both in number and in size, and possible associations require confirmation in larger studies.

The reported odds of colorectal cancer comparing the highest to lowest quartiles of IGF-1 in five cohort studies published prior to 2002 was 1.58 (95% CI: 1.11–2.27) [66], and is consistent with a more recent multivariate adjusted risk estimate of 1.35 (95% CI: 0.92–1.98, $p_{\text{trend}} = 0.05$) between upper and lower quartiles of free IGF-1 in a large cohort of postmenopausal women [46]. In this study, the effects of both insulin and free IGF-1 were attenuated to nonsignificance after mutual adjustment.

In a large pooled analysis of 3,700 prostate cancer cases and 5,200 controls from 12 prospective studies, the overall risk estimate for prostate cancer comparing the highest and lowest quintiles of IGF-1 was 1.38 (95% CI:1.19–1.60, $p_{\text{trend}} = < 0.001$) [120]. IGFBP-3 was also positively associated with cancer risk in this analysis; however, its effects were attenuated to nonsignificance after adjustment for IGF-1, suggesting that the association between IGFBP-3 and prostate cancer risk is indirect. In contrast, the effect of IGF-1 was virtually unchanged after adjustment for IGFBP-3. IGF-2 and IGFBP-2 were also examined for a small subsample of men in this analysis, but neither showed any association with the risk of prostate cancer.

Generally, a positive association between IGF-1 has been reported for premenopausal but not postmenopausal status [18]; however, the magnitude of the association between IGF-1 and risk of premenopausal breast cancer has become attenuated with passing time of publication, with higher risk estimates reported in earlier studies [128]. More recently, no association between plasma IGF-1, IGFBP-1, or IGFBP-3 and breast cancer development was observed among premenopausal women in the Nurses' Health Study II [129]. Conflicting results have likewise been reported among postmenopausal women. A meta-regression analysis of four cohort studies and one case–control study reported no overall associations for IGF-1 or IGF-3 [66, 122]. Yet, more recently, a modest positive association for both IGF-1 and IGFBP-3 was reported among women who developed breast cancer after age 50 in the EPIC study [130], with odds ratios (OR) of 1.38 (95% CI: 1.02–1.86) and 1.44 (95% CI: 1.04–1.98) comparing the highest and lowest quartiles of IGF-1 and IGFBP-3, respectively. Similarly, a modest but nonlinear positive association with postmenopausal breast cancer risk was observed for free IGF-1, but not total IGF-1 in the Women's Health Initiative Observational Study (WHIOS) [46]. This association was independent of endogenous estradiol levels, but was no longer significant after adjusting for insulin.

In direct contrast to the positive association observed for other cancer sites, an inverse association between IGF-1 levels and endometrial cancer has been reported in several case–control studies [131, 132, 133, 134] and one prospective study [54]. It should be noted that the inverse association reported in the prospective study was significant only for free IGF-1, and not total IGF-1. Furthermore, the association was stronger in overweight/obese women, compared to leaner women [91]. The explanation for this seemingly paradoxical association is not known, although several hypotheses have been proposed [91]. Further studies will be required to better understand the complex interrelationships between insulin, IGF-1, and estrogens, and how these exposures combine to influence cancer risk.

2.3 Hyperglycemia

Given that hyperglycemia and hyperinsulinemia typically occur simultaneously and are both associated with excess body fat, it is difficult to distinguish their unique importance in promoting carcinogenesis. Nevertheless, high levels of blood glucose are associated with an increased risk of endometrial [135, 136] and pancreatic cancers [90], and with a modestly elevated colorectal cancer risk [90], though different glycemia markers and diverse conditions at blood drawing impede direct comparisons between studies. Comparing the highest to lowest categories of glycemia, overall RRs of 1.98 (95% CI: 1.67–2.35) for pancreatic cancer and of 1.18 (95% CI: 1.07–1.31) for colorectal cancer (similar in both men and women) were recently estimated in a meta-analysis of prospective studies using the available maximally adjusted risk ratios [90].

Findings with respect to hyperglycemia and breast cancer have been mixed [86, 89, 136, 137, 138, 139]. For example, baseline fasting glucose levels were positively associated with breast cancer incidence only among postmenopausal ($\geq$65 years) women in a large population-based cohort study of Austrian women (RR: 1.62, 95% CI:1.12–2.34, comparing fasting glucose levels $\geq$7.0 mmol/L to 2.2–4.1 mmol/L) [139], but among premenopausal (<49 years) women only in a large Swedish cohort (RR: 2.13, 95% CI:1.2–4.1, $p_{\text{trend}} = 0.002$ across extreme quartiles) [136]. Glucose levels showed no association with risk in women from the Women's Health Initiative clinical trials [86].

Hyperglycemia has also been positively associated with some less prevalent cancers in a few large prospective cohorts [93, 136, 139]. For instance, a particularly strong positive association between fasting blood glucose and the incidence of liver cancer was observed among Austrian men (HR 4.58; 95% CI: 1.81–11.62, comparing values $\geq$7 mmol/L to <5.2 mmol/L) [139] Significant positive associations have also been reported for urinary tract cancers [136], malignant melanoma [136], non-Hodgkin's lymphoma [139], and kidney [93] cancers in men, and for bladder cancer in women [139]. In virtually all of these cases, adjustment for BMI had little effect on the associations, suggesting they are at least to some degree independent of body mass.

2.4 Adipokines: Adiponectin

Adiponectin is a peptide hormone secreted by adipose tissue that is present in high concentrations in the circulation [140, 141]. Although its exact physiological role has not yet been fully elucidated, it is postulated to play a key role in regulating energy intake and expenditure [142] and has been implicated in glucose metabolism and insulin sensitivity [143, 144].

In direct contrast to other adipokines, circulating levels of adiponectin are inversely correlated with BMI and adipose tissue mass [145, 146], and down-regulated in overweight/obesity and in insulin-resistant states [140, 146, 147]. Adiponectin levels demonstrate a strong inverse association with visceral adipose tissue, and are negatively correlated with fasting insulin levels [148] and with the development of insulin resistance [149].

Adiponectin has not yet been extensively examined in large epidemiological studies of cancer development, but available evidence supports a significant inverse association for risk of multiple cancers [142]. Such an observation has been reported for both pre- and postmenopausal breast cancer in several [150, 151, 152, 153, 154, 155], but not all [137, 155] studies. A risk reduction of approximately 30% (RR: 0.73, 95% CI: 0.55–0.98; $p_{\text{trend}} = 0.08$) was observed among postmenopausal women in the highest compared to lowest quartile of adiponectin levels in a large (1,477 cases) nested case–control study within the Nurses' Health Study (NHS) and NHSII cohorts [155]; however, no association was seen in premenopausal women. Findings in a more recent, albeit smaller, Swedish sample of both pre- and postmenopausal women also observed a stronger association in postmenopausal women; however, significant heterogeneity was not detected [137]. Another study demonstrated an association between higher levels (above the median >15.5 μg/ml) of adiponectin and increased breast cancer survival in a cohort of breast cancer survivors (HR 0.39, CI 0.15–0.95; $p_{\text{trend}} = 0.04$) [68].

Findings from investigations of adiponectin and colorectal cancer remain contradictory. A nearly 60% risk reduction was reported in the highest compared to lowest quintile of circulating adiponectin levels (RR: 0.42, 95% CI: 0.23–0.78, $p_{\text{trend}} = 0.01$) in a nested case–control study selected from the 18,225 men in the Health Professionals Follow-up Study [156]. This magnitude of risk reduction was robust and only slightly diminished after adjustment for BMI and other established colorectal cancer risk factors (RR=0.50, 95% CI: 0.26–0.97; $p_{\text{trend}} = 0.08$). In contrast, no significant associations were observed among men or women in the Northern Sweden Health and Disease Cohort [157], or in a cohort of Norwegian men, despite a large number of cases in both studies [158].

Only limited evidence is available with respect to adiponectin and the risk of developing other cancers. Comparing the highest to the lowest quartile of adiponectin was associated with a significant reduction in endometrial cancer cases (RR=0.56, 95% CI: 0.36–0.86, $p_{\text{trend}} = 0.006$) in the EPIC study [159]. The inverse association was even stronger among postmenopausal women (RR top vs. bottom tertile =0.44, 95% CI: 0.28–0.69, $p_{\text{trend}} = 0.0003$), although menopausal status was not a significant effect modifier of the observed relationship. High adiponectin levels were also inversely associated with the incidence of pancreatic cancer in a cohort of Finnish male smokers [160], such that men in the highest vs. lowest quintile of adiponectin concentrations had a 35% risk reduction (OR: 0.65, 95% CI: 0.39, 1.07, $p_{\text{trend}} = 0.04$). A significant inverse association between adiponectin and prostate cancer, independent of BMI and other well-established risk factors has been reported in case–control studies [161, 162], but was not confirmed in a subsequent prospective cohort study [163]. Further studies to better understand the role of adiponectin in the development and progression of obesity-related cancers are warranted.

2.5 *Inflammation, Obesity, and Cancer*

Several studies suggest that obesity is a state of chronic low-grade inflammation that is characterized by increased cytokine production, increased levels of acute phase reactants, and activation of inflammatory signaling pathways [164]. Excess accumulation of fat stimulates production of chemotactic factors (e.g., monocyte chemoattractant protein-1) triggering infiltration of macrophages [165]. Studies have shown that macrophage infiltration is associated with higher body weight [166], and that weight loss leads to a reduction in both inflammatory markers and macrophage content [167, 166].

Increased production of inflammatory cytokines from adipose tissue results in alteration of physiological functions of adipose tissue such as increased tumor necrosis factor-α (TNF-α), which is considered to play a critical role in developing insulin resistance and type 2 diabetes [45, 168]. Inflammation is also a key feature of the precancerous state, as described below.

Inflammation has been implicated in the development of several types of cancer [41, 169]. A nonspecific marker of inflammation, serum C-reactive protein (CRP), has been shown to be a predictor of colon cancer risk [170, 171]. Adipose tissue secretes several pro-inflammatory cytokines, such as interleukin-1 (IL-1), interleulkin-6 (IL-6), TNF-α [172], which stimulate the release of C-reactive protein (CRP) from the liver; these biomarkers (TNF-α, and CRP) have been linked to cancer risk [173]. Evidence for cancer-preventive effects of nonsteroidal anti-inflammatory drugs (NSAIDs) in population studies further supports the role of inflammatory processes in cancer development [174], although not all studies have found a significant association [175, 176].

Pro-inflammatory biomarkers (e.g., CRP, IL-6, serum amyloid A (SAA), and TNF-α) are increased in individuals with excess adiposity with some studies observing stronger associations with direct measures of adiposity compared to indirect ones [180, 181]. Several reviews of intervention studies have also reported significant associations between weight loss, physical activity, and reductions in inflammatory markers [182, 183, 184].

The relationship between obesity and inflammation is thus recognized as one mechanism that may account for the increased cancer risk among overweight/obese individuals [185, 186]. The reduction in risk associated with weight loss may also be explained by a concomitant decrease in inflammatory markers [187, 188, 189, 190].

Inflammation is a complex mechanism involving multiple pathways with pleiotropic effects on diverse cells and tissue types [169, 191]. Below we discuss the role of inflammatory biomarkers, CRP, SAA, TNF-α, and IL-6, which are all elevated in the obese state, on cancer risk.

2.6 C-Reactive Protein

CRP is an acute phase protein produced predominantly in liver, stimulated by pro-inflammatory cytokines such as IL-6 and TNF-α [192, 193, 194]. Evidence from epidemiological and intervention studies suggest significant associations between CRP and body weight. CRP is known to be positively associated with BMI in cross-sectional data [179], with weight change in intervention studies [190], and with weight gain in longitudinal data [195].

In breast cancer, prospective case–control studies have identified that high-baseline CRP levels are associated with subsequent risk for breast cancer in one [197], but not other, studies [173, 196, 198, 199]. This study reported a statistically significant relationship between breast cancer and CRP after adjusting for BMI, suggesting the effect of CRP may be independent of body weight [197].

However, the interpretation of these studies is challenging due to heterogeneity of study design. It is possible that menopausal status, which is an established moderator of the relationship between obesity and breast cancer [200, 201, 202], may have confounded the finding. There are currently no case–control studies that examined the effect of CRP specifically on postmenopausal cancer risk [190], and additional studies are required to examine the effect of CRP on breast cancer risk by menopausal status.

Although evidence is conflicting with regard to CRP and colorectal cancer risk, some evidence points to CRP as a risk factor for colorectal cancer [203]. In a review of eight prospective cohort studies (1,159 colorectal cancer cases and 37,896 controls), a one unit change in log-transformed CRP was associated with a 12% increased risk for colorectal cancer (relative risk (RR) =1.12, 95% confidence interval (CI), 1.01–1.25 [204]). Another meta-analysis of 10 prospective studies derived a random effects estimate of 1.09 (95% CI: 0.98–1.21) for each natural log increase in CRP [196]. Of the studies included in these reviews, some reported significant relationship between CRP and colorectal cancer adjusting for BMI, indicating a potential independent effect of CRP on colorectal cancer risk [170, 205, 206].

One nested case–control study in a cohort of male smokers suggested that the relationship between CRP and colorectal cancer risk was stronger among lean individuals (OR 4.6 [1.9–10.7] highest vs. lowest serum CRP quartile, $p_{\text{trend}} = 0.01$) than in heavier individuals (OR 2.0 [0.9–4.6] highest vs. lowest serum CRP quartile, $p_{\text{trend}} = 0.43$) [170]. It is possible that other obesity-related risk factors (e.g., insulin resistance) are more prominent risk factors for colorectal cancer among individuals with excess weight compared with inflammation; however, this study was limited by virtue of only examining smokers. In contrast to this finding, the chemopreventive effect of aspirin on colorectal adenoma was found to be stronger among obese compared to lean individuals, suggesting a stronger role of inflammation among obese individuals than those with normal weight [207]. Due to limited number of studies, future studies are required to understand the moderating effects of obesity.

It is not clear whether systemic inflammation associated with obesity affects prostate cancer risk [208]. Three prospective case–control studies identified nonsignificant effects of elevated CRP on prostate cancer risk [209, 210, 211], while meta-analyses have consistently identified an inverse relationship between NSAID use and prostate cancer risk [212, 213, 214]. Some have suggested that local inflammation could be associated with the development of prostate cancer; however, further well-designed studies are required to fully elucidate the role of inflammation in this cancer [210].

2.7 Interleukin-6

IL-6, a pleotrophic cytokine produced in various tissues including adipose tissue, is regulated by hormones (glucocorticoids), insulin, and catecholamines [237]. It is estimated that approximately one third of IL-6 is produced from adipose tissue in healthy individuals [238]. Lifestyle intervention studies support the association between adipose tissue and IL-6 level. A 2-year randomized controlled trial of diet and physical activity in 120 overweight postmenopausal women resulted in a decrease in circulating concentrations of IL-6 and CRP [240]. Among obese women on very-low-calorie diets ranging from 6 to 10 weeks, a decrease in IL-6 mRNA has been reported in some [241, 242], but not all, studies [243]. In a 15-week combined diet and exercise intervention in both men and women, a decrease in IL-6 mRNA was observed [244].

Limited prospective studies have examined IL-6 as a predictor of cancers. In a meta-analysis of four studies, IL-6 had a nonsignificant effect on overall cancer risk [196], but a nested case–control study including 2,438 older adults found that a 1-unit increase in IL-6 on the natural log-scale was associated with increased incidence of overall cancer HR=1.13, 95% CI= 0.94–1.37 [173].

In studies of breast cancer, two prospective case–control studies have reported nonsignificant associations between IL-6 level and breast cancer risk [173, 196]. Although epidemiological studies do not support the relationship between IL-6 and breast cancer, studies have shown that IL-6 interferes with estrogen synthesis of peripheral tissues [245] by modifying aromatase expression, estradiol 17β-hydroxysteroid dehydrogenase and estrone sulfatase [245], insulin resistance, and CRP [246]. Thus, it is possible that IL-6 may indirectly affect breast cancer development via the sex steroid hormone pathway.

The observed relationship between IL-6 and prostate cancer risk is also inconsistent. In a study of 22,071 male US physicians, higher levels of IL-6 were associated with increased risk in healthy weight men, but with lower risk in overweight individuals [211]. Another prospective case–control study reported an inverse relationship between IL-6 and prostate cancer risk [196]. However, some case–control studies have reported an elevated IL-6 level in patients with advanced or androgen refractory prostate cancer [247, 248]. Some prostate cancer cell lines, especially androgen-independent cancer cells lines, develop a self-regulated proliferation cycle by producing IL-6 and expressing IL-6 receptor [249, 250, 251]. Therefore, IL-6 may also potentially be involved in the development and progression of prostate cancer.

2.8 Serum Amyloid A

Serum amyloid A (SAA) is another acute-phase protein produced in response to pro-inflammatory cytokines (e.g., IL-1, IL-6, TNF-α) [215, 216]. The adipocyte was identified as the primary site of SAA production during the nonacute inflammatory phase, and the liver, the second [217]. Studies have shown that serum SAA is significantly associated with indicators of adiposity (BMI, percentage body fat, and subcutaneous adipocyte diameter), weight loss (negatively), biomarkers of glucose metabolism and systemic inflammation [218, 219, 220]. Serum SAA level decreased in response to diet-induced weight loss, which was correlated with SAA mRNA expression at subcutaneous adipose tissue [217]. In addition, significant relationships were identified between SAA levels and potential factors linking obesity and cancer, including CRP, IL-6, leptin, insulin, HbA1c, and HOMA-IR, in a sample of adults with and without type 2 diabetes [219].

To the best of our knowledge, no prospective studies have examined SAA and subsequent cancer incidence. However, previous studies have assessed SAA as a marker to detect cancer and its progression. Researchers have identified elevated SAA levels in patients of gastric [221], lung [222, 223, 224], prostate [225], colorectal [226], kidney [227], and endometrial [228] cancers compared to nondiseased populations. Weinstein et al. [229] examined SAA level in 236 patients with 13 different types of cancer and identified that SAA levels were consistently higher in individuals with metastatic compared with limited cancer. Other studies also reported an association of SAA with tumor progression [221, 230, 231, 232, 233]. Expression of SAA was found to increase with progression from normal, dysplasia, and neoplasia of epithelium [234], which may explain elevated SAA levels in cancer patients, especially those in advanced stages of disease.

However, a recent study in disease-free breast cancer survivors identified that elevated SAA was associated with reduced overall and cancer-specific survival regardless of age, BMI, or tumor stage [235]. Significant positive associations between indicators of obesity and SAA level were identified from a separate analysis from this study [236].

Therefore, growing evidence suggests that SAA is associated with dyslipidemia, insulin tolerance, and stimulation of proinflammatory cytokines, and that SAA may have similar effects as IL-6 and TNF-α on stimulating lypolysis [220]. However, additional studies are still needed to elucidate the potential carcinogenic effects of SAA and the role of obesity in the relationship between SAA and cancer.

2.9 Sex Steroid Hormones

Chronic positive energy balance and obesity involve alteration of metabolic and endocrine functions [252]. Production and bioavailability of sex hormones are one of the physiological conditions influenced by obesity [40]. Adipose tissue is a primary location for estrogen synthesis in overweight/obese postmenopausal women and men [40], and the increased volume of adipose tissue associated with obesity increases serum levels of estrogens (i.e., estrone and estradiol) [253, 254, 255]. One proposed mechanism for the association between obesity and estrogen-related cancers, such as postmenopausal breast cancer, is via elevated levels of circulating estrogens from peripheral aromatization of androgens in adipose tissue, whereby estrogens are formed by the aromatization of androstenedione and testosterone via the action of aromatase [55, 256, 257]. In premenopausal women, obesity is associated with increased testosterone and decreased progesterone, which may increase the risk for breast and endometrial cancer [40]. In addition, insulin resistance, which is associated with obesity (as discussed elsewhere in this chapter), can suppress the hepatic synthesis of sex-hormone binding globulin (SHBG), resulting in increased bioavailability of estrogens and androgens [40].

There is convincing evidence from experimental and epidemiological studies suggesting that obesity-related alterations in sex hormones account for several cancers, as described below. The following sections will briefly discuss how obesity alters sex hormones, and summarize current epidemiological evidence supporting the role of obesity-associated changes in estrogens, progesterone, androgens, and SHBG on cancer risk; potential biological mechanisms that explain this increased risk are described later in this chapter.

2.9.1 Estrogens

Obesity alters serum estrogens both directly, by increasing its production, and indirectly, through altering other regulators of estrogen such as insulin and leptin [40, 55]. Adipose tissue is a primary location for estrogen synthesis in men and postmenopausal women [40]; thus, obesity increases serum levels of estrogens (estradiol and estrone) [253, 254, 255]. A 1-year randomized-controlled exercise intervention study has shown that circulating estrogens decreased significantly among exercisers who lost at least 0.5 % body fat. After 12 months, among the 26 exercisers who lost more than 2% body fat, concentrations of estradiol, free estradiol, and estrone decreased by 13.7, 16.7, and 11.8%, respectively, supporting the relationship between adiposity and estrogens [258]. In addition, high insulin levels are associated with obesity and increased estrogen synthesis [259]. A review of nine cross-sectional studies identified a higher serum estradiol level among individuals with type 2 diabetes in both men and postmenopausal women compared to controls which remained significant after matching on BMI [260].

In postmenopausal women, epidemiological studies support a strong link between high serum estrogens, obesity, and breast cancer risk [40]. Large prospective studies of postmenopausal women have consistently reported a significant effect of serum estrogens on postmenopausal breast cancer risk [261, 262, 263]. A combined analysis of nested case–control data from nine cohort studies (663 breast cancer cases and 1,765 controls) showed a positive association between elevated serum concentrations of estrogens or androgens and postmenopausal breast cancer risk [303]. Further analysis from this pooled data showed that the association between BMI and breast cancer risk could be attributed almost entirely to increasing serum concentrations of total or bioavailable estradiol with increasing BMI [254].

Because of variable estrogen levels during the menstrual cycle [264], few studies have examined the relationship between premenopausal breast cancer and estrogen. In the Nurses' Health Study II, total and free estradiol levels during the follicular phase were associated with premenopausal breast cancer risk [265]. Case–control studies have reported higher estradiol levels among premenopausal breast cancer patients compared with controls [266, 267]. Although high estrogen in premenopausal women may be associated with increased risk of breast cancer [268], the role of obesity and its interaction with estrogen on risk of premenopausal breast cancer is unclear. Studies suggest that central obesity and weight gain during adulthood are positively associated with risk of premenopausal breast cancer [269, 270]. However, other studies have shown that BMI is inversely associated with premenopausal cancer risk [201, 271]. The relationship between BMI and estrogens is also not consistent in premenopausal women. Higher BMI was associated with increased salivary estrogen levels throughout the menstrual cycle in premenopausal women [272, 273]. A study of 636 premenopausal women found a non-significant trend of lower estradiol levels among women with higher BMI categories ($p_{\text{trend}} = 0.055$) [274]. This study found that SHBG accounted for most of the variation of estradiol explained by BMI, suggesting that the observed trend may be confounded by SHBG. Another study found nonsignificant associations between SHBG-bounded estradiol and weight [275].

High estrogen levels, and the balance between estrogen and progesterone among postmenopausal and premenopausal women, were investigated as a primary mechanism of obesity-induced endometrial cancer [40, 84]. In a case–control study, estrogens (estradiol and estrone) were significantly associated with endometrial cancer risk in postmenopausal women [276, 277]. This association was attenuated, but remained significant, after adjusting for BMI. In a prospective case–control study of postmenopausal women (124 cases), the odds ratio (OR) for endometrial cancer in the highest quartile vs. lowest were 4.13 for estradiol and 3.67 for estrone, adjusting for BMI, use of oral contraceptives, and hormone replacement therapy [278]. In addition, other sex hormones such as androstenedione, testosterone, Dehydroepiandrosterone sulfate (DHEAS), and SHBG were significantly associated with the risk of endometrial cancer, with DHEAS and SHBG remaining significant after adjusting for estrogen levels. Another prospective case–control study of 247 endometrial cancer cases further supported the relationship between obesity, sex hormones, and cancer risk, by demonstrating a significantly increased risk of endometrial cancer associated with elevated levels of free estradiol (OR=1.66; 95% CI 0.98–2.82; $p_{\text{trend}} = 0.001$) and testosterone (OR = 2.05; 95% CI 1.23–3.42; $p_{\text{trend}} = 0.005$) in postmenopausal women. These hormones were positively associated with BMI, and adjusting for BMI attenuated the significant associations of these hormones with endometrial cancer [279].

Limited studies have examined effects of estrogen on endometrial cancer risk among premenopausal women; however, the unopposed estrogen hypothesis, i.e., estrogen without sufficient progesterone, is considered to be responsible for increased endometrial cancer risk [55]. Within the range of 20–30 kg/m^2, BMI has negligible effects on free estradiol and progesterone levels in premenopausal women [253]. However, with obesity (BMI $\geq$30 kg/m^2), there is an increase in anovulatory menstrual cycles resulting from low progesterone [280]. Anovulation cycles due to persisting progesterone deficiency is characteristic of polycystic ovary syndrome or infertile women, and both of these groups are at increased risk of developing endometrial cancer [281, 282].

Elevated estrogen levels were also found to be associated with cancers other than the reproductive organs. A recent case–control study identified an OR of 1.8 for the highest vs. lowest estrone quartile for colorectal cancer, which became non-significant after adjusting for BMI [283]. Another report from a subsample of the WHI-OS found that endogenous estradiol level was positively associated with risk of colorectal cancer (Hazard ratio (HR) comparing high vs. low levels, 1.53; 95% CI = 1.05–2.22) adjusting for waist circumference, insulin, and IGF-1, suggesting an independent effect of estradiol on colon cancer risk [54]. In vitro studies reporting estrogen-stimulated cell proliferation on colon cancer cells and 17β-hydroxysteroid dehydrogenase expression in colon support the hypothesis that estrogens may affect colon cancer risk [284].

Paradoxically, exogenous sex hormone therapy is associated with decreased risk for colorectal cancer. A meta-analysis of 18 studies have identified that hormone replacement therapy was associated with approximately 20% reduced risk for colon and rectal cancers [285]. The WHI, a randomized controlled primary prevention trial, also found decreased risk in women taking combination drug of estrogen and progesterone (HR=0.63 (95% CI 0.43–0.92) [286]). In studies of postmenopausal breast cancer, hormone replacement therapy was identified as a modifier of the relationship between obesity, weight gain, and breast cancer risk [287, 288], and future studies of endogenous hormones and cancer risk may benefit from assessing the effects of hormone replacement therapy.

2.9.2 Progesterone

Physiological roles of progesterone include breast development, stimulation of stromal regeneration in the endometrium, and maintenance of pregnancy [289]. Obesity has a threshold effect on progesterone produced from the ovary before menopause. For individuals who are obese (BMI$\geq$30 kg/m^2), there is an increase in anovulatory menstrual cycles resulting from low progesterone [280].

Progesterone levels were found to be inversely associated with the risk of breast cancer in some nested case–control studies of premenopausal women [290, 291], but not all [265]. Progesterone deficiency (e.g., polycystic ovary syndrome or infertile women) was found to be associated with a nonsignificant increase in incidence of breast cancer [281, 282]. As previously described, obesity can result in progesterone deficiency, which may partially account for the obesity-related breast cancer risk. However, it is possible that the identified inverse relationship between progesterone and breast cancer may be confounded by other risk factors (e.g., nullparity and lactation) [292, 293]. Additional studies are necessary to determine the mechanisms through which progesterone and obesity affect breast cancer risk. In postmenopausal women, conversely, progesterone administration increases breast cancer risk. In the Women's Health Initiative hormone therapy trials, women randomized to conjugated equine estrogen plus progesterone had a 26% increased risk of developing breast cancer over a mean 5.6 years vs. women randomized to placebo [294]. In contrast, women without a uterus randomized to conjugated equine estrogen did not show an increased risk of developing breast cancer compared with those randomized to placebo, after a mean 7.1 years follow-up [295].

2.9.3 Androgens

Androgens, which include testosterone and its metabolites, are responsible for developing the male phenotype and maintaining reproductive function [296]. Obesity affects androgen levels, but there are gender differences in the association between obesity and androgen levels. In women, excess adiposity is associated with increased bioavailable androgens [297, 298], and exercise and weight loss interventions accompanied with fat loss have reported reduced androgen levels [258]. In contrast, obesity is associated with decreased total testosterone and free testosterone in men [299]. Men who are extremely obese are at high risk for hypogonadotrophic hypogonadism and infertility due to low testosterone [299, 300, 301, 302].

Case–control studies nested within prospective cohort studies have shown that testosterone level is positively associated with risk for postmenopausal breast cancer [262, 303, 304]. In addition, breast cancer risk was associated with DHEAS, a precursor of androstenendione and testosterone [261, 262, 304]. Although these studies did not investigate the effects of BMI, other studies have shown a positive association between BMI and free testosterone in postmenopausal women; thus, obesity may have contributed to the observed associations between testosterone and postmenopausal breast cancer risk.

Testosterone has also been found to be associated with premenopausal breast cancer risk. Two nested case–control studies in cohorts of premenopausal women have shown elevated testosterone to be associated with increased risk of breast cancer [265, 290]. The latter study stratified the sample by BMI, but did not find any differences across BMI categories, suggesting that testosterone is a risk factor independent of BMI status [265]. However, given that obesity is negatively associated with risk for breast cancer in premenopausal women [306], it is not clear how testosterone and adiposity are interrelated in the etiology of premenopausal breast cancer.

High androgen level increases the risk for endometrial cancer. A case–control study from a prospective cohort study ($n = 500{,}000$) found that total (OR = 1.44, highest vs lowest tertile) and free (OR = 2.05) testosterone were significantly associated with risk [279]. Free testosterone remained significant after adjusting for BMI. Another case–control study from New York (USA), Umea (Sweden), and Milan (Italy) also reported ORs of 1.74 (95% CI 0.88–3.46) and 2.15 (95% CI 1.05–4.40) for testosterone and androstenedione, respectively, after adjusting for BMI and other factors [278]. These studies suggest free testosterone as an independent risk factor for endometrial cancer in postmenopausal women. However, these studies also reported significant findings for other sex hormones including estradiol, estrone, DHEAS, and testosterone. Whether testosterone is an independent risk factor for endometrial cancer requires further investigation [278].

Although androgens are found to be involved in development and progress of prostate cancer in animal experiments, these findings are not supported by epidemiological studies of circulating androgens and prostate cancer risk [307]. In a review of studies that examined blood testosterone level and risk of prostate cancer, none of the studies reported significant findings on the relationship between free testosterone and prostate cancer risk [307]. A nested case–control study from combined cohorts of three European countries also found no support for the relationship between blood androgen levels and prostate cancer risk [308].

One potential reason to explain these nonsignificant findings is that serum testosterone level does not reflect the actual exposure of the prostate to dihydrotestosterone (bioactive form of testosterone), as testosterone is locally converted to dihydrotestosterone at the epithelium of the prostate by 5α-reductase [309]. Focusing on the local production of sex hormones in the testis may fill the gap between experimental and epidemiological studies.

2.9.4 Sex Hormone-Binding Globulin

SHBG produced from hepatocytes regulates the bioavailability of sex hormones [310]. Most serum estradiol and testosterone are bound to SHBG or albumin, and the unbound fraction of these sex hormones (approximately 2%) can bind to steroid hormone receptors [253]. Obesity and its related conditions (e.g., high insulin level) decreases hepatic synthesis of SHBG [311]. In vitro studies have identified that insulin [312, 313] as well as IGF-1 [312, 313] inhibits SHBG synthesis in hepatocytes. A recent meta-analysis has shown that metformin (insulin sensitizer) treatment was associated with approximately six times increased SHBG level, indicating a role for insulin in SHBG production [314].

Decreased SHBG due to excess adiposity alters the levels of bioavailable sex hormones. Low SHBG is associated with increased bioavailable estradiol in both men and women [40]. In women, low SHBG results in high bioavailable testosterone [55, 255, 315, 316]. In contrast, in men, decreased SHBG levels have minimal effects on bioavailable testosterone [255, 307, 315].

A meta-analysis of nine prospective case control studies has shown that high SHBG is associated with reduced risk for postmenopausal breast cancer [303]. In another prospective case–control study of postmenopausal women, serum SHBG was inversely associated with breast cancer risk only among women using postmenopausal hormone for less than 60 months, and the association between SHBG and breast cancer risk did not change by controlling for BMI, suggesting an independent effect of SHBG on breast cancer risk [317].

Two prospective case–control studies in premenopausal women found no direct effect of SHBG on breast cancer [265, 290]. However, the latter study identified an inverse association of SHBG with BMI, testosterone, and androstenedione, which were significantly associated with the premenopausal breast cancer risk [290]. This study also identified a significant association between SHBG, estradiol, and BMI; however, estradiol was not associated with premenopasual breast cancer risk, suggesting that reduced SHBG in obese premenopausal women may affect cancer risk through altering bioavailable androgen levels, but not estrogens.

SHBG may also be associated with cancers outside of the reproductive system. In a case–control study nested within the New York University Women's Health Study, a nonsignificant inverse association was observed between SHBG and colorectal cancer risk, which disappeared after controlling for BMI [283]. Since obesity is associated with various risk factors for cancers (insulin, leptin, inflammation), additional studies are required to determine whether SHBG has an independent effect on colorectal cancer.

3 Proposed Mechanistic Pathway(s) Leading to Cancer

Efforts to understand the specific pathways through which insulin, adipokines, sex steroid hormones, and inflammation influence cancer risk is an area of active and ongoing research. The specific molecular pathways linking these pathways to malignancy are beyond the scope of this chapter; however, a basic overview is provided below.

3.1 Insulin and the IGF System

It is postulated that the tumorigenic effects of insulin could be attributable to its direct effect on insulin receptors (IR) in preneoplastic target cells or mediated through closely related changes in IGF and their binding proteins [119]. A recent paper examining severe insulin resistance and hyperinsulinemia in a non-obese diabetic mouse model showed accelerated mammary gland development and breast cancer progression independent of obesity and inflammation, which was mediated via insulin, insulin receptor/IGF-1 receptor, and the PI3K/Akt pathway [318], supporting the postulated tumor-promoting effect of elevated circulating insulin levels.

Both insulin and IGF-1 signal through tyrosine kinase receptors (IR and IGF-1R, respectively) and use docking proteins to mediate their signal [319]. Activation of signaling pathways downstream of these receptors, including the phosphatidylinositol 3-kinase(PI3)/ Akt and Ras/mitogen-activated protein kinase (MAPK) systems [320, 321], promote cellular proliferation and inhibit apoptosis [322, 323, 324, 325, 326, 327, 328], favoring carcinogenesis through the stepwise accumulation of genetic mutations. Further, it is probable that the neoplastic behavior of transformed cells is also directly stimulated by high insulin levels, leading to more rapid proliferation and worse outcomes [321]. An overexpression of IR, IGF-1R, and hybrid receptors has been demonstrated in various types of cancer cells and tissue specimens [323, 329, 330, 331, 332].

Insulin and IGF-1 also stimulate the synthesis of sex hormones and inhibit sex hormone-binding globulin (SHBG), linking them with a well-established tumor-promoting pathway [40, 55, 333]. Lowered SHBG alters circulating levels of both estrogens and androgens, including rises in bioavailable estradiol in both men and women [40], as discussed above. Furthermore, laboratory and human studies point to multiple levels of crosstalk between the two systems, and provide compelling evidence that estrogens and IGFs act synergistically in the pathogenesis of certain cancers [334, 335, 336].

A recent paper investigated the link between the IGF-1 system and inflammation in two mouse models, and demonstrated that basal expression levels of inflammatory cytokines and cell adhesion molecules were upregulated in obese mice, and this was dependent on hepatic IGF-I expression [337]. This study also reported that in control mice obesity-induced changes to the hepatic microenvironment sustained tumor cell growth and increased incidence of hepatic metastases after inoculation of colon carcinoma cells, but not in mice with chronic IGF-1 deficiency [337].

Low levels of IGFBP-3 have also been postulated to increase cancer risk through increases in bioactive IGF-1; however, circulating levels appear increased or unchanged by obesity [40]. In contrast to mouse models, where IGF-1 correlate strongly with increasing body weight, a plateau effect is seen in humans where the total IGF-1 levels increase concomitantly with body weight up to a BMI of approximately 27 kg/m^2; but decline beyond this [119]. Some in vitro evidence suggests that IGFBP-3 may have bidirectional effects on tumor activity and act to enhance the proliferative effects of IGF-1 under some conditions [114, 338]. More recently, overexpression of other IGFBPs, including IGFBP-2 and -5, has also been associated with increased IGF-1 action in particular contexts, and efforts to elucidate the pathways implicated in this process are an area of ongoing investigation [321].

3.2 Glucose

In theory, high glucose levels associated with overweight/obesity could increase the risk of cancer by conferring a selective growth advantage on malignant cells. Recent findings suggest that glucose may have a role in regulating concentrations of IGFBP-1 independently of insulin [113]. It has also been suggested that hyperglycemia may impair the intracellular actions of ascorbic acid and compromise immune function [339] In addition, glucose-related pathways including auto-oxidation, oxidative phosphorylation, glycosylation, and the glucosamine pathways induce the formation of reactive oxygen species (ROS) [340]. The overproduction of ROS is associated with inflammatory processes and mitochondrial dysfunction [340], and signals several pathways known to induce cell damage [339, 341].

Furthermore, evidence that hyperglycemia is associated with increased risk of cancer progression independent of insulin has recently been demonstrated in a diabetic mouse model [342], where hepatocarcinogenesis was chemically induced in the offspring of mice with a heterozygous germ line mutation causing insulin-deficiency mated with normal C3H/HeJ mice with high sensitivity to liver carcinogenesis. Both the mean and total volumes of subsequent hepatocellular tumors in the insulin-deficient offspring were more than twofold larger than those in the normal (non-diabetic) offspring and showed a significantly lower frequency of apoptosis. The implications of these findings for human malignancy will require further study.

3.3 Adiponectin

A number of mechanisms have been postulated to explain the relationship between adiponectin and carcinogenesis, including both direct and indirect effects.

Adiponectin has antidiabetic, anti-inflammatory, and anti-atherogenic actions including stimulation of glucose utilization, fatty-acid oxidation, and inhibition of gluconeogenesis [143, 144], through binding to its two receptors: AdipoR1 and AdipoR2 [143, 343]. Binding of adiponectin to AdipoR1 (located in skeletal muscle and liver) activates AMPK pathways, while the AdipoR2 (expressed predominantly in the liver) activates peroxisome proliferator-activated receptor α (PPARα) pathways [344].

Overexpression of adiponectin in dyslipidemic, hyperglycemic, and hyperinsulinemic leptin-deficient mice has been shown to rescue the diabetic phenotype and reduce systemic inflammation and macrophage infiltration in adipose tissue [144, 345, 346, 347]. The insulin-sensitizing effect of adiponectin appears to be mediated by an increase in fatty acid oxidation via activation of AMPK [348] and also by upregulation of PPARα [144]. Additional anti-inflammatory effects of adiponectin include reduction of phagocytic activity, reduction of TNF-α secretion from macrophages [349, 350], and suppression of TNF-α -induced inflammatory changes in endothelial cells via inhibition of nuclear factor (NF)-κB phosphorylation, known to be involved in the development of malignancy [351, 352, 353]. Adiponectin also has effects on cell proliferation and cytokine production [354], and experiments both in vitro and in animal models suggest an interaction between adiponectin and estrogen receptors [355, 356, 357, 358]. In humans, adiponectin has been associated with an increase in tyrosine phosphorylation of insulin receptors in skeletal muscle and improved whole-body insulin resistance [359]. A recent paper reports that disruption of AdipoR1 suppressed the adiponectin-mediated increase in intracellular Ca(2+) concentration, and decreased the activation of CaMKK, AMPK and SIRT1 by adiponectin, decreased mitochondrial content and enzymes, decreased oxidative type I myofibers, and decreased oxidative stress-detoxifying enzymes in skeletal muscle, which were associated with insulin resistance and decreased exercise endurance [360].

Using a transgenic mouse model expressing human adiponectin in macrophages, one study reported that adiponectin expression was associated with reduced whole-animal body and fat-pad weight and an improved lipid accumulation in macrophages after exposure to a high-fat diet. Furthermore, these mice exhibited enhanced whole-body glucose tolerance and insulin sensitivity with reduced proinflammatory cytokines, MCP-1 and TNF-α [361].

Finally, in addition to its insulin-sensitizing and anti-inflammatory effects, adiponectin may have direct effects at the local tissue level. These include the activation of the AMPK system, which serves to help regulate growth arrest and apoptosis

[362, 363], decreased production of reactive oxygen species (ROS) [364], and the inhibition of angiogenesis as well as proapoptotic effects through the activation of the caspase cascade [365].

3.4 Inflammation

Inflammatory cytokines interact with complex mechanisms with a number of overlaps in their functions. For this reason, the following section will briefly review the role of NF-κB in cancer (a transcriptional factor activated by many proinflammatory cytokines), inflammation affecting other cancer risk factors (insulin resistance), and specific moderation of tumor cells by inflammatory cytokines.

Inflammatory cytokines activate three major transcription factors, NF-κB, STAT1 and STAT3 [366], and the activation of NF-κB [169] is considered a major player linking inflammation and cancer. Many proinflammatory cytokines including TNF-α activate NF-κB [367, 368, 369], which regulates transcription of genes encoding inflammatory cytokines such as TNF- α, IL-6, and IL-1β [370]. Inhibiting NK-κB was shown to reduce inflammatory cytokines such as IL-6 and IL-1β and alleviate obesity-induced insulin resistance [370, 372].

Although inflammation is recognized as mainly interfering with tumor promotion and progression, some studies suggest that it plays a role in tumor initiation. Activation of NF-κB signaling pathway stimulates production of inducible nitric oxide synthase (iNOS) [373], which leads to DNA damage [374]. Macrophages present at the inflammation cite produce reactive oxygen and nitrogen species [375], and macrophage migration inhibitory factor produced from macrophage and T cells [376] suppresses the expression of tumor suppressor genes [377], which may result in impaired DNA repair and genomic instability.

Experimental studies have shown that the NF-κB signaling pathway contributes to cancer promotion and progression [378]. In a mouse model of colitis-associated cancer, blocking NF-κB activation in enterocytes was associated with decreased tumor incidence, supporting its role in tumor promotion [379]. Inhibition of NF-κB activation in myeloid cells using IkappaB kinase (IKκ)-beta ablation decreased size and number of colitis-associated cancers [379], while neutralizing serum IL-6 resulted in a similar inhibition of tumor progression [380]. The underlying mechanisms of NF-κB in tumor promotion and progression may include regulation of genes related to cell survival [367] and apoptosis [381].

In addition to these direct effects, inflammation modifies other risk factors for cancer. For instance, inflammation is considered to play a major role in insulin resistance [382], a major contributor for carcinogenesis [1]. (see section of insulin resistance). Activation of NF-κB by IL-6 leads to insulin resistance, and inhibition of IL-6 and its downstream target IKκ-β were found to improve insulin resistance in mice [370]. SAA was found to increase lipolysis in cultured adipose tissue and increase IL-6 production in endothelial cells [220].

Lastly, inflammatory cytokines have been found to have specific roles in some cancers. Increased expression IL-6 and aromatase activity in breast cancer tissue suggests induction of aromatase by IL-6 in [383]. For example, IL-6 was found to interfere with androgen receptor-mediated signaling, leading to androgen-independent growth of prostate cancer cells [384], and inhibition of IL-6 has been shown to increase sensitivity of androgen-independent prostate cancer cells to chemotherapeutic agents [385].

3.5 Sex Steroid Hormones

3.5.1 Estrogens

Obesity and its related conditions (e.g., systemic inflammation and insulin resistance) are associated with increased serum estrogens. Excess adipose tissue increases the major site of estrogen biosynthesis resulting in increased production [40]. Cytokines, such as IL-6 and TNFα, can stimulate aromatase activity [245, 386, 387], and leptin, a product of adipocytes, has been shown to stimulate estrogen production through the increase of aromatase expression and activity in adipose stromal cells [40]. One study demonstrated that chronic estrogen administration in ovariectomized rats downregulated resistin, leptin, and adiponectin, and was associated with reduced adiposity [388].

Elevated estrogens trigger various cellular signaling pathways hypothesized to be associated with cancer development and progression [389]. First, estrogens, via the direct activation of estrogen receptors, stimulates cell signaling pathways (e.g., MAPK, PI3K/Akt pathways) that lead to cell proliferation and inhibit apoptosis of breast cancer cell lines [390, 391, 392]. Increased cell cycle increases the possibility of DNA mutation and proliferation of abnormal cells [393]. Second, metabolites of estrogens (especially catechol estrogen-3,4-quinones) have carcinogenic effects due to their ability to initiate DNA mutations [186, 394, 395, 396]. Finally, estrogens are considered to promote carcinogenesis by moderating other factors. In endometrial tissue, estrogens stimulate local production of IGF-1, which in turn stimulates cell proliferation [40]. Although the precise mechanisms are yet to be determined, in vitro studies have shown that insulin stimulates ovarian production of sex hormones through activation of insulin receptors [259].

3.5.2 Progesterone

Progesterone is known to have opposing effects to estrogen, which are considered to reduce the risk for endometrial cancer. Progesterone stimulates expression of IGFBP-1 [397, 398], which counteracts IGF-1 in the endometrium [399]. Progesterone also stimulates local production of 17β-hydroxysteroid dehydrogenase and estrogen sulfotransferase, which coverts estradiol to less bioactive form and promotes its excretion [400, 401].

In contrast to endometrial cancer, it is hypothesized that progesterone has both positive and negative effects on breast cancer [402]. In vivo studies have reported that progesterone and activation of progesterone receptor promoted development of mammary cancer and carcinogen-induced tumorigenesis in rodent models [403, Kordon, 1993, p. 509, 404, 405, 406]. These in vivo findings are supported by increased breast cancer risk among users of combination therapy of estrogen and progesterone [286, 408, 409], while estrogen alone has lesser or no affect on risk [407]. However, as previously described, there is less support from epidemiological studies showing increased endogenous progesterone level as a risk factor for breast cancer. The precise mechanism requires further investigation.

3.5.3 Androgens

Androgens have similar effects as growth-stimulating substances such as IGF-1 and IL-6 [410], which is thought to account for the role of androgens in carcinogenesis. In vivo studies have shown that prolonged exposure to androgens can induce spontaneous and growth of chemically induced cancers [411, 412, 413, 414–416]. In breast cancer, high testosterone may stimulate breast cancer cells through direct binding to androgen receptors, promoting cell proliferation and indirectly by increasing testosterone available to produce estrogen [417].

3.5.4 Sex Steroid Hormone-Binding Globulin

Sex steroid hormone-binding globulin (SHBG) is involved with cancers through its control of androgen and estrogen bioavailability. However, there is also increasing evidence for a direct effect of SHBG on breast cancer. In ER-positive breast cancer cells, SHBG binds to SHBG-receptor, activates cyclic adenosine monophosphate, and inhibits estradiol-stimulated cell signals related to cell proliferation and apoptosis [418, 419, 420]. Because the ER-mediated pathway activated by estradiol is considered a primary mechanism to explain the anti-apoptotic effect of estradiol in breast cancer cells [421], the ability of SHBG to intervene on this pathway, may have a substantial effect on breast cancer cell growth.

4 Summary

Epidemiological evidence supports the pro-carcinogenic effects of alterations in the sex steroid hormone, inflammatory, and insulin/IGF pathways in the overweight/obese states. Further studies into the biochemical and cellular effects of these candidates will clarify downstream effects of obesity-induced alterations in these biomarkers. It is clear that the obesity–carcinogenesis link is complex and multifactorial, and further studies are needed to clarify mechanistic pathways involved in this process.

References

1 Renehan AG, Roberts DL et al (2008) Obesity and cancer: pathophysiological and biological mechanisms. Arch Physiol Biochem 114(1):71–83

2 WHO (2006) Definition and diagnosis of diabetes mellitus and intermediate hyperglycemia: report of a WHO/IDF consultation. WHO, Geneva

3 Calle EE, Rodriguez C et al (2005) Overweight, obesity, and mortality from cancer in a prospectively studied cohort of US adults. N Engl J Med 348:1625–1638
4 IARC Working Group on the Evaluation of Cancer-Preventive Agents (2002) Weight control and physical activity (IARC Handbooks of Cancer Prevention, vol 6). IARC, Lyon
5 Matthews DR, Hosker JP et al (1985) Homeostasis model assessment: insulin resistance and beta-cell function from fasting plasma glucose and insulin concentrations in man. Diabetologia 28(7):412–419
6 Roberts DL, Dive C et al (2010) Biological mechanisms linking obesity and cancer risk: new perspectives. Annu Rev Med 61:301–316
7 Goodpaster BH (2002) Measuring body fat distribution and content in humans. Curr Opin Clin Nutr Metab Care 5(5):481–487
8 Mazess RB, Barden HS et al (1990) Dual-energy x-ray absorptiometry for total-body and regional bone-mineral and soft-tissue composition. Am J Clin Nutr 51(6):1106–1112
9 Kuk JL, Church TS et al (2006) Does measurement site for visceral and abdominal subcutaneous adipose tissue alter associations with the metabolic syndrome? Diabetes Care 29(3):679–684
10 Pi-Sunyer FX (2000) Obesity: criteria and classification. Proc Nutr Soc 59(4):505–509
11 van der Kooy K, Seidell JC (1993) Techniques for the measurement of visceral fat: a practical guide. Int J Obes Relat Metab Disord 17(4):187–196
12 Eknoyan G (2008) Adolphe Quetelet (1796–1874)–the average man and indices of obesity. Nephrol Dial Transplant 23(1):47–51
13 Willet, W (ed) (1998) Nutritional epidemiology. Oxford University Press, New York, NY
14 Calle EE, Thun MJ et al (1999) Body-mass index and mortality in a prospective cohort of US adults. N Engl J Med 341(15):1097–1105
15 Freedman DM, Ron E et al (2006) Body mass index and all-cause mortality in a nationwide US cohort. Int J Obes (London) 30(5):822–829
16 Pischon T, Boeing H et al (2008) General and abdominal adiposity and risk of death in Europe. N Engl J Med 359(20):2105–2120
17 Joint World Health Organization/Food and Agriculture Organization Expert Consultation (2003) Diet, nutrition and the prevention of chronic diseases, WHO technical report series no.916. WHO, Generva
18 Pischon T, Nothlings U et al (2008) Obesity and cancer. Proc Nutr Soc 67(2): 128–145
19 World Health Organization (2000) Obesity: preventing and managing the global epidemic, Technical report series no.894. World Health Organization, Geneva
20 Expert Panel on the Identification Evaluation and Treatment of Overweight in Adults (1998) Clinical guidelines on the identification, evaluation, and treatment of overweight and obesity in adults: executive summary. Am J Clin Nutr 68(4):899–917
21 Deurenberg P, Weststrate JA et al (1991) Body mass index as a measure of body fatness: age- and sex-specific prediction formulas. Br J Nutr 65(2):105–114
22 Garrow JS, Webster J (1985) Quetelet's index (W/H2) as a measure of fatness. Int J Obes 9(2):147–153
23 Baumgartner RN, Heymsfield SB et al (1995) Human body composition and the epidemiology of chronic disease. Obes Res 3(1):73–95
24 Bouchard C, Bray GA et al (1990) Basic and clinical aspects of regional fat distribution. Am J Clin Nutr 52(5):946–950
25 Despres JP (2006) Is visceral obesity the cause of the metabolic syndrome? Ann Med 38(1):52–63
26 Janssen I, Katzmarzyk PT et al (2004) Waist circumference and not body mass index explains obesity-related health risk. Am J Clin Nutr 79(3):379–384
27 Janssen I, Katzmarzyk PT et al (2002) Body mass index, waist circumference, and health risk: evidence in support of current National Institutes of Health guidelines. Arch Intern Med 162(18):2074–2079

28 Despres JP, Moorjani S et al (1990) Regional distribution of body fat, plasma lipoproteins, and cardiovascular disease. Arteriosclerosis 10(4):497–511
29 Kuk JL, Katzmarzyk PT et al (2006) Visceral fat is an independent predictor of all-cause mortality in men. Obesity 14(2):336–341
30 Bjorntorp P (1992) Abdominal fat distribution and disease: an overview of epidemiological data. Ann Med 24(1):15–18
31 Lean ME, Han TS et al (1995) Waist circumference as a measure for indicating need for weight management. BMJ 311(6998):158–161
32 Wallace TM, Matthews DR (2002) The assessment of insulin resistance in man. Diabet Med 19(7):527–534
33 Muniyappa R, Lee S et al (2008) Current approaches for assessing insulin sensitivity and resistance in vivo: advantages, limitations, and appropriate usage. Am J Physiol Endocrinol Metab 294(1):E15–E26
34 Expert committee on the diagnosis and classification of diabetes mellitus (2003) Report of the expert committee on the diagnosis and classification of diabetes mellitus. Diabetes Care 26(Suppl 1):S5–S20
35 American Diabetes Association (2010) ADA executive summary: standards of medical care in diabetes. Diabetes Care 33:S4–S10
36 Katz A, Nambi SS et al (2000) Quantitative insulin sensitivity check index: a simple, accurate method for assessing insulin sensitivity in humans. J Clin Endocrinol Metab 85(7): 2402–2410
37 Mather KJ, Hunt AE et al (2001) Repeatability characteristics of simple indices of insulin resistance: implications for research applications. J Clin Endocrinol Metab 86(11): 5457–5464
38 Radikova Z (2003) Assessment of insulin sensitivity/resistance in epidemiological studies. Endocr Regul 37(3):189–194
39 WHO (2006). Obesity and overweight. WHO Fact Sheets Fact Sheet no. 311.
40 Calle E, Kaaks R (2004) Overweight, obesity and cancer: epidemiological evidence and proposed mechanisms. Nat Rev Cancer 4(8):579–591
41 Coussens LM, Werb Z (2002) Inflammation and cancer. Nature 420(6917):860–867
42 Despres JP, Lemieux S et al (1995) The insulin resistance-dyslipidemic syndrome: contribution of visceral obesity and therapeutic implications. Int J Obes Relat Metab Disord 19(Suppl 1):S76–S86
43 Fox CS, Massaro JM et al (2007) Abdominal visceral and subcutaneous adipose tissue compartments: association with metabolic risk factors in the Framingham Heart Study. Circulation 116(1):39–48
44 Reaven GM (1995) Pathophysiology of insulin resistance in human disease. Physiol Rev 75:473
45 van Kruijsdijk RC, van der Wall E et al (2009) Obesity and cancer: the role of dysfunctional adipose tissue. Cancer Epidemiol Biomarkers Prev 18(10):2569–2578
46 Gunter MJ, Hoover DR et al (2009) Insulin, insulin-like growth factor-I, and risk of breast cancer in postmenopausal women. J Natl Cancer Inst 101(1):48–60
47 Kaaks R (1996) Nutrition, hormones, and breast cancer: is insulin the missing link? Cancer Causes Control 7(6):605–625
48 Larsson SC, Mantzoros CS et al (2007) Diabetes mellitus and risk of breast cancer: a meta-analysis. Int J Cancer 121(4):856–862
49 Lawlor DA, Smith GD et al (2004) Hyperinsulinaemia and increased risk of breast cancer: findings from the British Women's Heart and Health Study. Cancer Causes Control 15(3):267–275
50 Stoll BA (1999) Western nutrition and the insulin resistance syndrome: a link to breast cancer. Eur J Clin Nutr 53(2):83–87
51 Weiderpass E, Gridley G et al (1997) Risk of endometrial and breast cancer in patients with diabetes mellitus. Int J Cancer 71(3):360–363

52 Wolf I, Sadetzki S et al (2005) Diabetes mellitus and breast cancer. Lancet Oncol 6(2): 103–111
53 Yang G, Lu G et al (2001) Population-based, case-control study of blood C-peptide level and breast cancer risk. Cancer Epidemiol Biomarkers Prev 10(11):1207–1211
54 Gunter MJ, Hoover DR et al (2008) A prospective evaluation of insulin and insulin-like growth factor-I as risk factors for endometrial cancer. Cancer Epidemiol Biomarkers Prev 17(4):921–929
55 Kaaks R, Lukanova A et al (2002) Obesity, endogenous hormones, and endometrial cancer risk: a synthetic review. Cancer Epidemiol Biomarkers Prev 11(12): 1531–1543
56 Lukanova A, Zeleniuch-Jacquotte A et al (2004) Prediagnostic levels of C-peptide, IGF-I, IGFBP -1, -2 and -3 and risk of endometrial cancer. Int J Cancer 108(2):262–268
57 Giovannucci E (1995) Insulin and colon cancer. Cancer Causes Control 6(2):164–179
58 Jenab M, Riboli E et al (2007) Serum C-peptide, IGFBP-1 and IGFBP-2 and risk of colon and rectal cancers in the European prospective investigation into cancer and nutrition. Int J Cancer 121(2):368–376
59 Ma J, Giovannucci E et al (2004) A prospective study of plasma C-peptide and colorectal cancer risk in men. J Natl Cancer Inst 96(7):546–553
60 McKeown-Eyssen G (1994) Epidemiology of colorectal cancer revisited: are serum triglycerides and/or plasma glucose associated with risk? Cancer Epidemiol Biomarkers Prev 3(8):687–695
61 Wei EK, Ma J et al (2005) A prospective study of C-peptide, insulin-like growth factor-I, insulin-like growth factor binding protein-1, and the risk of colorectal cancer in women. Cancer Epidemiol Biomarkers Prev 14(4):850–855
62 Weiderpass E, Partanen T et al (1998) Occurrence, trends and environment etiology of pancreatic cancer. Scand J Work Environ Health 24(3):165–174
63 Albanes D, Weinstein SJ et al (2009) Serum Insulin, Glucose, Indices of Insulin Resistance, and Risk of Prostate Cancer. J Natl Cancer Inst 101(18):1272–1279
64 Hsing AW, Gao YT et al (2003) Insulin resistance and prostate cancer risk. J Natl Cancer Inst 95(1):67–71
65 Stocks T, Lukanova A et al (2007) Insulin resistance is inversely related to prostate cancer: a prospective study in Northern Sweden. Int J Cancer 120(12):2678–2686
66 Renehan AG, Zwahlen M et al (2004) Insulin-like growth factor (IGF)-I, IGF binding protein-3, and cancer risk: systematic review and meta-regression analysis. Lancet 363(9418): 1346–1353
67 Colangelo LA, Gapstur SM et al (2002) Colorectal cancer mortality and factors related to the insulin resistance syndrome. Cancer Epidemiol Biomarkers Prev 11(4):385–391
68 Duggan C, Irwin ML et al (2010) Associations of insulin resistance and adiponectin with mortality in women with breast cancer. J Clin Oncol (in press)
69 Goodwin PJ, Ennis M et al (2002) Fasting insulin and outcome in early-stage breast cancer: results of a prospective cohort study. J Clin Oncol 20(1):42–51
70 Amling CL, Riffenburgh RH et al (2004) Pathologic variables and recurrence rates as related to obesity and race in men with prostate cancer undergoing radical prostatectomy. J Clin Oncol 22(3):439–445
71 Gapstur SM, Gann PH et al (2000) Abnormal glucose metabolism and pancreatic cancer mortality. JAMA 283(19):2552–2558
72 Ryan AM, Healy LA et al (2008) Barrett esophagus: prevalence of central adiposity, metabolic syndrome, and a proinflammatory state. Ann Surg 247(6):909–915
73 Siegel AB, Zhu AX (2009) Metabolic syndrome and hepatocellular carcinoma: two growing epidemics with a potential link. Cancer 115(24):5651–5661
74 Grundy SM, Brewer HB Jr et al (2004) Definition of metabolic syndrome: report of the National Heart, Lung, and Blood Institute/American Heart Association conference on scientific issues related to definition. Circulation 109(3):433–438

75 Reaven GM (1988) Banting lecture 1988: role of insulin resistance in human disease. Diabetes 37:1595
76 Larsson SC, Orsini N et al (2005) Diabetes mellitus and risk of colorectal cancer: a meta-analysis. J Natl Cancer Inst 97(22):1679–1687
77 Friberg E, Orsini N et al (2007) Diabetes mellitus and risk of endometrial cancer: a meta-analysis. Diabetologia 50(7):1365–1374
78 Michels KB, Solomon CG et al (2003) Type 2 diabetes and subsequent incidence of breast cancer in the Nurses' Health Study. Diabetes Care 26(6):1752–1758
79 Mink PJ, Shahar E et al (2002) Serum insulin and glucose levels and breast cancer incidence: the atherosclerosis risk in communities study. Am J Epidemiol 156(4):349–352
80 Huxley R, Ansary-Moghaddam A et al (2005) Type-II diabetes and pancreatic cancer: a meta-analysis of 36 studies. Br J Cancer 92(11):2076–2083
81 Chuang SC, Vecchia CL et al (2008) Liver cancer: descriptive epidemiology and risk factors other than HBV and HCV infection. Cancer Lett 286(1):9–14
82 Donadon V, Balbi M et al (2008) Association between hepatocellular carcinoma and type 2 diabetes mellitus in Italy: potential role of insulin. World J Gastroenterol 14(37): 5695–5700
83 Mori M, Saitoh S et al (2000) A review of cohort studies on the association between history of diabetes mellitus and occurrence of cancer. Asian Pac J Cancer Prev 1(4):269–276
84 Coughlin SS, Calle EE et al (2004) Diabetes mellitus as a predictor of cancer mortality in a large cohort of US adults. Am J Epidemiol 159(12):1160–1167
85 Del Giudice ME, Fantus IG et al (1998) Insulin and related factors in premenopausal breast cancer risk. Breast Cancer Res Treat 47(2):111–120
86 Kabat GC, Kim M et al (2009) Repeated measures of serum glucose and insulin in relation to postmenopausal breast cancer. Int J Cancer 125(11):2704–2710
87 Verheus M, Peeters PH et al (2006) Serum C-peptide levels and breast cancer risk: results from the European Prospective Investigation into Cancer and Nutrition (EPIC). Int J Cancer 119(3):659–667
88 Eliassen AH, Tworoger SS et al (2007) Circulating insulin and c-peptide levels and risk of breast cancer among predominately premenopausal women. Cancer Epidemiol Biomarkers Prev 16(1):161–164
89 Muti P, Quattrin T et al (2002) Fasting glucose is a risk factor for breast cancer: a prospective study. Cancer Epidemiol Biomarkers Prev 11(11):1361–1368
90 Pisani P (2008) Hyper-insulinaemia and cancer, meta-analyses of epidemiological studies. Arch Physiol Biochem 114(1):63–70
91 Gunter MJ, Hoover DR et al (2008) Insulin, insulin-like growth factor-I, endogenous estradiol, and risk of colorectal cancer in postmenopausal women. Cancer Res 68(1): 329–337
92 Cust AE, Allen NE et al (2007) Serum levels of C-peptide, IGFBP-1 and IGFBP-2 and endometrial cancer risk; results from the European prospective investigation into cancer and nutrition. Int J Cancer 120(12):2656–2664
93 Jee SH, Ohrr H et al (2005) Fasting serum glucose level and cancer risk in Korean men and women. JAMA 293(2):194–202
94 Stolzenberg-Solomon RZ, Graubard BI et al (2005) Insulin, glucose, insulin resistance, and pancreatic cancer in male smokers. JAMA 294(22):2872–2878
95 Borugian MJ, Spinelli JJ et al (2007) Prediagnostic C-peptide and risk of prostate cancer. Cancer Epidemiol Biomarkers Prev 16(10):2164–5
96 Chen C, Lewis SK et al (2005) Prostate carcinoma incidence in relation to prediagnostic circulating levels of insulin-like growth factor I, insulin-like growth factor binding protein 3, and insulin. Cancer 103(1):76–84
97 Hubbard JS, Rohrmann S et al (2004) Association of prostate cancer risk with insulin, glucose, and anthropometry in the Baltimore longitudinal study of aging. Urology 63(2): 253–258

98 Stattin P, Bylund A et al (2000) Plasma insulin-like growth factor-I, insulin-like growth factor-binding proteins, and prostate cancer risk: a prospective study. J Natl Cancer Inst 92(23):1910–1917
99 Ma J, Li H et al (2008) Prediagnostic body-mass index, plasma C-peptide concentration, and prostate cancer-specific mortality in men with prostate cancer: a long-term survival analysis. Lancet Oncol 9(11):1039–1047
100 Currie CJ, Poole CD et al (2009) The influence of glucose-lowering therapies on cancer risk in type 2 diabetes. Diabetologia 52(9):1766–1777
101 Evans JM, Donnelly LA et al (2005) Metformin and reduced risk of cancer in diabetic patients. BMJ 330(7503):1304–5
102 Li D, Yeung SC et al. ((2009)) Antidiabetic therapies affect risk of pancreatic cancer. Gastroenterology 137(2):482–488
103 Libby G, Donnelly LA et al (2009) New users of metformin are at low risk of incident cancer: a cohort study among people with type 2 diabetes. Diabetes Care 32(9):1620–1625
104 Wright JL, Stanford JL (2009) Metformin use and prostate cancer in Caucasian men: results from a population-based case-control study. Cancer Causes Control 20(9):1617–1622
105 Zhou G, Myers R et al (2001) Role of AMP-activated protein kinase in mechanism of metformin action. J Clin Invest 108(8):1167–1174
106 Zakikhani M, Dowling R et al (2006) Metformin is an AMP kinase-dependent growth inhibitor for breast cancer cells. Cancer Res 66(21):10269–10273
107 Hirsch HA, Iliopoulos D et al (2009) Metformin selectively targets cancer stem cells, and acts together with chemotherapy to block tumor growth and prolong remission. Cancer Res 69(19):7507–7511
108 Kisfalvi K, Eibl G et al (2009) Metformin disrupts crosstalk between G protein-coupled receptor and insulin receptor signaling systems and inhibits pancreatic cancer growth. Cancer Res 69(16):6539–6545
109 Jiralerspong S, Palla SL et al (2009) Metformin and pathologic complete responses to neoadjuvant chemotherapy in diabetic patients with breast cancer. J Clin Oncol 27(20): 3297–3302
110 Jones JI, Clemmons DR (1995) Insulin-like growth factors and their binding proteins: biological actions. Endocr Rev 16(1):3–34
111 Yakar S, Wu Y et al (2002) The role of circulating IGF-I: lessons from human and animal models. Endocrine 19(3):239–248
112 Villafuerte BC, Fine JB et al (2000) Expressions of leptin and insulin-like growth factor-I are highly correlated and region-specific in adipose tissue of growing rats. Obes Res 8(9): 646–655
113 Arafat AM, Weickert MO et al (2009) The role of insulin-like growth factor (IGF) binding Protein-2 in the Insulin-Mediated decrease in IGF-I bioactivity. J Clin Endocrinol Metab 94(12):5093–5101
114 Firth SM, Baxter RC (2002) Cellular actions of the insulin-like growth factor binding proteins. Endocr Rev 23(6):824–854
115 Pollak M (2007) Insulin, insulin-like growth factors, insulin resistance, and neoplasia. Am J Clin Nutr 86(Suppl):820S–822S
116 Chapman IM, Hartman ML et al (1998) Recovery of growth hormone release from suppression by exogenous insulin-like growth factor I (IGF-I): evidence for a suppressive action of free rather than bound IGF-I. J Clin Endocrinol Metab 83(8):2836–2842
117 Hartman ML, Clayton PE et al (1993) A low dose euglycemic infusion of recombinant human insulin-like growth factor I rapidly suppresses fasting-enhanced pulsatile growth hormone secretion in humans. J Clin Invest 91(6):2453–2462
118 Kaaks R, Lukanova A (2001) Energy balance and cancer: the role of insulin and insulin-like growth factor-I. Proc Nutr Soc 60(1):91–106
119 Renehan AG, Frystyk J et al (2006) Obesity and cancer risk: the role of the insulin-IGF axis. Trends Endocrinol Metab 17(8):328–336

120 Roddam AW, Allen NE et al (2008) Insulin-like growth factors, their binding proteins, and prostate cancer risk: analysis of individual patient data from 12 prospective studies. Ann Intern Med 149(7):461–471, W83–88
121 Rowlands MA, Gunnell D et al (2009) Circulating insulin-like growth factor peptides and prostate cancer risk: a systematic review and meta-analysis. Int J Cancer 124(10):2416–2429
122 Renehan AG, Egger M et al (2005) IGF-I, IGF binding protein-3 and breast cancer risk: comparison of 3 meta-analyses. Int J Cancer 115(6):1006–1007 author reply 1008
123 Shi R, Yu H et al (2004) IGF-I and breast cancer: a meta-analysis. Int J Cancer 111(3): 418–423
124 Wolpin BM, Michaud DS et al (2007) Circulating insulin-like growth factor axis and the risk of pancreatic cancer in four prospective cohorts. Br J Cancer 97(1):98–104
125 Wolpin BM, Michaud DS et al (2007) Circulating insulin-like growth factor binding protein-1 and the risk of pancreatic cancer. Cancer Res 67(16):7923–7928
126 Siahpush SH, Vaughan TL et al (2007) Longitudinal study of insulin-like growth factor, insulin-like growth factor binding protein-3, and their polymorphisms: risk of neoplastic progression in Barrett's esophagus. Cancer Epidemiol Biomarkers Prev 16(11): 2387–2395
127 Sohda M, Kato H et al (2004) The role of insulin-like growth factor 1 and insulin-like growth factor binding protein 3 in human esophageal cancer. Anticancer Res 24(5A):3029–3034
128 Renehan AG, Harvie M et al (2006) Insulin-like growth factor (IGF)-I, IGF binding protein-3, and breast cancer risk: eight years on. Endocr Relat Cancer 13(2):273–278
129 Schernhammer ES, Holly JM et al (2006) Insulin-like growth factor-I, its binding proteins (IGFBP-1 and IGFBP-3), and growth hormone and breast cancer risk in The Nurses Health Study II. Endocr Relat Cancer 13(2):583–592
130 Rinaldi S, Peeters PH et al (2006) IGF-I, IGFBP-3 and breast cancer risk in women: the European prospective investigation into cancer and nutrition (EPIC). Endocr Relat Cancer 13(2):593–605
131 Augustin LS, Dal Maso L et al (2004) Association between components of the insulin-like growth factor system and endometrial cancer risk. Oncology 67(1):54–59
132 Lacey JV Jr, Potischman N et al (2004) Insulin-like growth factors, insulin-like growth factor-binding proteins, and endometrial cancer in postmenopausal women: results from a U.S. case-control study. Cancer Epidemiol Biomarkers Prev 13(4):607–612
133 Oh JC, Wu W et al (2004) Increased plasma levels of insulin-like growth factor 2 and insulin-like growth factor binding protein 3 are associated with endometrial cancer risk. Cancer Epidemiol Biomarkers Prev 13(5):748–752
134 Petridou E, Koukoulomatis P et al (2003) Endometrial cancer and the IGF system: a case-control study in Greece. Oncology 64(4):341–345
135 Cust AE, Kaaks R et al (2007) Plasma adiponectin levels and endometrial cancer risk in pre- and postmenopausal women. J Clin Endocrinol Metab 92(1):255–263
136 Stattin P, Bjor O et al (2007) Prospective study of hyperglycemia and cancer risk. Diabetes Care 30(3):561–567
137 Cust AE, Stocks T et al (2009) The influence of overweight and insulin resistance on breast cancer risk and tumour stage at diagnosis: a prospective study. Breast Cancer Res Treat 113(3):567–576
138 Kabat GC, Kim M et al (2009) A longitudinal study of the metabolic syndrome and risk of postmenopausal breast cancer. Cancer Epidemiol Biomarkers Prev 18(7):2046–2053
139 Rapp K, Schroeder J et al (2006) Fasting blood glucose and cancer risk in a cohort of more than 140,000 adults in Austria. Diabetologia 49(5):945–952
140 Arita Y, Kihara S et al (1999) Paradoxical decrease of an adipose-specific protein, adiponectin, in obesity. Biochem Biophys Res Commun 257(1):79–83
141 Maeda K, Okubo K et al (1996) cDNA cloning and expression of a novel adipose specific collagen-like factor, apM1 (AdiPose Most abundant Gene transcript 1). Biochem Biophys Res Commun 221(2):286–289

142 Barb D, Williams CJ et al (2007) Adiponectin in relation to malignancies: a review of existing basic research and clinical evidence. Am J Clin Nutr 86(3):s858–s866
143 Kadowaki T, Yamauchi T et al (2006) Adiponectin and adiponectin receptors in insulin resistance, diabetes, and the metabolic syndrome. J Clin Invest 116(7):1784–1792
144 Yamauchi T, Kamon J et al (2003) Globular adiponectin protected ob/ob mice from diabetes and ApoE-deficient mice from atherosclerosis. J Biol Chem 278(4):2461–2468
145 Ryan AS, Nicklas BJ et al (2003) Adiponectin levels do not change with moderate dietary induced weight loss and exercise in obese postmenopausal women. Int J Obes Relat Metab Disord 27(9):1066–1071
146 Weyer C, Funahashi T et al (2001) Hypoadiponectinemia in obesity and type 2 diabetes: close association with insulin resistance and hyperinsulinemia. J Clin Endocrinol Metab 86(5):1930–1935
147 Chandran M, Phillips SA et al (2003) Adiponectin: more than just another fat cell hormone? Diabetes Care 26(8):2442–2450
148 Hotta K, Funahashi T et al (2000) Plasma concentrations of a novel, adipose-specific protein, adiponectin, in type 2 diabetic patients. Arterioscler Thromb Vasc Biol 20(6): 1595–1599
149 Yamamoto Y, Hirose H et al (2004) Adiponectin, an adipocyte-derived protein, predicts future insulin resistance: two-year follow-up study in Japanese population. J Clin Endocrinol Metab 89(1):87–90
150 Chen DC, Chung YF et al (2006) Serum adiponectin and leptin levels in Taiwanese breast cancer patients. Cancer Lett 237(1):109–114
151 Korner A, Pazaitou-Panayiotou K et al (2007) Total and high-molecular-weight adiponectin in breast cancer: in vitro and in vivo studies. J Clin Endocrinol Metab 92(3):1041–1048
152 Mantzoros C, Petridou E et al (2004) Adiponectin and breast cancer risk. J Clin Endocrinol Metab 89(3):1102–1107
153 Miyoshi Y, Funahashi T et al (2003) Association of serum adiponectin levels with breast cancer risk. Clin Cancer Res 9(15):5699–5704
154 Tian YF, Chu CH et al (2007) Anthropometric measures, plasma adiponectin, and breast cancer risk. Endocr Relat Cancer 14(3):669–677
155 Tworoger SS, Eliassen AH et al (2007) Plasma adiponectin concentrations and risk of incident breast cancer. J Clin Endocrinol Metab 92(4):1510–1516
156 Wei EK, Giovannucci E et al (2005) Low plasma adiponectin levels and risk of colorectal cancer in men: a prospective study. J Natl Cancer Inst 97(22):1688–1694
157 Stocks T, Lukanova A et al (2008) Components of the metabolic syndrome and colorectal cancer risk; a prospective study. Int J Obes 32(2):304–314
158 Lukanova A, Soderberg S et al (2006) Serum adiponectin is not associated with risk of colorectal cancer. Cancer Epidemiol Biomarkers Prev 15(2):401–402
159 Cust AE, Kaaks R et al (2007) Metabolic syndrome, plasma lipid, lipoprotein and glucose levels, and endometrial cancer risk in the European Prospective Investigation into Cancer and Nutrition (EPIC). Endocr Relat Cancer 14(3):755–767
160 Stolzenberg-Solomon RZ, Weinstein S et al (2008) Prediagnostic adiponectin concentrations and pancreatic cancer risk in male smokers. Am J Epidemiol 168(9):1047–1055
161 Goktas S, Yilmaz MI et al (2005) Prostate cancer and adiponectin. Urology 65(6):1168–1172
162 Michalakis K, Williams CJ et al (2007) Serum adiponectin concentrations and tissue expression of adiponectin receptors are reduced in patients with prostate cancer: a case control study. Cancer Epidemiol Biomarkers Prev 16(2):308–313
163 Baillargeon J, Platz EA et al (2006) Obesity, adipokines, and prostate cancer in a prospective population-based study. Cancer Epidemiol Biomarkers Prev 15(7):1331–1335
164 Wellen KE, Hotamisligil GS (2005) Inflammation, stress, and diabetes. J Clin Invest 115(5):1111–1119
165 Xu H, Barnes GT et al (2003) Chronic inflammation in fat plays a crucial role in the development of obesity-related insulin resistance. J Clin Invest 112(12):1821–1830

166 Weisberg SP, McCann D et al (2003) Obesity is associated with macrophage accumulation in adipose tissue. J Clin Invest 112(12):1796–1808
167 Cancello R, Henegar C et al (2005) Reduction of macrophage infiltration and chemoattractant gene expression changes in white adipose tissue of morbidly obese subjects after surgery-induced weight loss. Diabetes 54(8):2277–2286
168 Hotamisligil GS, Arner P et al (1995) Increased adipose tissue expression of tumor necrosis factor-alpha in human obesity and insulin resistance. J Clin Invest 95(5):2409–2415
169 Balkwill F, Coussens LM (2004) Cancer: an inflammatory link. Nature 431(7007):405–406
170 Gunter MJ, Stolzenberg-Solomon R et al (2006) A prospective study of serum C-reactive protein and colorectal cancer risk in men. Cancer Res 66(4):2483–2487
171 Helzlsouer KJ, Erlinger TP et al (2006) C-reactive protein levels and subsequent cancer outcomes: results from a prospective cohort study. Eur J Cancer 42(6):704–707
172 Tilg H, Moschen AR (2006) Adipocytokines: mediators linking adipose tissue, inflammation and immunity. Nat Rev Immunol 6(10):772–783
173 Il'yasova D, Colbert LH et al (2005) Circulating levels of inflammatory markers and cancer risk in the health aging and body composition cohort. Cancer Epidemiol Biomarkers Prev 14(10):2413–2418
174 Ulrich CM, Bigler J et al (2006) Non-steroidal anti-inflammatory drugs for cancer prevention: promise, perils and pharmacogenetics. Nat Rev Cancer 6(2):130–140
175 Cuzick J, Otto F et al (2009) Aspirin and non-steroidal anti-inflammatory drugs for cancer prevention: an international consensus statement. Lancet Oncol 10(5):501–507
176 Harris R, Chlebowski R et al (2003) Breast cancer and nonsteroidal anti-inflammatory drugs: prospective results from the Women's Health Initiative. Cancer Research 63:6096–6101
177 Das UN (2001) Is obesity an inflammatory condition? Nutrition 17(11–12):953–966
178 Park HS, Park JY et al (2005) Relationship of obesity and visceral adiposity with serum concentrations of CRP, TNF-alpha and IL-6. Diabetes Res Clin Pract 69(1):29–35
179 Visser M, Bouter LM et al (1999) Elevated C-reactive protein levels in overweight and obese adults. JAMA 282(22):2131–2135
180 Belza A, Toubro S et al (2009) Effect of diet-induced energy deficit and body fat reduction on high-sensitive CRP and other inflammatory markers in obese subjects. Int J Obes (London) 33(4):456–464
181 Campbell KL, Campbell PT et al (2008) No reduction in C-reactive protein following a 12-month randomized controlled trial of exercise in men and women. Cancer Epidemiol Biomarkers Prev 17(7):1714–1718
182 Forsythe LK, Wallace JM et al (2008) Obesity and inflammation: the effects of weight loss. Nutr Res Rev 21(2):117–133
183 Nicklas BJ, You T et al (2005) Behavioural treatments for chronic systemic inflammation: effects of dietary weight loss and exercise training. CMAJ 172(9):1199–1209
184 Selvin E, Paynter NP et al (2007) The effect of weight loss on C-reactive protein: a systematic review. Arch Intern Med 167(1):31–39
185 McTiernan A (2005) Obesity and cancer: the risks, science, and potential management strategies. Oncology (Williston Park) 19(7):871–881 discussion 881–882, 885–886
186 Roberts DL, Dive C et al (2009) Biological mechanisms linking obesity and cancer risk: new perspectives. Annu Rev Med 61:301–316
187 Campbell KL, McTiernan A (2007) Exercise and biomarkers for cancer prevention studies. J Nutr 137(1 Suppl):161S–169S
188 Fair AM, Montgomery K (2009) Energy balance, physical activity, and cancer risk. Methods Mol Biol 472:57–88
189 McTiernan A (2008) Mechanisms linking physical activity with cancer. Nat Rev Cancer 8(3):205–211
190 Neilson HK, Friedenreich CM et al (2009) Physical activity and postmenopausal breast cancer: proposed biologic mechanisms and areas for future research. Cancer Epidemiol Biomarkers Prev 18(1):11–27

191 Lin WW, Karin M (2007) A cytokine-mediated link between innate immunity, inflammation, and cancer. J Clin Invest 117(5):1175–1183
192 Bataille R, Klein B (1992) C-reactive protein levels as a direct indicator of interleukin-6 levels in humans in vivo. Arthritis Rheum 35(8):982–984
193 Heinrich PC, Castell JV et al (1990) Interleukin-6 and the acute phase response. Biochem J 265(3):621–636
194 Pepys MB, Hirschfield GM (2003) C-reactive protein: a critical update. J Clin Invest 111(12):1805–1812
195 Fogarty AW, Glancy C et al (2008) A prospective study of weight change and systemic inflammation over 9 y. Am J Clin Nutr 87(1):30–35
196 Heikkila K, Harris R et al (2009) Associations of circulating C-reactive protein and interleukin-6 with cancer risk: findings from two prospective cohorts and a meta-analysis. Cancer Causes Control 20(1):15–26
197 Siemes C, Visser LE et al (2006) C-reactive protein levels, variation in the C-reactive protein gene, and cancer risk: the Rotterdam Study. J Clin Oncol 24(33):5216–5222
198 Allin KH, Bojesen SE et al (2009) Baseline C-reactive protein is associated with incident cancer and survival in patients with cancer. J Clin Oncol 27(13):2217–2224
199 Zhang SM, Lin J et al (2007) C-reactive protein and risk of breast cancer. J Natl Cancer Inst 99(11):890–894
200 Carmichael AR, Bates T (2004) Obesity and breast cancer: a review of the literature. Breast 13(2):85–92
201 Cleary MP, Maihle NJ (1997) The role of body mass index in the relative risk of developing premenopausal versus postmenopausal breast cancer. Proc Soc Exp Biol Med 216(1):28–43
202 Franceschi S, Favero A et al (1996) Body size indices and breast cancer risk before and after menopause. Int J Cancer 67(2):181–186
203 Heikkila K, Ebrahim S et al (2007) A systematic review of the association between circulating concentrations of C reactive protein and cancer. J Epidemiol Community Health 61(9): 824–833
204 Tsilidis KK, Branchini C et al (2008) C-reactive protein and colorectal cancer risk: a systematic review of prospective studies. Int J Cancer 123(5):1133–1140
205 Erlinger TP, Platz EA et al (2004) C-reactive protein and the risk of incident colorectal cancer. JAMA 291(5):585–590
206 Otani T, Iwasaki M et al (2006) Plasma C-reactive protein and risk of colorectal cancer in a nested case-control study: Japan Public Health Center-based prospective study. Cancer Epidemiol Biomarkers Prev 15(4):690–695
207 Kim S, Baron JA et al (2006) Aspirin may be more effective in preventing colorectal adenomas in patients with higher BMI (United States). Cancer Causes Control 17(10):1299–1304
208 Sutcliffe S, Platz EA (2007) Inflammation in the etiology of prostate cancer: an epidemiologic perspective. Urol Oncol 25(3):242–249
209 Pierce BL, Biggs ML et al (2009) C-reactive protein, interleukin-6, and prostate cancer risk in men aged 65 years and older. Cancer Causes Control 20(7):1193–1203
210 Platz EA, De Marzo AM et al. (2004) No association between pre diagnostic plasma C-reactive protein concentration and subsequent prostate cancer. Prostate 59(4):393–400. J Urol 171(2 Pt 2):S36–S40
211 Stark JR, Li H et al (2009) Circulating prediagnostic interleukin-6 and C-reactive protein and prostate cancer incidence and mortality. Int J Cancer 124(11):2683–2689
212 Harris RE, Beebe-Donk J et al (2005) Aspirin, ibuprofen, and other non-steroidal anti-inflammatory drugs in cancer prevention: a critical review of non-selective COX-2 blockade (review). Oncol Rep 13(4):559–583
213 Jacobs EJ, Rodriguez C et al (2005) A large cohort study of aspirin and other nonsteroidal anti-inflammatory drugs and prostate cancer incidence. J Natl Cancer Inst 97(13):975–980
214 Mahmud S, Franco E et al (2004) Prostate cancer and use of nonsteroidal anti-inflammatory drugs: systematic review and meta-analysis. Br J Cancer 90(1):93–99

215 Raynes JG, Eagling S et al (1991) Acute-phase protein synthesis in human hepatoma cells: differential regulation of serum amyloid A (SAA) and haptoglobin by interleukin-1 and interleukin-6. Clin Exp Immunol 83(3):488–491
216 Schultz DR, Arnold PI (1990) Properties of four acute phase proteins: C-reactive protein, serum amyloid A protein, alpha 1-acid glycoprotein, and fibrinogen. Semin Arthritis Rheum 20(3):129–147
217 Sjoholm K, Palming J et al (2005) A microarray search for genes predominantly expressed in human omental adipocytes: adipose tissue as a major production site of serum amyloid A. J Clin Endocrinol Metab 90(4):2233–2239
218 Poitou C, Coussieu C et al (2006) Serum amyloid A: a marker of adiposity-induced low-grade inflammation but not of metabolic status. Obesity (Silver Spring) 14(2):309–318
219 Sjoholm K, Lundgren M et al (2009) Association of serum amyloid A levels with adipocyte size and serum levels of adipokines: differences between men and women. Cytokine 48(3):260–266
220 Yang RZ, Lee MJ et al (2006) Acute-phase serum amyloid A: an inflammatory adipokine and potential link between obesity and its metabolic complications. PLoS Med 3(6):e287
221 Chan DC, Chen CJ et al (2007) Evaluation of serum amyloid A as a biomarker for gastric cancer. Ann Surg Oncol 14(1):84–93
222 Benson MD, Eyanson S et al (1986) Serum amyloid A in carcinoma of the lung. Cancer 57(9):1783–1787
223 Khan N, Cromer CJ et al (2004) Clinical utility of serum amyloid A and macrophage migration inhibitory factor as serum biomarkers for the detection of nonsmall cell lung carcinoma. Cancer 101(2):379–384
224 Nel AE, Strachan AF et al (1985) Acute phase response in bronchiectasis and bronchus carcinoma. Respiration 47(3):196–200
225 Kaneti J, Winikoff Y et al (1984) Importance of serum amyloid A (SAA) level in monitoring disease activity and response to therapy in patients with prostate cancer. Urol Res 12(5): 239–241
226 Glojnaric I, Casl MT et al (2001) Serum amyloid A protein (SAA) in colorectal carcinoma. Clin Chem Lab Med 39(2):129–133
227 Kimura M, Tomita Y et al (2001) Significance of serum amyloid A on the prognosis in patients with renal cell carcinoma. Cancer 92(8):2072–2075
228 Cocco E, Bellone S et al (2009) Serum amyloid A (SAA): a novel biomarker for uterine serous papillary cancer. Br J Cancer 101(2):335–341
229 Weinstein PS, Skinner M et al (1984) Acute-phase proteins or tumour markers: the role of SAA, SAP, CRP and CEA as indicators of metastasis in a broad spectrum of neoplastic diseases. Scand J Immunol 19(3):193–198
230 Findeisen P, Zapatka M et al (2009) Serum amyloid A as a prognostic marker in melanoma identified by proteomic profiling. J Clin Oncol 27(13):2199–2208
231 Le L, Chi K et al (2005) Identification of serum amyloid A as a biomarker to distinguish prostate cancer patients with bone lesions. Clin Chem 51(4):695–707
232 Ramankulov A, Lein M et al (2008) Serum amyloid A as indicator of distant metastases but not as early tumor marker in patients with renal cell carcinoma. Cancer Lett 269(1):85–92
233 Raynes JG, Cooper EH (1983) Comparison of serum amyloid A protein and C-reactive protein concentrations in cancer and non-malignant disease. J Clin Pathol 36(7):798–803
234 Gutfeld O, Prus D et al (2006) Expression of serum amyloid A, in normal, dysplastic, and neoplastic human colonic mucosa: implication for a role in colonic tumorigenesis. J Histochem Cytochem 54(1):63–73
235 Pierce BL, Ballard-Barbash R et al (2009) Elevated biomarkers of inflammation are associated with reduced survival among breast cancer patients. J Clin Oncol 27(21):3437–3444
236 Pierce BL, Neuhouser ML et al (2009) Correlates of circulating C-reactive protein and serum amyloid A concentrations in breast cancer survivors. Breast Cancer Res Treat 114(1): 155–167

237 Vicennati V, Vottero A et al (2002) Hormonal regulation of interleukin-6 production in human adipocytes. Int J Obes Relat Metab Disord 26(7):905–911
238 Mohamed-Ali V, Goodrick S et al (1997) Subcutaneous adipose tissue releases interleukin-6, but not tumor necrosis factor-alpha, in vivo. J Clin Endocrinol Metab 82(12):4196–4200
239 Clement K, Viguerie N et al (2004) Weight loss regulates inflammation-related genes in white adipose tissue of obese subjects. Faseb J 18(14):1657–1669
240 Esposito K, Pontillo A et al (2003) Effect of weight loss and lifestyle changes on vascular inflammatory markers in obese women: a randomized trial. JAMA 289(14): 1799–1804
241 Arvidsson E, Viguerie N et al (2004) Effects of different hypocaloric diets on protein secretion from adipose tissue of obese women. Diabetes 53(8):1966–1971
242 Bastard JP, Jardel C et al (2000) Elevated levels of interleukin 6 are reduced in serum and subcutaneous adipose tissue of obese women after weight loss. J Clin Endocrinol Metab 85(9):3338–3342
243 Salas-Salvado J, Bullo M et al (2006) Subcutaneous adipose tissue cytokine production is not responsible for the restoration of systemic inflammation markers during weight loss. Int J Obes (London) 30(12):1714–1720
244 Bruun JM, Helge JW et al (2006) Diet and exercise reduce low-grade inflammation and macrophage infiltration in adipose tissue but not in skeletal muscle in severely obese subjects. Am J Physiol Endocrinol Metab 290(5):E961–E967
245 Purohit A, Newman SP et al (2002) The role of cytokines in regulating estrogen synthesis: implications for the etiology of breast cancer. Breast Cancer Res 4(2):65–69
246 Bastard JP, Maachi M et al (2006) Recent advances in the relationship between obesity, inflammation, and insulin resistance. Eur Cytokine Netw 17(1):4–12
247 Drachenberg DE, Elgamal AA et al (1999) Circulating levels of interleukin-6 in patients with hormone refractory prostate cancer. Prostate 41(2):127–133
248 Shariat SF, Andrews B et al (2001) Plasma levels of interleukin-6 and its soluble receptor are associated with prostate cancer progression and metastasis. Urology 58(6):1008–1015
249 Chung TD, Yu JJ et al (1999) Characterization of the role of IL-6 in the progression of prostate cancer. Prostate 38(3):199–207
250 Okamoto M, Lee C et al (1997) Interleukin-6 as a paracrine and autocrine growth factor in human prostatic carcinoma cells in vitro. Cancer Res 57(1):141–146
251 Siegall CB, Schwab G et al (1990) Expression of the interleukin 6 receptor and interleukin 6 in prostate carcinoma cells. Cancer Res 50(24):7786–7788
252 International Agency for Research on Cancer (2002) IARC handbooks of cancer prevention, vol 6, Weight control and physical activity. IARC Press, Lyon
253 Key TJ, Allen NE et al (2001) Energy balance and cancer: the role of sex hormones. Proc Nutr Soc 60(1):81–89
254 Key TJ, Appleby PN et al (2003) Body mass index, serum sex hormones, and breast cancer risk in postmenopausal women. J Natl Cancer Inst 95(16):1218–1226
255 Tchernof A, Despres JP (2000) Sex steroid hormones, sex hormone-binding globulin, and obesity in men and women. Horm Metab Res 32(11–12):526–536
256 Harvie M, Howell A (2006) Energy balance adiposity and breast cancer – energy restriction strategies for breast cancer prevention. Obes Rev 7(1):33–47
257 Lorincz AM, Sukumar S (2006) Molecular links between obesity and breast cancer. Endocr Relat Cancer 13(2):279–292
258 McTiernan A, Tworoger SS et al (2004) Effect of exercise on serum androgens in postmenopausal women: a 12-month randomized clinical trial. Cancer Epidemiol Biomarkers Prev 13(7):1099–1105
259 Poretsky L, Cataldo NA et al (1999) The insulin-related ovarian regulatory system in health and disease. Endocr Rev 20(4):535–582
260 Ding EL, Song Y et al (2006) Sex differences of endogenous sex hormones and risk of type 2 diabetes: a systematic review and meta-analysis. JAMA 295(11):1288–1299

261 Hankinson SE, Willett WC et al (1998) Plasma sex steroid hormone levels and risk of breast cancer in postmenopausal women. J Natl Cancer Inst 90(17):1292–1299
262 Manjer J, Johansson R et al (2003) Postmenopausal breast cancer risk in relation to sex steroid hormones, prolactin and SHBG (Sweden). Cancer Causes Control 14(7):599–607
263 Thomas HV, Key TJ et al (1997) A prospective study of endogenous serum hormone concentrations and breast cancer risk in post-menopausal women on the island of Guernsey. Br J Cancer 76(3):401–405
264 Goebelsmann U, Mishell D (1979) The menstrual cycle. In D. Mishell and V. Davajan (eds) Reproductive endocrinology, infertility and contraception. FA Davis, Philadeiphia PA P67–89.
265 Eliassen AH, Missmer SA et al (2006) Endogenous steroid hormone concentrations and risk of breast cancer among premenopausal women. J Natl Cancer Inst 98(19): 1406–1415
266 Rosenberg CR, Pasternack BS et al (1994) Premenopausal estradiol levels and the risk of breast cancer: a new method of controlling for day of the menstrual cycle. Am J Epidemiol 140(6):518–525
267 Thomas HV, Key TJ et al (1997) A prospective study of endogenous serum hormone concentrations and breast cancer risk in premenopausal women on the island of Guernsey. Br J Cancer 75(7):1075–1079
268 Key TJ, Verkasalo PK (1999) Endogenous hormones and the aetiology of breast cancer. Breast Cancer Res 1(1):18–21
269 Sonnenschein E, Toniolo P et al (1999) Body fat distribution and obesity in pre- and postmenopausal breast cancer. Int J Epidemiol 28(6):1026–1031
270 Wenten M, Gilliland FD et al (2002) Associations of weight, weight change, and body mass with breast cancer risk in Hispanic and non-Hispanic white women. Ann Epidemiol 12(6):435–4
271 Ursin G, Longnecker MP et al (1995) A meta-analysis of body mass index and risk of premenopausal breast cancer. Epidemiology 6(2):137–141
272 Emaus A, Espetvedt S et al (2008) 17-beta-estradiol in relation to age at menarche and adult obesity in premenopausal women. Hum Reprod 23(4):919–927
273 Furberg AS, Jasienska G et al (2005) Metabolic and hormonal profiles: HDL cholesterol as a plausible biomarker of breast cancer risk. The Norwegian EBBA Study. Cancer Epidemiol Biomarkers Prev 14(1):33–40
274 Verkasalo PK, Thomas HV et al (2001) Circulating levels of sex hormones and their relation to risk factors for breast cancer: a cross-sectional study in 1092 pre- and postmenopausal women. Cancer Causes Control 12:47–59
275 Dorgan JF, Reichman ME et al (1995) The relation of body size to plasma levels of estrogens and androgens in premenopausal women (Maryland, United States). Cancer Causes Control 6(1):3–8
276 Austin H, Austin JM Jr et al (1991) Endometrial cancer, obesity, and body fat distribution. Cancer Res 51(2):568–572
277 Potischman N, Hoover RN et al (1996) Case-control study of endogenous steroid hormones and endometrial cancer. J Natl Cancer Inst 88(16):1127–1135
278 Lukanova A, Lundin E et al (2004) Circulating levels of sex steroid hormones and risk of endometrial cancer in postmenopausal women. Int J Cancer 108(3):425–432
279 Allen NE, Key TJ et al (2008) Endogenous sex hormones and endometrial cancer risk in women in the European Prospective Investigation into Cancer and Nutrition (EPIC). Endocr Relat Cancer 15(2):485–497
280 Sherman BM, Korenman SG (1974) Measurement of serum LH, FSH, estradiol and progesterone in disorders of the human menstrual cycle: the inadequate luteal phase. J Clin Endocrinol Metab 39(1):145–149
281 Modan B, Ron E et al (1998) Cancer incidence in a cohort of infertile women. Am J Epidemiol 147(11):1038–1042

282 Wild S, Pierpoint T et al (2000) Long-term consequences of polycystic ovary syndrome: results of a 31 year follow-up study. Hum Fertil (Cambridge) 3(2):101–105
283 Clendenen TV, Koenig KL et al (2009) Postmenopausal levels of endogenous sex hormones and risk of colorectal cancer. Cancer Epidemiol Biomarkers Prev 18(1):275–281
284 English MA, Stewart PM et al (2001) Estrogen metabolism and malignancy: analysis of the expression and function of 17beta-hydroxysteroid dehydrogenases in colonic cancer. Mol Cell Endocrinol 171(1-2):53–60
285 Grodstein F, Newcomb PA et al (1999) Postmenopausal hormone therapy and the risk of colorectal cancer: a review and meta-analysis. Am J Med 106(5):574–582
286 Rossouw JE, Anderson GL et al (2002) Risks and benefits of estrogen plus progestin in healthy postmenopausal women: principal results From the Women's Health Initiative randomized controlled trial. JAMA 288(3):321–333
287 Feigelson HS, Jonas CR et al (2004) Weight gain, body mass index, hormone replacement therapy, and postmenopausal breast cancer in a large prospective study. Cancer Epidemiol Biomarkers Prev 13(2):220–224
288 Lahmann PH, Schulz M et al (2005) Long-term weight change and breast cancer risk: the European prospective investigation into cancer and nutrition (EPIC). Br J Cancer 93(5): 582–589
289 Graham JD, Clarke CL (1997) Physiological action of progesterone in target tissues. Endocr Rev 18(4):502–519
290 Kaaks R, Berrino F et al (2005) Serum sex steroids in premenopausal women and breast cancer risk within the European Prospective Investigation into Cancer and Nutrition (EPIC). J Natl Cancer Inst 97(10):755–765
291 Micheli A, Muti P et al (2004) Endogenous sex hormones and subsequent breast cancer in premenopausal women. Int J Cancer 112(2):312–318
292 Newcomb PA, Storer BE et al (1994) Lactation and a reduced risk of premenopausal breast cancer. N Engl J Med 330(2):81–87
293 Parsa P, Parsa B (2009) Effects of reproductive factors on risk of breast cancer: a literature review. Asian Pac J Cancer Prev 10(4):545–550
294 Chlebowski RT, Hendrix SL et al (2003) Influence of estrogen plus progestin on breast cancer and mammography in healthy postmenopausal women: the Women's Health Initiative Randomized Trial. JAMA 289(24):3243–3253
295 Stefanick ML, Anderson GL et al (2006) Effects of conjugated equine estrogens on breast cancer and mammography screening in postmenopausal women with hysterectomy. JAMA 295(14):1647–1657
296 Claessens F, Denayer S et al (2008) Diverse roles of androgen receptor (AR) domains in AR-mediated signaling. Nucl Recept Signal 6:e008
297 McTiernan A, Rajan KB et al (2003) Adiposity and sex hormones in postmenopausal breast cancer survivors. J Clin Oncol 21(10):1961–1966
298 McTiernan A, Wu L et al (2006) Relation of BMI and physical activity to sex hormones in postmenopausal women. Obesity (Silver Spring) 14(9):1662–1677
299 Mah PM, Wittert GA (2009) Obesity and testicular function. Mol Cell Endocrinol 316(2):180–186
300 Amatruda JM, Harman SM et al (1978) Depressed plasma testosterone and fractional binding of testosterone in obese males. J Clin Endocrinol Metab 47(2):268–271
301 Despres JP, Lemieux I et al (2008) Abdominal obesity and the metabolic syndrome: contribution to global cardiometabolic risk. Arterioscler Thromb Vasc Biol 28(6):1039–1049
302 Strain GW, Zumoff B et al (1982) Mild Hypogonadotropic hypogonadism in obese men. Metabolism 31(9):871–875
303 Key T, Appleby P et al (2002) Endogenous sex hormones and breast cancer in postmenopausal women: reanalysis of nine prospective studies. J Natl Cancer Inst 94(8):606–616
304 Missmer S, Eliassen A et al (2004) Endogenous estrogen, androgen, and progesterone concentrations and breast cancer risk among postmenopausal women. J Natl Cancer Inst 96(24):1856–1865

305 Eliassen AH, Colditz GA et al (2006) Adult weight change and risk of postmenopausal breast cancer. JAMA 296(2):193–201
306 London SJ, Colditz GA et al (1989) Prospective study of relative weight, height, and risk of breast cancer. JAMA 262(20):2853–2858
307 Kaaks R, Lukanova A et al (2000) Plasma androgens, IGF-1, body size, and prostate cancer risk: a synthetic review. Prostate Cancer Prostatic Dis 3(3):157–172
308 Stattin P, Lumme S et al (2004) High levels of circulating testosterone are not associated with increased prostate cancer risk: a pooled prospective study. Int J Cancer 108(3): 418–424
309 Crawford ED (2009) Understanding the epidemiology, natural history, and key pathways involved in prostate cancer. Urology 73(5 Suppl):S4–S10
310 Dunn JF, Nisula BC et al (1981) Transport of steroid hormones: binding of 21 endogenous steroids to both testosterone-binding globulin and corticosteroid-binding globulin in human plasma. J Clin Endocrinol Metab 53(1):58–68
311 Pugeat M, Nader N et al (2009) Sex hormone-binding globulin gene expression in the liver: Drugs and the metabolic syndrome. Mol Cell Endocrinol 316(1):53–59
312 Crave JC, Lejeune H et al (1995) Differential effects of insulin and insulin-like growth factor I on the production of plasma steroid-binding globulins by human hepatoblastoma-derived (Hep G2) cells. J Clin Endocrinol Metab 80(4):1283–1289
313 Singh A, Hamilton-Fairley D et al (1990) Effect of insulin-like growth factor-type I (IGF-I) and insulin on the secretion of sex hormone binding globulin and IGF-I binding protein (IBP-I) by human hepatoma cells. J Endocrinol 124(2):R1–R3
314 Barba M, Schunemann HJ et al (2009) The effects of metformin on endogenous androgens and SHBG in women: a systematic review and meta-analysis. Clin Endocrinol (Oxford) 70(5):661–670
315 Kokkoris P, Pi-Sunyer FX (2003) Obesity and endocrine disease. Endocrinol Metab Clin North Am 32(4):895–914
316 Pugeat M, Crave JC et al (1991) Pathophysiology of sex hormone binding globulin (SHBG): relation to insulin. J Steroid Biochem Mol Biol 40(4-6):841–849
317 Tworoger SS, Missmer SA et al (2005) Plasma sex hormone concentrations and subsequent risk of breast cancer among women using postmenopausal hormones. J Natl Cancer Inst 97(8):595–602
318 Novosyadlyy R, Lann DE et al (2010) Insulin-mediated acceleration of breast cancer development and progression in a nonobese model of type 2 diabetes. Cancer Res 70(2): 741–751
319 Hotamisligil GS, Peraldi P et al (1996) IRS-1-mediated inhibition of insulin receptor tyrosine kinase activity in TNF-alpha- and obesity-induced insulin resistance. Science 271(5249):665–668
320 Hursting SD, Lashinger LM et al (2007) Energy balance and carcinogenesis: underlying pathways and targets for intervention. Curr Cancer Drug Targets 7(5):484–491
321 Pollak M (2008) Insulin, insulin-like growth factors and neoplasia. Best Pract Res Clin Endocrinol Metab 22(4):625–638
322 Finlayson CA, Chappell J et al (2003) Enhanced insulin signaling via Shc in human breast cancer. Metabolism 52(12):1606–1611
323 Frasca F, Pandini G et al (2008) The role of insulin receptors and IGF-I receptors in cancer and other diseases. Arch Physiol Biochem 114(1):23–37
324 Ish-Shalom D, Christoffersen CT et al (1997) Mitogenic properties of insulin and insulin analogues mediated by the insulin receptor. Diabetologia 40(Suppl 2):S25–S31
325 Khandwala HM, McCutcheon IE et al (2000) The effects of insulin-like growth factors on tumorigenesis and neoplastic growth. Endocr Rev 21(3):215–244
326 Lawlor MA, Alessi DR (2001) PKB/Akt: a key mediator of cell proliferation, survival and insulin responses? J Cell Sci 114(Pt 16):2903–2910
327 Prisco M, Romano G et al (1999) Insulin and IGF-I receptors signaling in protection from apoptosis. Horm Metab Res 31(2–3):80–89

328 Van der Burg BB, Rutterman GR et al (1988) Mitogenic stimulation of human breast cancer cells in a growth-defined medium: synergistic action of insulin and estrogen. J Cell Physiol 134:101–108
329 Belfiore A, Frittitta L et al (1996) Insulin receptors in breast cancer. Ann N Y Acad Sci 784:173–188
330 Blakesley VA, Stannard BS et al (1997) Role of the IGF-I receptor in mutagenesis and tumor promotion. J Endocrinol 152(3):339–344
331 Cox ME, Gleave ME et al (2009) Insulin receptor expression by human prostate cancers. Prostate 69(1):33–40
332 Papa V, Belfiore A (1996) Insulin receptors in breast cancer: biological and clinical role. J Endocrinol Invest 19(5):324–333
333 Tamimi RM, Byrne C et al (2007) Endogenous hormone levels, mammographic density, and subsequent risk of breast cancer in postmenopausal women. J Natl Cancer Inst 99(15): 1178–1187
334 Fagan DH, Yee D (2008) Crosstalk between IGF1R and estrogen receptor signaling in breast cancer. J Mammary Gland Biol Neoplasia 13(4):423–429
335 Yee D, Lee AV (2000) Crosstalk between the insulin-like growth factors and estrogens in breast cancer. J Mammary Gland Biol Neoplasia 5(1):107–115
336 Yu H, Shu XO et al (2003) Joint effect of insulin-like growth factors and sex steroids on breast cancer risk. Cancer Epidemiol Biomarkers Prev 12(10):1067–1073
337 Wu Y, Brodt P et al (2010) Insulin-like growth factor-I regulates the liver microenvironment in obese mice and promotes liver metastasis. Cancer Res 70(1):57–67
338 Grimberg A, Cohen P (2000) Role of insulin-like growth factors and their binding proteins in growth control and carcinogenesis. J Cell Physiol 183(1):1–9
339 Vigneri P, Frasca F et al (2009) Diabetes and cancer. Endocr Relat Cancer 16(4):1103–1123
340 Brownlee M (2001) Biochemistry and molecular cell biology of diabetic complications. Nature 414(6865):813–820
341 Becker S, Dossus L et al (2009) Obesity related hyperinsulinaemia and hyperglycaemia and cancer development. Arch Physiol Biochem 115(2):86–96
342 Yamasaki K, Hayashi Y et al (2009) Insulin-independent promotion of chemically induced hepatocellular tumor development in genetically diabetic mice. Cancer Sci 101(1):65–72
343 Vasseur F (2006) Adiponectin and its receptors: partners contributing to the "vicious circle" leading to the metabolic syndrome? Pharmacol Res 53(6):478–481
344 Yamauchi T, Nio Y et al (2007) Targeted disruption of AdipoR1 and AdipoR2 causes abrogation of adiponectin binding and metabolic actions. Nat Med 13(3):332–339
345 Combs TP, Berg AH et al (2001) Endogenous glucose production is inhibited by the adipose-derived protein Acrp30. J Clin Invest 108(12):1875–1881
346 Combs TP, Pajvani UB et al (2004) A transgenic mouse with a deletion in the collagenous domain of adiponectin displays elevated circulating adiponectin and improved insulin sensitivity. Endocrinology 145(1):367–383
347 Kim JY, van de Wall E et al (2007) Obesity-associated improvements in metabolic profile through expansion of adipose tissue. J Clin Invest 117(9):2621–2637
348 Yamauchi T, Kamon J et al (2002) Adiponectin stimulates glucose utilization and fatty-acid oxidation by activating AMP-activated protein kinase. Nat Med 8(11):1288–1295
349 Ouchi N, Kihara S et al (2001) Adipocyte-derived plasma protein, adiponectin, suppresses lipid accumulation and class A scavenger receptor expression in human monocyte-derived macrophages. Circulation 103(8):1057–1063
350 Yokota T, Oritani K et al (2000) Adiponectin, a new member of the family of soluble defense collagens, negatively regulates the growth of myelomonocytic progenitors and the functions of macrophages. Blood 96(5):1723–1732
351 Ouchi N, Kihara S et al (2000) Adiponectin, an adipocyte-derived plasma protein, inhibits endothelial NF-kappaB signaling through a cAMP-dependent pathway. Circulation 102(11):1296–1301

352 Ouchi N, Walsh K (2007) Adiponectin as an anti-inflammatory factor. Clin Chim Acta 380 (1–2):24–30
353 Wang Y, Lam KS et al (2005) Adiponectin inhibits cell proliferation by interacting with several growth factors in an oligomerization-dependent manner. J Biol Chem 280(18):18341–18347
354 Fenton JI, Birmingham JM et al (2008) Adiponectin blocks multiple signaling cascades associated with leptin-induced cell proliferation in Apc Min/+ colon epithelial cells. Int J Cancer 122(11):2437–2445
355 Grossmann ME, Nkhata KJ et al (2008) Effects of adiponectin on breast cancer cell growth and signaling. Br J Cancer 98(2):370–379
356 Kang JH, Lee YY et al (2005) Adiponectin induces growth arrest and apoptosis of MDA-MB-231 breast cancer cell. Arch Pharm Res 28(11):1263–1269
357 Pfeiler GH, Buechler C et al (2008) Adiponectin effects on human breast cancer cells are dependent on 17-beta estradiol. Oncol Rep 19(3):787–793
358 Wang Y, Lam JB et al (2006) Adiponectin modulates the glycogen synthase kinase-3beta/beta-catenin signaling pathway and attenuates mammary tumorigenesis of MDA-MB-231 cells in nude mice. Cancer Res 66(23):11462–11470
359 Stefan N, Vozarova B et al (2002) Plasma adiponectin concentration is associated with skeletal muscle insulin receptor tyrosine phosphorylation, and low plasma concentration precedes a decrease in whole-body insulin sensitivity in humans. Diabetes 51(6):1884–1888
360 Iwabu M, Yamauchi T et al (2010) Adiponectin and AdipoR1 regulate PGC-1alpha and mitochondria by Ca(2+) and AMPK/SIRT1. Nature 464(7293):1313–1319
361 Luo N, Liu J et al Macrophage adiponectin expression improves insulin sensitivity and protects against inflammation and atherosclerosis. Diabetes 59(4):791–799 year: 2010
362 Igata M, Motoshima H et al (2005) Adenosine monophosphate-activated protein kinase suppresses vascular smooth muscle cell proliferation through the inhibition of cell cycle progression. Circ Res 97(8):837–844
363 Inoki K, Zhu T et al (2003) TSC2 mediates cellular energy response to control cell growth and survival. Cell 115(5):577–590
364 Ouedraogo R, Wu X et al (2006) Adiponectin suppression of high-glucose-induced reactive oxygen species in vascular endothelial cells: evidence for involvement of a cAMP signaling pathway. Diabetes 55(6):1840–1846
365 Brakenhielm E, Veitonmaki N et al (2004) Adiponectin-induced antiangiogenesis and antitumor activity involve caspase-mediated endothelial cell apoptosis. Proc Natl Acad Sci USA 101(8):2476–2481
366 Yoshimura A (2006) Signal transduction of inflammatory cytokines and tumor development. Cancer Sci 97(6):439–447
367 Karin M, Greten FR (2005) NF-kappaB: linking inflammation and immunity to cancer development and progression. Nat Rev Immunol 5(10):749–759
368 Maeda S, Omata M (2008) Inflammation and cancer: role of nuclear factor-kappaB activation. Cancer Sci 99(5):836–842
369 Pikarsky E, Porat RM et al (2004) NF-kappaB functions as a tumour promoter in inflammation-associated cancer. Nature 431(7007):461–466
370 Cai D, Yuan M et al (2005) Local and systemic insulin resistance resulting from hepatic activation of IKK-beta and NF-kappaB. Nat Med 11(2):183–190
371 Yuan M, Konstantopoulos N et al (2001) Reversal of obesity- and diet-induced insulin resistance with salicylates or targeted disruption of Ikkbeta. Science 293(5535): 1673–1677
372 Arkan MC, Hevener AL et al (2005) IKK-beta links inflammation to obesity-induced insulin resistance. Nat Med 11(2):191–198
373 Xie QW, Kashiwabara Y et al (1994) Role of transcription factor NF-kappa B/Rel in induction of nitric oxide synthase. J Biol Chem 269(7):4705–4708

374 Kawanishi S, Hiraku Y et al (2006) Oxidative and nitrative DNA damage in animals and patients with inflammatory diseases in relation to inflammation-related carcinogenesis. Biol Chem 387(4):365–372
375 Pollard JW (2004) Tumour-educated macrophages promote tumour progression and metastasis. Nat Rev Cancer 4(1):71–78
376 Calandra T, Bucala R (1997) Macrophage migration inhibitory factor (MIF): a glucocorticoid counter-regulator within the immune system. Crit Rev Immunol 17(1):77–88
377 Hudson JD, Shoaibi MA et al (1999) A proinflammatory cytokine inhibits p53 tumor suppressor activity. J Exp Med 190(10):1375–1382
378 Balkwill F, Mantovani A (2001) Inflammation and cancer: back to Virchow? Lancet 357(9255):539–545
379 Greten FR, Eckmann L et al (2004) IKKbeta links inflammation and tumorigenesis in a mouse model of colitis-associated cancer. Cell 118(3):285–296
380 Becker C, Fantini MC et al (2004) TGF-beta suppresses tumor progression in colon cancer by inhibition of IL-6 trans-signaling. Immunity 21(4):491–501
381 Van Antwerp DJ, Martin SJ et al (1996) Suppression of TNF-alpha-induced apoptosis by NF-kappaB. Science 274(5288):787–789
382 Ferrante AW Jr (2007) Obesity-induced inflammation: a metabolic dialogue in the language of inflammation. J Intern Med 262(4):408–414
383 Purohit A, Ghilchik MW et al (1995) Aromatase activity and interleukin-6 production by normal and malignant breast tissues. J Clin Endocrinol Metab 80(10):3052–3058
384 Chen T, Wang LH et al (2000) Interleukin 6 activates androgen receptor-mediated gene expression through a signal transducer and activator of transcription 3-dependent pathway in LNCaP prostate cancer cells. Cancer Res 60(8):2132–2135
385 Smith PC, Hobisch A et al (2001) Interleukin-6 and prostate cancer progression. Cytokine Growth Factor Rev 12(1):33–40
386 Macdiarmid F, Wang D et al (1994) Stimulation of aromatase activity in breast fibroblasts by tumor necrosis factor alpha. Mol Cell Endocrinol 106(1–2):17–21
387 Reed MJ, Coldham NG et al (1992) Interleukin-1 and interleukin-6 in breast cyst fluid: their role in regulating aromatase activity in breast cancer cells. J Endocrinol 132(3):R5–R8
388 D'Eon TM, Souza SC et al (2005) Estrogen regulation of adiposity and fuel partitioning. Evidence of genomic and non-genomic regulation of lipogenic and oxidative pathways. J Biol Chem 280(43):35983–35991
389 Cheskis BJ, Greger JG et al (2007) Signaling by estrogens. J Cell Physiol 213(3):610–617
390 Campbell RA, Bhat-Nakshatri P et al (2001) Phosphatidylinositol 3-kinase/AKT-mediated activation of estrogen receptor alpha: a new model for anti-estrogen resistance. J Biol Chem 276(13):9817–9824
391 Castoria G, Migliaccio A et al (2001) PI3-kinase in concert with Src promotes the S-phase entry of oestradiol-stimulated MCF-7 cells. EMBO J 20(21):6050–6059
392 Migliaccio A, Di Domenico M et al (1996) Tyrosine kinase/p21ras/MAP-kinase pathway activation by estradiol-receptor complex in MCF-7 cells. EMBO J 15(6):1292–1300
393 Feigelson HS, Henderson BE (1996) Estrogens and breast cancer. Carcinogenesis 17(11):2279–2284
394 Cavalieri E, Chakravarti D et al (2006) Catechol estrogen quinones as initiators of breast and other human cancers: implications for biomarkers of susceptibility and cancer prevention. Biochim Biophys Acta 1766(1):63–78
395 Yager JD, Liehr JG (1996) Molecular mechanisms of estrogen carcinogenesis. Annu Rev Pharmacol Toxicol 36:203–232
396 Yue W, Santen RJ et al (2003) Genotoxic metabolites of estradiol in breast: potential mechanism of estradiol induced carcinogenesis. J Steroid Biochem Mol Biol 86(3–5):477–486
397 Gao JG, Mazella J et al (1994) Activation of the human IGFBP-1 gene promoter by progestin and relaxin in primary culture of human endometrial stromal cells. Mol Cell Endocrinol 104(1):39–46

398 Liu HC, He ZY et al (1997) Hormonal regulation of expression of messenger RNA encoding insulin-like growth factor binding proteins in human endometrial stromal cells cultured in vitro. Mol Hum Reprod 3(1):21–26
399 Frost RA, Mazella J et al (1993) Insulin-like growth factor binding protein-1 inhibits the mitogenic effect of insulin-like growth factors and progestins in human endometrial stromal cells. Biol Reprod 49(1):104–111
400 Clarke CL, Adams JB et al (1982) Induction of estrogen sulfotransferase in the human endometrium by progesterone in organ culture. J Clin Endocrinol Metab 55(1):70–75
401 Kitawaki J, Yamamoto T et al (1988) Induction of estradiol dehydrogenase activity in human uterine endometrium by synthetic steroids. J Endocrinol Invest 11(5):351–354
402 Hankinson SE (2005) Endogenous hormones and risk of breast cancer in postmenopausal women. Breast Dis 24:3–15
403 Nagasawa H, Aoki M et al (1988) Medroxyprogesterone acetate enhances spontaneous mammary tumorigenesis and uterine adenomyosis in mice. Breast Cancer Res Treat 12(1):59–66
404 Aldaz CM, Liao QY et al (1996) Allelotypic and cytogenetic characterization of chemically induced mouse mammary tumors: high frequency of chromosome 4 loss of heterozygosity at advanced stages of progression. Mol Carcinog 17(3):126–133
405 Lydon JP, Ge G et al (1999) Murine mammary gland carcinogenesis is critically dependent on progesterone receptor function. Cancer Res 59(17):4276–4284
406 Pazos P, Lanari C et al (1992) Mammary carcinogenesis induced by N-methyl-N-nitrosourea (MNU) and medroxyprogesterone acetate (MPA) in BALB/c mice. Breast Cancer Res Treat 20(2):133–138
407 Beral V (2003) Breast cancer and hormone-replacement therapy in the Million Women Study. Lancet 362(9382):419–427
408 Chen WY, Hankinson SE et al (2004) Association of hormone replacement therapy to estrogen and progesterone receptor status in invasive breast carcinoma. Cancer 101(7): 1490–1500
409 Hankinson SE, Colditz GA et al (2004) Towards an integrated model for breast cancer etiology: the lifelong interplay of genes, lifestyle, and hormones. Breast Cancer Res 6(5):213–218
410 Santos AF, Huang H et al (2004) The androgen receptor: a potential target for therapy of prostate cancer. Steroids 69(2):79–85
411 Bosland MC, Ford H et al (1995) Induction at high incidence of ductal prostate adenocarcinomas in NBL/Cr and Sprague-Dawley Hsd:SD rats treated with a combination of testosterone and estradiol-17 beta or diethylstilbestrol. Carcinogenesis 16(6):1311–1317
412 Leav I, Ho SM et al (1988) Biochemical alterations in sex hormone-induced hyperplasia and dysplasia of the dorsolateral prostates of Noble rats. J Natl Cancer Inst 80(13):1045–1053
413 Noble RL (1977) The development of prostatic adenocarcinoma in Nb rats following prolonged sex hormone administration. Cancer Res 37(6):1929–1933
414 Pollard M, Luckert PH et al (1982) Induction of prostate adenocarcinomas in Lobund Wistar rats by testosterone. Prostate 3(6):563–568
415 Pollard M, Luckert PH (1986) Promotional effects of testosterone and high fat diet on the development of autochthonous prostate cancer in rats. Cancer Lett 32(2):223–227
416 Pollard M, Luckert PH et al (1989) The promotional effect of testosterone on induction of prostate-cancer in MNU-sensitized L-W rats. Cancer Lett 45(3):209–212
417 Nicolas Diaz-Chico B, German Rodriguez F et al (2007) Androgens and androgen receptors in breast cancer. J Steroid Biochem Mol Biol 105(1–5):1–15
418 Catalano MG, Frairia R et al (2005) Sex hormone-binding globulin antagonizes the anti-apoptotic effect of estradiol in breast cancer cells. Mol Cell Endocrinol 230(1–2):31–37
419 Fortunati N, Becchis M et al (1999) Sex hormone-binding globulin, its membrane receptor, and breast cancer: a new approach to the modulation of estradiol action in neoplastic cells. J Steroid Biochem Mol Biol 69(1–6):473–479

420 Fortunati N, Catalano MG (2006) Sex hormone-binding globulin (SHBG) and estradiol crosstalk in breast cancer cells. Horm Metab Res 38(4):236–240
421 Razandi M, Pedram A et al (2000) Plasma membrane estrogen receptors signal to antiapoptosis in breast cancer. Mol Endocrinol 14(9):1434–1447

Chapter 7
Mechanisms Underlying the Effects of Physical Activity on Cancer

Andrew Rundle

Abstract There are numerous biological mechanisms that have been proposed to explain how physical activity might prevent cancer, including effects on body size, sex hormone levels, insulin resistance, immune surveillance, inflammation, and oxidative stress. There is very little human epidemiologic data supporting or refuting proposed mechanistic hypotheses. Thus at this point in time, our understanding of the mechanisms through which physical activity impacts cancer incidence is more theoretical than practical. The International Agency for Research on Cancer (IARC) has determined that there is sufficient evidence to conclude that physical activity is protective against cancers of the colon and breast. Using these cancers as a lens, this chapter will review and critique major areas of the mechanistic literature on physical activity and suggest other mechanistic hypotheses that might explain the effects of physical activity.

1 Introduction

There are numerous biological mechanisms that have been proposed to explain how physical activity might prevent cancer. While not an exhaustive list, proposed mechanisms have included effects on body size, sex hormone levels, insulin resistance, immune surveillance, DNA methylation, inflammation, and oxidative stress. Figure 7.1 attempts to organize many of the various proposed mechanisms by showing their relationships to physical activity and where they might influence the multistage process of carcinogenesis. The figure is not exhaustive in diagramming all of the proposed mechanisms, and this chapter will provide a critique of many of these proposals. It is very common for reports of epidemiologic studies of physical activity and cancer incidence to devote a section of the Discussion to speculating about possible mechanisms. However, molecular epidemiologic studies that test

A. Rundle (✉)
Department of Epidemiology, Mailman School of Public Health, Columbia University, New York, NY, USA
e-mail: agr3@columbia.edu

A. McTiernan (ed.), *Physical Activity, Dietary Calorie Restriction, and Cancer*, Energy Balance and Cancer 3, DOI 10.1007/978-1-4419-7551-5_7,

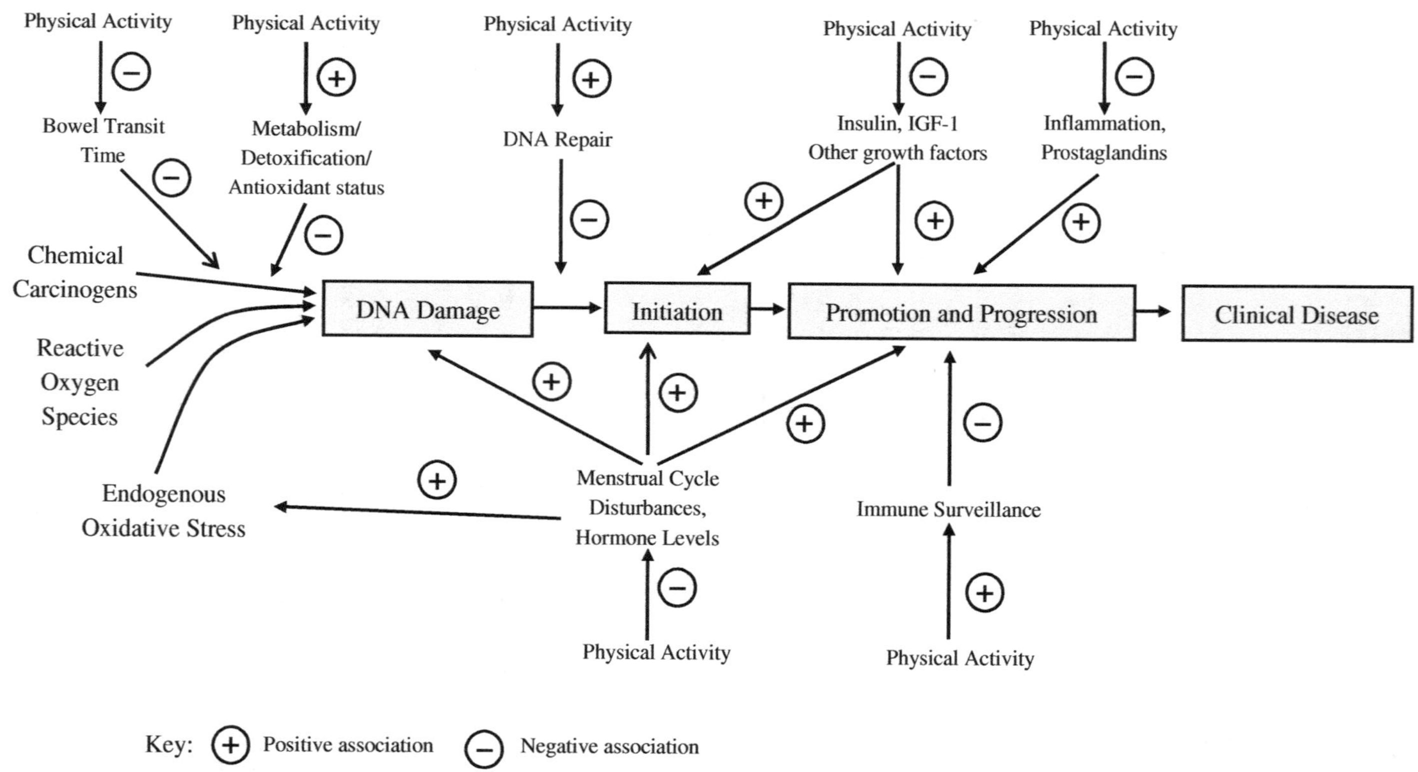

Fig. 7.1 Summary of many of the proposed mechanisms linking physical activity to lower cancer risk

possible mechanisms as part of epidemiologic analysis of physical activity and cancer are rare in the literature [1, 2, 3]. Thus there is very little human epidemiologic data supporting or refuting proposed mechanistic hypotheses.

The elucidation of mechanisms through which physical activity influences cancer risk is important for the design of public health interventions to prevent cancer, and is important from the basic science perspective of understanding how cancer arises. For cancers where traditional epidemiology has already provided sufficient data to accept the link as being causal, a mechanistic understanding would be useful in identifying new targets for pharmacological or other interventions. Additionally, biomarkers representing critical elements in the mechanistic pathway would be useful as surrogate outcomes in intervention trials to test various physical activity-based prevention programs [4, 5, 6]. To maximize the effectiveness of public health intervention programs, it is important to understand the role of frequency, timing and level of exertion, and a mechanistic understanding would help calibrate such interventions [4, 6, 7]. For cancers where traditional epidemiology has not provided consistent data on the role of physical activity, tests of mechanistic hypotheses would generate biological data useful in the process of causal inference [4, 6].

The two cancers, breast and colon, for which the International Agency for Research on Cancer (IARC) has reported that there was sufficient evidence for a determination that there was a protective effect of physical activity, are also cancers for which obesity is an established cause [8]. It is thus tempting to assume that physical activity primarily exerts its effects by facilitating weight control and preventing obesity; however, the available data suggest that this is not the case. This chapter will review the mechanistic literature on physical activity, obesity, and these cancers; will discuss other proposed mechanisms; and suggest other mechanistic hypotheses that might explain the effects of physical activity.

2 Breast Cancer

2.1 Obesity and Sex Hormone Levels

Obesity is a cause of postmenopausal breast cancer, and physical activity is more strongly protective against postmenopausal as opposed to premenopausal breast cancer. There is substantial evidence that obesity influences postmenopausal breast cancer risk by increasing circulating estradiol levels [9]. Estradiol binds to nuclear estrogen receptors and induces cell proliferation and reduces apoptosis [10, 11]. Additionally, estrogen metabolism can produce genotoxic metabolites that form unstable DNA-adducts leading to DNA damage through depurination [11, 12, 13, 14, 15]. Furthermore, redox cycling of estrogen quinones produces reactive oxygen species that can also damage DNA [12, 16, 17]. Thus estrogen may play a role in the initiation, promotion, and progression of breast cancer [11].

In postmenopausal women not using hormone replacement therapy, circulating estrogens are primarily derived from aromatization of androgens in the peripheral tissues, particularly adipose tissue [18, 19]. Prospective studies of obesity and postmenopausal breast cancer risk have shown that serum estradiol levels mediate the association between obesity and cancer risk [9]. That is, in these studies serum-free estradiol levels are associated with body mass index (BMI); and after control for inter-individual variation in serum hormone levels, BMI is no longer associated with breast cancer risk [9]. Further substantiating the key role of serum hormone levels in the obesity–postmenopausal breast cancer link, obesity is associated with only estrogen receptor positive/progesterone receptor positive (ER+/PR+) breast cancer [20]. That is, obesity is only associated with breast tumors that are responsive to serum sex hormones [20]. Generally however, epidemiologic studies assessing associations between physical activity and breast cancer have controlled for BMI and found protective effects even after accounting for differences in body size [8, 21]. This suggests that physical activity's effects on body fat or body size do not represent the primarily mechanistic pathway connecting activity to lower breast cancer risk.

The direct effects of exercise on blood hormone levels and urinary estrogen metabolite levels have been evaluated in postmenopausal women [22, 23]. A recent intervention study in postmenopausal women showed that physical activity could lower serum sex hormone levels, but mainly among those who lost body fat during the trial [23]. Overall compared to light stretching, 45 min a day of moderate exercise, five times a week, caused reductions in body weight, body fat, serum estrone, estradiol, and free estradiol. The effects on serum hormones were statistically significant after 3 months of the intervention, but not after 12 months. The effects on serum hormones were primarily observed among women who lost body fat during the intervention, and in this subgroup the effects were significant after both 3 and 12 months of intervention. There was no significant effect of the intervention on urinary levels of 2-hydroxyestrone (2-OHE_1), 16-α-hydroxyestrone (16-α-OHE_1), or their ratio [22]. This trial suggests that exercise in postmenopausal women has minimal effects on serum hormone levels unless there is concurrent weight loss.

In premenopausal women disturbances in the menstrual cycle have been reported in recreationally active women and in athletes [24, 25]. The most severe disturbance is amenorrhea, involving complete follicular and luteal suppression, most commonly reported by athletes in sports requiring a slender physique, such as gymnastics [24]. Luteal phase defects are a less severe menstrual disturbance reported to be common among women who are highly recreationally active [26]. A study of 24 recreational joggers (average distance per week was 32 km) over a 3-month period found that 42% of the women predominantly exhibited menstrual cycles with luteal phase defects and 16% had menstrual cycles that were predominantly anovulatory [26]. Forty six percent of the exercising women had inconsistent menstrual status with intermittent presentations of ovulatory, luteal phase defects, and anovulatory cycles [26]. An analysis from the Nurses' Health Study II found in premenopausal women that total physical activity was inversely associated with luteal estradiol, free estradiol, and estrone, but that these associations disappeared when women with anovulatory or irregular cycles were removed from the analysis [25]. Reproductive factors associated with inter-individual differences in the number of menstrual cycles are associated with both pre- and postmenopausal breast cancer

[27]. Thus an effect of physical activity on the number of cycles or their length may represent a mechanism through which physical activity affects breast cancer risk. However, it is not yet clear if the population prevalence of women engaged in sufficient amounts of activity to cause menstrual cycle disturbance is sufficient to account for the link between activity and breast cancer.

Several intervention studies have assessed the effect of physical activity and exercise training on estrogen metabolite levels in premenopausal women [28, 29–31, 32, 33, 34]. A recent intervention study of 15 weeks of aerobic exercise observed no effects on training on 2-OHE$_1$, 16-α-OHE$_1$, 2-hydroxyestradiol (2-OHE$_2$), 4-hydroxyestrone (4-OHE$_1$), or 4-hydroxyestradiol (4-OHE$_2$) [33]. Similarly a 12-week aerobic intervention study observed no effect on 2-OHE1, 16-α-OHE$_1$, or the ratio of 2-OHE1 to 16-α-OHE$_1$ [28]. A series of three publications reported on the effects of 5 days of aerobic exercise training on estrogen metabolites, and observed no significant changes in follicular phase metabolites, but did see decreases in 2-hydroxyestrogens during the luteal phase [29–31]. Another study observed a training effect on the ratio of urinary 2-OHE1/16-α-OHE$_1$ ratio among those women in the lowest tertile of 2/16 ratio prior to training [34].

Additional evidence that the effect of physical activity is not predominantly mediated by effects on serum sex hormone levels is seen in studies that have assessed breast cancer risk by the hormone receptor status of the tumor. While studies have shown that higher BMI is only associated with ER+/PR+ breast cancer, the protective effect of physical activity appears to be consistent across tumors regardless of receptor status [1, 2, 3]. These studies have been interpreted variously to suggest that physical activity does not affect breast cancer risk via a hormone-related mechanism, or that it affects risk by both hormonal and nonhormone-dependent mechanisms.

In sum, the current literature provides little evidence that physical activity influences breast cancer risk primarily through effects on body fat which in turn influence serum hormone levels. The evidence that physical activity affects serum sex hormone levels and/or estrogen metabolism through pathways that are independent of effects on adiposity is also currently rather weak.

2.2 Other Possible Mechanisms

2.2.1 Insulin, Insulin Resistance, and Insulin-Like Growth Factors (IGF)

Numerous reviews have suggested that insulin resistance and the resulting hormonal and metabolic changes may promote tumor development and affect breast cancer risk (for instance, see [35, 36]). Insulin resistance is a condition in which the effectiveness of insulin in regulating blood glucose levels is reduced or lost and is closely related to obesity [37]. Insulin resistance causes increases in blood glucose levels and in response the pancreas increases insulin production, resulting in hyperinsulinemia [38, 39]. In turn, impaired glucose tolerance and insulin resistance are risk factors for type 2 diabetes [38, 40]. Thus obesity is an underlying causal factor in insulin resistance, impaired glucose tolerance, and type 2 diabetes. Weight loss and physical activity improve insulin sensitivity; and clinical consensus statements from the American Diabetes Association, the North American Association for the Study of Obesity, and the American Society for Clinical Nutrition promote physical activity to prevent diabetes [41]. Even in the absence of weight loss or gains in fitness, physical activity can substantially improve insulin resistance [42, 43, 44, 45, 46]. Thus, to the extent that insulin-resistance-related pathways affect breast cancer risk, these pathways may represent a route through which physical activity can affect breast cancer risk independent of changes in BMI or body fat.

Elevated insulin levels have numerous downstream effects suggested to affect cancer risk [47, 48]. Chronically elevated levels of insulin cause a reduction in insulin-like growth factor-binding proteins (IGFBP) and increases in free insulin-like growth factor 1 (IGF-1) [47, 48]. In vitro studies have shown that insulin and IGF-1 cause cell proliferation and inhibit apoptosis [39, 49, 50, 51, 52]. Furthermore, experimental animal models using either tumor xenographs or chemical carcinogens show that insulin promotes mammary tumor growth [53, 54, 55, 56]. Additionally, elevated insulin and IGF-1 levels inhibit the synthesis of sex hormone-binding globulin (SHBG), and this effect is thought to underlie the inverse association between BMI and SHBG [35, 48, 57]. SHBG levels influence the relative availability of bound and free, bio-available sex hormones [35, 48, 57].

However, despite the various, and complex, inter-relationships between insulin, IGF-1, and IGFBP and their plausible relationship to breast cancer, there is not strong evidence that they underlie the protective effect of physical activity. A recent literature review found mixed evidence for indicators of type 2 diabetes and insulin resistance being associated with postmenopausal breast incidence [35]. Analyses from the Nurses Health Study II found suggestive evidence that breast cancer risk was inversely associated with blood insulin levels [58], while a cohort study in Italy found that breast cancer risk was nonsignificantly positively associated with blood insulin levels [59]. A recent meta-analysis of markers of hyperinsulinemia and breast cancer found that the pooled analysis of available cohort studies showed no association with breast cancer risk [36].

As noted above, physical activity is most consistently associated with postmenopausal breast cancer, and multiple meta-analyses and reviews of the literature have failed to find an association between elevated IGF-1 levels, IGFBP-3 levels, and postmenopausal breast cancer [60, 61, 62]. Furthermore, studies of postmenopausal women have observed either no associations between physical activity and IGF-1 [63, 64, 65, 66] or a positive association [67]. The IGF-1 meta-analyses have found elevated IGF-1 levels to be associated with premenopausal breast cancer, suggesting a pathway through which physical activity may affect premenopausal breast cancer [60, 61, 62]. However, studies have found either null or positive associations between physical activity and IGF-1 levels in premenopausal women [25, 68, 69]. The picture is further complicated by the results of a 11-week training study that suggested the effects of exercise on the IGF system depended on whether the individual was untrained or well trained prior to the intervention [70]. Overall, it does not appear that levels of circulating IGF-1 and IGFBP-3 mediate the effects of physical activity on breast cancer [35].

2.2.2 Enhanced Defenses Against Reactive Oxygen Species

Another possible mechanism underlying the effects of physical activity on breast cancer is the ability of physical activity to induce the body's endogenous antioxidant systems. Reactive oxygen species are thought to contribute to carcinogenesis, both during initiation and promotion [71, 72]. Oxygen radicals can damage DNA directly, for instance, through 8-hydroxylation of guanine, yielding the mutagenic lesion 8-hydroxy-2′-deoxyguanosine (8-OHdG) [73, 74]. Exercise causes increased oxygen demand with contracting muscles requiring as much as 100-fold more oxygen than while in the resting state, and this increased consumption produces elevated levels of reactive oxygen species [75, 76, 77], which can damage DNA [78, 79, 80]. However, regular exercise appears to cause an adaptive response that induces endogenous antioxidant enzyme systems and lowers oxidative stress [33, 79, 81, 82, 83, 84, 85, 86]. Endogenous antioxidant enzymes of interest include the glutathione system (glutathione peroxidase, glutathione reductase, glutathione) [84, 87, 88, 89, 90, 91, 92, 93, 94], catalase [84, 90, 91], and superoxide dismutase [84, 90, 91, 92]. The net effect of this adaptive response may reduce oxidative damage caused by reactive oxygen species from external environmental exposures and the redox cycling of estrogen quinones [6, 95].

In considering the role of endogenous antioxidant enzyme induction, it is important to note that there appear to be nonlinear dose response curves between activity and enzyme induction [96]. Differential effects have been noted, which appear to depend on whether the activity is acute or chronic, is performed by trained or untrained individuals, and is of moderate or exhaustive intensity [6]. For instance, Miyazaki and colleagues have shown that bouts of exhaustive exercise cause increases in lipid peroxidation, indicative of increased oxidative stress [84]. However, training increased glutathione peroxidase and superoxide dismutase activity, and training reduced the levels of lipid peroxidation caused by subsequent bouts of exhaustive exercise [84]. Similarly in a cross-sectional study, hours per week of moderate intensity activity were positively associated with glutathione levels, while hours of vigorous intensity activity were not [93]. Inspection of the reported activity patterns suggested that some of those reporting vigorous activities were "weekend warriors" engaging in occasional bouts of vigorous activity, while others were engaged in regular exercise programs [93]. The combination of trained and untrained individuals engaging in vigorous activity may have obscured any observable effects on glutathione levels.

Thus far, there has been limited research on breast cancer risk associated with markers of oxidative stress or expression of endogenous antioxidant enzyme systems [97, 98, 99, 100]. The Long Island Breast Cancer study found that urinary levels of 15-F_{2t}-Isoprostane were associated with breast cancer case–control status, but that isoprostane levels were not associated with lifetime average recreational physical activity [100]. However, in the same study, when women treated with radiation therapy prior to enrollment into the study were excluded from analyses, high urinary 8-OHdG levels, a biomarker of oxidative DNA damage, were inversely associated with breast cancer [73, 100]. The prospective Shanghai Women's Health Study found that urinary isoprostane levels were positively associated with breast cancer risk in overweight women and negatively associated with breast cancer risk in women with a BMI $\leq$23 [97].

Only the Long Island Breast Cancer has integrated physical activity into analyses of oxidative stress and breast cancer risk and focused on average lifetime recreational activity [100]. Considering the potential for nonlinear relationships between activity and antioxidant enzyme induction, any further research should carefully measure patterns of activity (regular or training versus sporadic bouts) and should carefully distinguish between moderate and vigorous activity [6]. This recommendation to highly specify the type and context of physical activity to maximize our ability to observe associations with induction of endogenous antioxidant systems reduces the prior probability that this pathway actually underlies the protective effect of physical activity on breast cancer. Physical activity measured relatively crudely, in a variety of ways, has been shown to be associated with lower risk of breast cancer, and it appears that the lower risk is not restricted to the patterns of activity thought most likely to protect against oxidative stress.

2.2.3 Immune Function

Reviews on physical activity and breast cancer risk and cancer in general commonly propose that physical activity-related increases in immune function may mediate associations between activity and cancer risk [8, 101, 102]. The tumor immunosurveillance theory posits that the immune system is constantly vigilant for tumor development, and that tumors that do develop are rare exceptions which have escaped surveillance [103, 104]. Evidence for this theory is seen in the higher tumor incidence observed among those who are immunocompromised [105]. However, tumors prevalent among the immunocompromised are those associated with viral infections, not the common epithelial tumors of the breast, lung, colon, or prostate, and not the tumors associated with sedentary lifestyles [103, 104, 105]. Furthermore, the literature ascribes various roles to the different elements of the immune system in preventing carcinogenesis and/or playing a role in its pathogenesis [7, 103, 104, 106]. Macrophages and neutrophils, which have phagocytic and cytotoxic properties, are capable of destroying tumor cells, and these inflammatory cells are commonly found to be infiltrating tumors [103, 106]. However, it is unclear whether these cells are acting to attack the tumor or are involved in tumor promotion [103, 106]. It has been suggested that, via inflammatory effects, these cells may play a role in tumor initiation and progression [103, 106, 104]. Numerous tumors including cancers of the lung, colon, pancreas, esophagus, and bladder are associated with persistent inflammatory conditions [107, 104]. Data from the Women's Health Initiative showing that a higher white blood cell count is associated with increased breast cancer risk has been interpreted as evidence for inflammation having a role in breast cancer etiology [106]. In this study physical activity was associated with lower white blood cell count, suggesting, following the logic of the authors, that physical activity is protective against inflammation [106]. Since inflammation when acute can have therapeutic effects and when chronic can have pathological effects, physical activity might act by reducing unhealthful inflammation [107]

Natural Killer (NK) cells represent another component of the immune system and often linked to immune surveillance theory [103]. NK cells have cytotoxic properties and have been shown to kill tumor cells [7, 103, 104, 108]. A prospective study in Japan found that individuals whose blood exhibited low in vitro natural cytotoxic activity against a leukemia cell line had a significantly higher risk of developing cancer in all sites over 11 years of follow-up [108]. This was the first epidemiologic evidence among individuals without obvious immune-compromised status that inter-individual variation in immunologic defenses plays a role in preventing common cancers.

Animal studies have shown that physical activity can enhance various elements of the immune system [109, 110, 111, 112, 113]. In human studies the effects of physical activity on immune function appear to depend on the context of the activity, be it of moderate intensity or exhaustive or part of a regular exercise program or sporadic [6]. Strenuous bouts of activity have been associated with increased upper respiratory infections and with reductions in NK cell counts, while cross-sectional comparisons of athletes and nonathletes have found higher NK activity in athletes [114]. As with effects on endogenous antioxidant systems, the apparent J-shaped response curve makes studies on physical activity, immune function, and cancer outcomes difficult. Thus far, there is little available evidence that the protective role of physical activity on breast cancer operates through alterations in immune function. That breast cancer rates do not increase among the immune-compromised suggests that inter-individual variation in immune surveillance does not play a substantial role in breast cancer etiology.

3 New Directions

Recent animal studies by Thompson and colleagues suggest new avenues of research for understanding how physical activity reduces breast cancer risk [115, 116]. Their studies of chemically induced mammary carcinogenesis in Sprague-Dawley rats showed that physical activity significantly reduced the incidence of mammary tumors and the average number of tumors per animal [116]. Analyses of the tumors that were present found that the tumors from physically active animals had lower expression of cyclin D1 and higher expression of p21, indicating lower cellular proliferation in the tumors [116]. Additionally, the tumors from the active animals had lower expression of Bcl-2, an inhibitor of apoptosis, and higher expression of Bax, a promoter of apoptosis [116]. In a second similar study with Sprague-Dawley rats, physical activity was found to cause higher expression of Bax in the tumors, a greater ratio of Bax to Bcl-2, and lower expression of vascular endothelial growth factor (VEGF) [115]. There are some data to suggest that physical activity increases Bax expression in humans [117, 118], notably in colonic crypts (see below) [119]. These animal studies warrant follow-up with human studies to determine whether physical activity predicts the expression of these proteins in breast tumors.

4 Colon Cancer

As in the case of breast cancer, obesity is an established cause of colon cancer. Yet studies linking physical activity to lower risk of colon cancer generally control for BMI, suggesting that the effect of physical activity is independent of physical activity's role in maintaining a healthy body weight [8, 120, 121, 122]. Other mechanisms that are commonly suggested include decreases in bowel transit time, effects on insulin and IGF-1, changes in bile acid metabolism, and decreases in prostaglandin E_2 expression [7, 121, 122]. Far less work has been done to test hypothesized mechanisms in the context of colon cancer than in breast cancer, and there has not been as strong a push to conduct physical activity intervention trials to evaluate mechanistic theories [120]. Additionally, few studies of physical activity and colon cancer have included intermediate biomarkers to test mechanistic hypotheses.

4.1 Other Possible Mechanisms

4.1.1 Decreased Bowel Transit Time

One of the earliest and most commonly proposed mechanisms to explain the protective effect of physical activity was that physical activity stimulated the passage of fecal matter through colon [7, 122]. The idea was that decreased transit time reduced the contact between the colonic mucosa and food mutagens and bile acids [7, 122]. However, studies have not provided consistent or strong data that physical activity actually affects transit time [123, 124, 125, 126, 127, 128, 129] and, despite perhaps an intuitive appeal, there is little available data on transit time and colon cancer risk [130, 131]. Two studies have studied bowel transit times in populations with differing risks of colon cancer and found similar transit times in the populations [130, 131].

4.1.2 Prostaglandin E_2

Increased E series prostaglandin production has been implicated in colon cancer development [7]. Prostaglandin E_2 (PGE_2) has been found to influence several processes involved in carcinogenesis, including cell proliferation, immune surveillance, angiogenesis, and inhibition of apoptosis [132, 133]. Human colonic cancer cells overexpress prostaglandins, and it has been shown that the colonic mucosa of individuals with colorectal polyps or cancer express higher levels of prostaglandin E_2 than the mucosa of controls [134, 135, 136]. Further evidence for the role of prostaglandins is seen in the protective effect that aspirin and other nonsteroidal anti-inflammatory drugs (NSAIDs) have on colon cancer [137, 138]. Aspirin and other NSAIDs inhibit prostaglandin synthesis by inhibiting the cyclooxygenases, which synthesize prostaglandins from arachidonic acid [138].

There is some evidence to suggest that physical activity may alter PGE_2 expression in the gastroenterological tract. A recent study of $APC^{Min/+}$ mice found that voluntary exercise on a running wheel was associated with lower expression of prostaglandin E_2 in small intestinal tumors [139]. A study of human rectal mucosa found that prostaglandin E_2 expression was inversely associated with MET-Hours of recreational physical activity reported in the past month [140]. However, a 12-month randomized controlled trial of moderate to vigorous aerobic activity in 95 men and 89 women had no effect on PGE_2 levels in colon biopsies [141]. While the available literature is still limited, the available studies do not provide strong evidence that physical activity affects colon cancer risk through effects on PGE_2.

4.1.3 Insulin and Insulin-Like Growth Factors

As in breast cancer, it has been hypothesized that insulin and insulin-like growth factors, particularly insulin-like growth factor -1 (IGF-1), play important roles in the development of colon cancer [47, 142]. In vitro studies show that both normal and malignant colorectal cells express IGF-1 receptors, and treatment with IGF-1 inhibits apoptosis and stimulates progression through the cell cycle [47, 143, 144]. As such, IGF-1 is thought to promote cell-turnover and the accumulation of genetic mutations [47]. Similarly, insulin increases the growth of normal and malignant colonic cells, although the mechanisms for this activity are less well characterized [47, 144, 145]. Insulin downregulates the production of IGFBP 1 and 2, increasing levels of free active IGF-1 [47, 146]. Insulin also increases the level of farnesylated ras protein, an action which is thought to prime the signal transduction pathway that mediates the effects of several growth factors, including IGF-1 [147, 148, 149]. Several prospective studies of blood insulin levels and other markers of hyperinsulinemia have found that higher circulating insulin levels are associated with colorectal cancer [36, 150, 151, 152, 153]. Additionally, prospective epidemiologic data from the Physicians' Health Study and the Nurses' Health Study show that high plasma levels of IGF-1 and low levels of IGFBP-3 are associated with higher risk of colorectal cancer and high-risk adenomas [154, 155].

As noted above, physical activity lowers plasma insulin levels and increases insulin sensitivity, with the effects of a bout of physical activity on insulin sensitivity lasting for several days. This suggests a very plausible mechanism through which physical activity might impact colon cancer risk. However, studies assessing whether inter-individual variation in insulin levels mediates associations between physical activity and colon cancer have not been published. It would be of great interest to determine within cohort studies that have found a protective effect of activity on colon cancer whether inter-individual variation in insulin levels mediates the association between activity and colon cancer risk. In regards to the IGF-1 system, as noted above, evidence regarding how physical activity influences the

IGF-1 and its binding proteins system is inconsistent. Some studies show little to no effect on IGF-1 and/or IGFBP-3 [1, 25, 63, 64, 65, 66, 69, 156, 157, 158, 159, 160, 161, 162], others show reductions in IGF-1 levels [158, 162, 163] and/or increases in IGFBP-3 [156, 163] and others show increases in IGF-1 [67, 68]. As such, the available evidence supporting effects on the IGF-1 system as being the link between physical activity and lower colon cancer risk appears fairly speculative.

4.1.4 Immune Function

As with breast cancer, the potential effects of activity on immune function and surveillance are often cited as mechanisms through which physical activity may influence colon cancer risk [7, 122]. The colon has a unique population of lymphocytes, the intraepithelial lymphocytes, which reside between the intestinal epithelial cells [164]. Intraepithelial lymphocytes are the first population of lymphoid cells to encounter antigens and pathogens in the diet, and are thought to play an important role in mucosal immunity [157]. Animal studies suggest that these lymphocytes have a natural killer function and are active against tumor cells [165], and intraepithelial lymphocytes are thought to play a role in the innate immune response to colon cancer in humans [166, 167]. Thus far, however, there appear to have been no studies conducted on the effects of physical activity on intraepithelial lymphocytes function or count. As described above, the higher cytotoxic capacity of blood samples has been shown to predict lower cancer risk at all sites, and physical activity has been found to have varying effects on cytotoxic NK cells.

As with breast cancer, studies have used total white blood cell count as an indicator of nonspecific inflammation and assessed the risk of colon cancer in relation to white blood cell count. Analyses of within the Women's Health Initiative found that higher total white blood cell counts were associated with increased risk of colorectal cancer, but did not present results separately for the colon and rectum [106]. A Korean cohort study found that higher total white blood cell count was associated with incidence and death from colon cancer, but not rectal cancer [168]. As noted above, in the Women's Health Initiative physical activity was associated with lower white blood cell counts, suggesting that physical activity prevents inflammation [106]. There are several inflammatory conditions of the colon that are associated with increased risk of colon cancer [107]. If physical activity is able to moderate inflammatory processes and inflammatory immune cells so that inflammation is therapeutic rather than pathological, this might represent a viable protective mechanism [103, 107].

In general, the potential for physical activity to impact colon cancer risk through effects on immune surveillance has not been extensively researched [7]. In considering this potential mechanism it is important to recognize that, similar to breast cancer rates, colon cancer rates are not elevated among individuals with suppressed immune function [103, 104, 105]. Rather than focusing on immune surveillance theory, studies on the effects of physical activity on inflammation and the immune system components involved in inflammation may yield important information regarding how physical activity prevents colon cancer.

5 New Directions

McTiernan and colleagues have recently completed a 12-month randomized controlled exercise intervention trial in which colonic epithelial cell biopsies were taken before randomization and after the 12-month intervention [120]. In intent to treat analyses, the intervention was associated with changes in colon crypt architecture, with border line significant increases in crypt height in men and women. Among men in the intervention group achieving higher levels of physical activity or increases in V_{O2} Max, there were significant reductions in markers of cell proliferation in the colonic crypts [120]. Further analyses from this study found some evidence that among men, exercise resulted in increased colonic crypt expression of Bax, a protein promoting apoptosis [119]. This work is congruent with studies in rats showing that exercise is associated with higher expression of Bax in mammary tumors [115, 116]. Studies such as this, assessing the architecture of colonic crypts and the expression of proteins thought to be related to carcinogenesis, are likely to substantially further our understanding of how physical activity affects colon cancer.

6 Conclusions

At this point in time, our understanding of the mechanisms through which physical activity impacts cancer incidence is more theoretical than practical. A multitude of theories have been proposed, but there are relatively little data with which to concretely substantiate or refute them. For some theories, such as the role of IGF-1 in postmenopausal breast cancer, findings across studies greatly reduce the prior probability that the theory is correct [35]. The work on obesity, serum sex hormone levels, and postmenopausal breast cancer, where inter-individual variation in sex hormone levels related to differences in body size statistically explains the association between obesity and breast cancer risk, serves as a useful analytical model for future work [9]. However, little to no research using intermediate biomarkers representing proposed mechanistic pathways have been conducted in the context of physical activity and breast or colon cancer. Using this model to study physical activity, insulin levels and colon cancer could be a very useful approach. The work assessing whether the protective effect of physical activity varies by hormone receptor status provides another model for future study designs [1, 3]. It would be of great interest to follow up the animal study results and determine whether the protective effect of physical activity varies by expression level of Bax, Bcl-2, and VEGF in breast tumors.

As noted in the introduction to this chapter, understanding the underlying mechanisms for breast and colon cancer are important for designing and implementing public health prevention programs [7]. Mechanistic studies are also important for cancers for which IARC has not yet determined the evidence for a causal link to sedentary lifestyles as being compelling [4, 169]. There is increasing epidemiological evidence that physical activity prevents endometrial cancer and data demonstrating a biological pathway would be useful for causal inference [4].

There is also epidemiologic data that physical activity prevents lung cancer [170]. However, given the overwhelming effects of cigarette smoking and that smoking and physical activity are likely to be inversely associated, data on mechanistic pathways would substantially aid in causal inference [6]. Epidemiologic studies incorporating intermediate biomarkers into their design are sorely needed, as are more studies of physical activity interventions using biomarkers as outcomes [5, 6].

References

1. Adams SA, Matthews CE et al (2006) Association of physical activity with hormone receptor status: the Shanghai Breast Cancer Study. Cancer Epidemiol Biomarkers Prev 15(6): 1170–1178
2. Bardia A, Hartmann LC et al (2006) Recreational physical activity and risk of postmenopausal breast cancer based on hormone receptor status. Arch Intern Med 166(22): 2478–2483
3. Enger SM, Ross RK et al (2000) Body size, physical activity, and breast cancer hormone receptor status: results from two case-control studies. Cancer Epidemiol Biomarkers Prev 9(7):681–687
4. Cust AE, Armstrong BK et al (2007) Physical activity and endometrial cancer risk: a review of the current evidence, biologic mechanisms and the quality of physical activity assessment methods. Cancer Causes Control 18(3):243–258
5. McTiernan A (2003) Intervention studies in exercise and cancer prevention. Med Sci Sports Exerc 35(11):1841–1845
6. Rundle A (2005) Molecular epidemiology of physical activity and cancer. Cancer Epidemiol Biomarkers Prev 14(1):227–236
7. Quadrilatero J, Hoffman-Goetz L (2003) Physical activity and colon cancer. A systematic review of potential mechanisms. J Sports Med Phys Fitness 43(2):121–138
8. Bianchini F, Kaaks R et al (2002) Weight control and physical activity in cancer prevention. Obes Rev 3(1):5–8
9. Key TJ, Appleby PN et al (2003) Body mass index, serum sex hormones, and breast cancer risk in postmenopausal women. J Natl Cancer Inst 95(16):1218–1226
10. Russo J, Russo IH (2006) The role of estrogen in the initiation of breast cancer. J Steroid Biochem Mol Biol 102(1–5):89–96
11. Yager JD, Davidson NE (2006) Estrogen carcinogenesis in breast cancer. N Engl J Med 354(3):270–282
12. Cavalieri E, Frenkel K et al (2000) Estrogens as endogenous genotoxic agents–DNA adducts and mutations. J Natl Cancer Inst Monogr 27:75–93
13. Liehr JG, Gladek A et al (1991) DNA adduct formation in liver and kidney of male Syrian hamsters treated with estrogen and/or alpha-naphthoflavone. Carcinogenesis 12(3): 385–389
14. Saeed M, Rogan E et al (2007) Formation of depurinating N3Adenine and N7Guanine adducts by MCF-10F cells cultured in the presence of 4-hydroxyestradiol. Int J Cancer 120(8):1821–1824
15. Yue W, Santen RJ et al (2003) Genotoxic metabolites of estradiol in breast: potential mechanism of estradiol induced carcinogenesis. J Steroid Biochem Mol Biol 86(3–5):477–486
16. Liehr JG (1990) Genotoxic effects of estrogens. Mutat Res 238(3):269–276
17. Liehr JG (2000) Is estradiol a genotoxic mutagenic carcinogen?. Endocr Rev 21(1):40–54
18. Longcope C, Pratt JH et al (1978) Aromatization of androgens by muscle and adipose tissue in vivo. J Clin Endocrinol Metab 46(1):146–152
19. Siiteri PK (1987) Adipose tissue as a source of hormones. Am J Clin Nutr 45(1 Suppl): 277–282

20. Suzuki R, Orsini N et al (2009) Body weight and incidence of breast cancer defined by estrogen and progesterone receptor status–a meta-analysis. Int J Cancer 124(3):698–712
21. Monninkhof EM, Elias SG et al (2007) Physical activity and breast cancer: a systematic review. Epidemiology 18(1):137–157
22. Atkinson C, Lampe JW et al (2004) Effects of a moderate intensity exercise intervention on estrogen metabolism in postmenopausal women. Cancer Epidemiol Biomarkers Prev 13(5):868–874
23. McTiernan A, Tworoger SS et al (2004) Effect of exercise on serum estrogens in postmenopausal women: a 12-month randomized clinical trial. Cancer Res 64(8):2923–2928
24. De Souza MJ (2003) Menstrual disturbances in athletes: a focus on luteal phase defects. Med Sci Sports Exerc 35(9):1553–1563
25. Tworoger SS, Missmer SA et al (2007) Physical activity and inactivity in relation to sex hormone, prolactin, and insulin-like growth factor concentrations in premenopausal women – exercise and premenopausal hormones. Cancer Causes Control 18(7):743–752
26. De Souza MJ, Miller BE et al (1998) High frequency of luteal phase deficiency and anovulation in recreational women runners: blunted elevation in follicle-stimulating hormone observed during luteal-follicular transition. J Clin Endocrinol Metab 83(12): 4220–4232
27. Kelsey JL, Gammon MD et al (1993) Reproductive factors and breast cancer. Epidemiol Rev 15(1):36–47
28. Campbell KL, Westerlind KC et al (2007) Effects of aerobic exercise training on estrogen metabolism in premenopausal women: a randomized controlled trial. Cancer Epidemiol Biomarkers Prev 16(4):731–739
29. De Cree C, Ball P et al (1997) Effects of a training program on resting plasma 2-hydroxycatecholestrogen levels in eumenorrheic women. J Appl Physiol 83(5):1551–1556
30. De Cree C, Ball P et al (1997) Responses of catecholestrogen metabolism to acute graded exercise in normal menstruating women before and after training. J Clin Endocrinol Metab 82(10):3342–3348
31. De Cree C, Van Kranenburg G et al (1997) 4-Hydroxycatecholestrogen metabolism responses to exercise and training: possible implications for menstrual cycle irregularities and breast cancer. Fertil Steril 67(3):505–516
32. Pasagian-Macaulay A, Meilahn EN et al (1996) Urinary markers of estrogen metabolism 2- and 16 alpha-hydroxylation in premenopausal women. Steroids 61(8):461–467
33. Schmitz KH, Warren M et al (2008) Exercise effect on oxidative stress is independent of change in estrogen metabolism. Cancer Epidemiol Biomarkers Prev 17(1):220–223
34. Westerlind KC, Williams NI (2007) Effect of energy deficiency on estrogen metabolism in premenopausal women. Med Sci Sports Exerc 39(7):1090–1097
35. Neilson HK, Friedenreich CM et al (2009) Physical activity and postmenopausal breast cancer: proposed biologic mechanisms and areas for future research. Cancer Epidemiol Biomarkers Prev 18(1):11–27
36. Pisani P (2008) Hyper-insulinaemia and cancer, meta-analyses of epidemiological studies. Arch Physiol Biochem 114(1):63–70
37. Abate N (1996) Insulin resistance and obesity. The role of fat distribution pattern. Diabetes Care 19(3):292–294
38. Fletcher B, Gulanick M et al (2002) Risk factors for type 2 diabetes mellitus. J Cardiovasc Nurs 16(2):17–23
39. Hursting SD, Lashinger LM et al (2008) Reducing the weight of cancer: mechanistic targets for breaking the obesity-carcinogenesis link. Best Pract Res Clin Endocrinol Metab 22(4):659–669
40. Hussain A, Claussen B et al (2007) Prevention of type 2 diabetes: a review. Diabetes Res Clin Pract 76(3):317–326
41. Klein S, Sheard NF et al (2004) Weight management through lifestyle modification for the prevention and management of type 2 diabetes: rationale and strategies. A statement of the

American Diabetes Association, the North American Association for the Study of Obesity, and the American Society for Clinical Nutrition. Am J Clin Nutr 80(2):257–263
42. Angelopoulos TJ, Schultz RM et al (2002) Significant enhancements in glucose tolerance and insulin action in centrally obese subjects following ten days of training. Clin J Sport Med 12(2):113–118
43. Brown MD, Moore GE et al (1997) Improvement of insulin sensitivity by short-term exercise training in hypertensive African American women. Hypertension 30(6):1549–1553
44. Dengel DR, Pratley RE et al (1996) Distinct effects of aerobic exercise training and weight loss on glucose homeostasis in obese sedentary men. J Appl Physiol 81(1):318–325
45. Oshida Y, Yamanouchi K et al (1989) Long-term mild jogging increases insulin action despite no influence on body mass index or VO2 max. J Appl Physiol 66(5):2206–2210
46. Reitman JS, Vasquez B et al (1984) Improvement of glucose homeostasis after exercise training in non-insulin-dependent diabetes. Diabetes Care 7(5):434–441
47. Giovannucci E (2001) Insulin, insulin-like growth factors and colon cancer: a review of the evidence. J Nutr 131(11 Suppl):3109S–20S
48. Kaaks R, Lukanova A et al (2002) Obesity, endogenous hormones, and endometrial cancer risk: a synthetic review. Cancer Epidemiol Biomarkers Prev 11(12):1531–1543
49. D'Ambrosio C, Valentinis B et al (1997) Protective effect of the insulin-like growth factor I receptor on apoptosis induced by okadaic acid. Cancer Res 57(15):3264–3271
50. Ish-Shalom D, Christoffersen CT et al (1997) Mitogenic properties of insulin and insulin analogues mediated by the insulin receptor. Diabetologia 40(Suppl 2):S25–S31
51. Khandwala HM, McCutcheon IE et al (2000) The effects of insulin-like growth factors on tumorigenesis and neoplastic growth. Endocr Rev 21(3):215–244
52. Prisco M, Romano G et al (1999) Insulin and IGF-I receptors signaling in protection from apoptosis. Horm Metab Res 31(2–3):80–89
53. Cocca C, Gutierrez A et al (2003) Suppression of mammary gland tumorigenesis in diabetic rats. Cancer Detect Prev 27(1):37–46
54. Heuson JC, Legros N (1970) Effect of insulin and of alloxan diabetes on growth of the rat mammary carcinoma in vivo. Eur J Cancer 6(4):349–351
55. Shafie SM, Grantham FH (1981) Role of hormones in the growth and regression of human breast cancer cells (MCF-7) transplanted into athymic nude mice. J Natl Cancer Inst 67(1):51–56
56. Shafie SM, Hilf R (1981) Insulin receptor levels and magnitude of insulin-induced responses in 7,12-dimethylbenz(a)anthracene-induced mammary tumors in rats. Cancer Res 41(3): 826–829
57. Fair AM, Montgomery K (2009) Energy balance, physical activity, and cancer risk. Methods Mol Biol 472:57–88
58. Eliassen AH, Tworoger SS et al (2007) Circulating insulin and c-peptide levels and risk of breast cancer among predominately premenopausal women. Cancer Epidemiol Biomarkers Prev 16(1):161–164
59. Muti P, Quattrin T et al (2002) Fasting glucose is a risk factor for breast cancer: a prospective study. Cancer Epidemiol Biomarkers Prev 11(11):1361–1368
60. Fletcher O, Gibson L et al (2005) Polymorphisms and circulating levels in the insulin-like growth factor system and risk of breast cancer: a systematic review. Cancer Epidemiol Biomarkers Prev 14(1):2–19
61. Renehan AG, Egger M et al (2005) IGF-I, IGF binding protein-3 and breast cancer risk: comparison of 3 meta-analyses. Int J Cancer 115(6):1006–1007 author reply 1008
62. Renehan AG, Zwahlen M et al (2004) Insulin-like growth factor (IGF)-I, IGF binding protein-3, and cancer risk: systematic review and meta-regression analysis. Lancet 363(9418): 1346–1353
63. Chang S, Wu X et al (2002) Plasma concentrations of insulin-like growth factors among healthy adult men and postmenopausal women: associations with body composition, lifestyle, and reproductive factors. Cancer Epidemiol Biomarkers Prev 11(8):758–766

64. DeLellis K, Rinaldi S et al (2004) Dietary and lifestyle correlates of plasma insulin-like growth factor-I (IGF-I) and IGF binding protein-3 (IGFBP-3): the multiethnic cohort. Cancer Epidemiol Biomarkers Prev 13(9):1444–1451
65. McTiernan A, Sorensen B et al (2005) No effect of exercise on insulin-like growth factor 1 and insulin-like growth factor binding protein 3 in postmenopausal women: a 12-month randomized clinical trial. Cancer Epidemiol Biomarkers Prev 14(4):1020–1
66. Milliken LA, Going SB et al (2003) Effects of exercise training on bone remodeling, insulin-like growth factors, and bone mineral density in postmenopausal women with and without hormone replacement therapy. Calcif Tissue Int 72(4):478–484
67. Barnes BB, Chang-Claude J et al (2009) Cancer risk factors associated with insulin-like growth factor (IGF)-I and IGF-binding protein-3 levels in healthy women: effect modification by menopausal status. Cancer Causes Control 20(10):1985–1996
68. Slattery ML, Baumgartner KB et al (2005) Genetic, anthropometric, and lifestyle factors associated with IGF-1 and IGFBP-3 levels in Hispanic and non-Hispanic white women. Cancer Causes Control 16(10):1147–1157
69. Voskuil DW, Bueno de Mesquita HB et al (2001) Determinants of circulating insulin-like growth factor (IGF)-I and IGF binding proteins 1-3 in premenopausal women: physical activity and anthropometry (Netherlands). Cancer Causes Control 12(10):951–958
70. Rosendal L, Langberg H et al (2002) Physical capacity influences the response of insulin-like growth factor and its binding proteins to training. J Appl Physiol 93(5):1669–1675
71. Cerutti PA (1985) Prooxidant states and tumor promotion. Science 227(4685):375–381
72. Frenkel K (1992) Carcinogen-mediated oxidant formation and oxidative DNA damage. Pharmacol Ther 53(1):127–166
73. Loft S, Fischer-Nielsen A et al (1993) 8-Hydroxydeoxyguanosine as a urinary biomarker of oxidative DNA damage. J Toxicol Environ Health 40(2–3):391–404
74. Teebor GW, Frenkel K et al (1982) Identification of radiation-induced thymine derivatives in DNA. Adv Enzyme Regul 20:39–54
75. Ji LL, Leeuwenburgh C et al (1998) Oxidative stress and aging. Role of exercise and its influences on antioxidant systems. Ann N Y Acad Sci 854:102–117
76. Powers SK, Ji LL et al (1999) Exercise training-induced alterations in skeletal muscle antioxidant capacity: a brief review. Med Sci Sports Exerc 31(7):987–997
77. Sen CK (1999) Glutathione homeostasis in response to exercise training and nutritional supplements. Mol Cell Biochem 196(1–2):31–42
78. Hartmann A, Plappert U et al (1994) Does physical activity induce DNA damage?. Mutagenesis 9(3):269–272
79. Niess AM, Hartmann A et al (1996) DNA damage after exhaustive treadmill running in trained and untrained men. Int J Sports Med 17(6):397–403
80. Tsai K, Hsu TG et al (2001) Oxidative DNA damage in human peripheral leukocytes induced by massive aerobic exercise. Free Radic Biol Med 31(11):1465–1472
81. Asami S, Hirano T et al (1998) Reduction of 8-hydroxyguanine in human leukocyte DNA by physical exercise. Free Radic Res 29(6):581–584
82. Goon JA, Aini AH et al (2009) Effect of Tai Chi exercise on DNA damage, antioxidant enzymes, and oxidative stress in middle-age adults. J Phys Act Health 6(1):43–54
83. Kasai H, Iwamoto-Tanaka N et al (2001) Life style and urinary 8-hydroxydeoxyguanosine, a marker of oxidative DNA damage: effects of exercise, working conditions, meat intake, body mass index, and smoking. Jpn J Cancer Res 92(1):9–15
84. Miyazaki H, Oh-ishi S et al (2001) Strenuous endurance training in humans reduces oxidative stress following exhausting exercise. Eur J Appl Physiol 84(1–2):1–6
85. Radak Z, Pucsuk J et al (2000) Changes in urine 8-hydroxydeoxyguanosine levels of super-marathon runners during a four-day race period. Life Sci 66(18):1763–1767
86. Sato Y, Nanri H et al (2003) Increase of human MTH1 and decrease of 8-hydroxydeoxyguanosine in leukocyte DNA by acute and chronic exercise in healthy male subjects. Biochem Biophys Res Commun 305(2):333–338

87. Elosua R, Molina L et al (2003) Response of oxidative stress biomarkers to a 16-week aerobic physical activity program, and to acute physical activity, in healthy young men and women. Atherosclerosis 167(2):327–334
88. Evelo CT, Palmen NG et al (1992) Changes in blood glutathione concentrations, and in erythrocyte glutathione reductase and glutathione S-transferase activity after running training and after participation in contests. Eur J Appl Physiol Occup Physiol 64(4):354–358
89. Karolkiewicz J, Szczesniak L et al (2003) Oxidative stress and antioxidant defense system in healthy, elderly men: relationship to physical activity. Aging Male 6(2):100–105
90. Mena P, Maynar M et al (1991) Erythrocyte free radical scavenger enzymes in bicycle professional racers. Adaptation to training. Int J Sports Med 12(6):563–566
91. Ohno H, Yahata T et al (1988) Physical training and fasting erythrocyte activities of free radical scavenging enzyme systems in sedentary men. Eur J Appl Physiol Occup Physiol 57(2):173–176
92. Robertson JD, Maughan RJ et al (1991) Increased blood antioxidant systems of runners in response to training load. Clin Sci (London) 80(6):611–618
93. Rundle AG, Orjuela M et al (2005) Preliminary studies on the effect of moderate physical activity on blood levels of glutathione. Biomarkers 10(5):390–400
94. Tessier F, Margaritis I et al (1995) Selenium and training effects on the glutathione system and aerobic performance. Med Sci Sports Exerc 27(3):390–396
95. Lenton KJ, Therriault H et al (1999) Glutathione and ascorbate are negatively correlated with oxidative DNA damage in human lymphocytes. Carcinogenesis 20(4):607–613
96. Poulsen HE, Weimann A et al (1999) Methods to detect DNA damage by free radicals: relation to exercise. Proc Nutr Soc 58(4):1007–1014
97. Dai Q, Gao YT et al (2009) Oxidative stress, obesity, and breast cancer risk: results from the Shanghai Women's Health Study. J Clin Oncol 27(15):2482–2488
98. Dziaman T, Huzarski T et al (2009) Elevated level of 8-oxo-7, 8-dihydro-2′-deoxyguanosine in leukocytes of BRCA1 mutation carriers compared to healthy controls. Int J Cancer 125(9):2209–2213
99. Frenkel K, Karkoszka J et al (1998) Serum autoantibodies recognizing 5-hydroxymethyl-2′-deoxyuridine, an oxidized DNA base, as biomarkers of cancer risk in women. Cancer Epidemiol Biomarkers Prev 7(1):49–57
100. Rossner P Jr, Gammon MD et al (2006) Relationship between urinary 15-F2t-isoprostane and 8-oxodeoxyguanosine levels and breast cancer risk. Cancer Epidemiol Biomarkers Prev 15(4):639–644
101. Irwin ML (2006) Randomized controlled trials of physical activity and breast cancer prevention. Exerc Sport Sci Rev 34(4):182–193
102. McTiernan A (2008) Mechanisms linking physical activity with cancer. Nat Rev Cancer 8(3):205–211
103. Jakobisiak M, Lasek W et al (2003) Natural mechanisms protecting against cancer. Immunol Lett 90(2–3):103–122
104. Nakachi K, Hayashi T et al (2004) Perspectives on cancer immuno-epidemiology. Cancer Sci 95(12):921–929
105. Penn I (2000) Cancers in renal transplant recipients. Adv Ren Replace Ther 7(2):147–156
106. Margolis KL, Rodabough RJ et al (2007) Prospective study of leukocyte count as a predictor of incident breast, colorectal, endometrial, and lung cancer and mortality in postmenopausal women. Arch Intern Med 167(17):1837–1844
107. Aggarwal BB, Shishodia S et al (2006) Inflammation and cancer: how hot is the link?. Biochem Pharmacol 72(11):1605–1621
108. Imai K, Matsuyama S et al (2000) Natural cytotoxic activity of peripheral-blood lymphocytes and cancer incidence: an 11-year follow-up study of a general population. Lancet 356(9244):1795–1799
109. Hoffman-Goetz L, May KM et al (1994) Exercise training and mouse mammary tumour metastasis. Anticancer Res 14(6B):2627–2631

110. Jadeski L, Hoffman-Goetz L (1996) Exercise and in vivo natural cytotoxicity against tumour cells of varying metastatic capacity. Clin Exp Metastasis 14(2):138–144
111. Jonsdottir IH, Asea A et al (1996) Voluntary chronic exercise augments in vivo natural immunity in rats. J Appl Physiol 80(5):1799–1803
112. MacNeil B, Hoffman-Goetz L (1993) Chronic exercise enhances in vivo and in vitro cytotoxic mechanisms of natural immunity in mice. J Appl Physiol 74(1):388–395
113. Woods JA, Davis JM et al (1993) Exercise increases inflammatory macrophage antitumor cytotoxicity. J Appl Physiol 75(2):879–886
114. Nieman DC (1997) Exercise immunology: practical applications. Int J Sports Med 18(Suppl 1):S91–S100
115. Zhu Z, Jiang W et al (2009) Energetics and mammary carcinogenesis: effects of moderate-intensity running and energy intake on cellular processes and molecular mechanisms in rats. J Appl Physiol 106(3):911–918
116. Zhu Z, Jiang W et al (2008) Effect of nonmotorized wheel running on mammary carcinogenesis: circulating biomarkers, cellular processes, and molecular mechanisms in rats. Cancer Epidemiol Biomarkers Prev 17(8):1920–1929
117. Atamaniuk J, Stuhlmeier KM et al (2008) Effects of ultra-marathon on circulating DNA and mRNA expression of pro- and anti-apoptotic genes in mononuclear cells. Eur J Appl Physiol 104(4):711–717
118. Kerksick C, Taylor Lt et al (2008) Gender-related differences in muscle injury, oxidative stress, and apoptosis. Med Sci Sports Exerc 40(10):1772–1780
119. Campbell KL, McTiernan A et al (2007) Effect of a 12-month exercise intervention on the apoptotic regulating proteins Bax and Bcl-2 in colon crypts: a randomized controlled trial. Cancer Epidemiol Biomarkers Prev 16(9):1767–1774
120. McTiernan A, Yasui Y et al (2006) Effect of a 12-month exercise intervention on patterns of cellular proliferation in colonic crypts: a randomized controlled trial. Cancer Epidemiol Biomarkers Prev 15(9):1588–1597
121. Nilsen TI, Romundstad PR et al (2008) Recreational physical activity and cancer risk in subsites of the colon (the Nord-Trondelag Health Study). Cancer Epidemiol Biomarkers Prev 17(1):183–188
122. Samad AK, Taylor RS et al (2005) A meta-analysis of the association of physical activity with reduced risk of colorectal cancer. Colorectal Dis 7(3):204–213
123. Bingham SA, Cummings JH (1989) Effect of exercise and physical fitness on large intestinal function. Gastroenterology 97(6):1389–1399
124. Coenen C, Wegener M et al (1992) Does physical exercise influence bowel transit time in healthy young men?. Am J Gastroenterol 87(3):292–295
125. Koffler KH, Menkes A et al (1992) Strength training accelerates gastrointestinal transit in middle-aged and older men. Med Sci Sports Exerc 24(4):415–419
126. Oettle GJ (1991) Effect of moderate exercise on bowel habit. Gut 32(8):941–944
127. Robertson G, Meshkinpour H et al (1993) Effects of exercise on total and segmental colon transit. J Clin Gastroenterol 16(4):300–303
128. Scott D, Scott B (1994) Should an athlete eat straight after training?–A study of intestinal transit time and its relationship to prior exercise. Br J Sports Med 28(1):22–24
129. Sesboue B, Arhan P et al (1995) Colonic transit in soccer players. J Clin Gastroenterol 20(3):211–214
130. Cummings JH, Branch WJ et al (1982) Colon cancer and large bowel function in Denmark and Finland. Nutr Cancer 4(1):61–66
131. Glober GA, Kamiyama S et al (1977) Bowel transit-time and stool weight in populations with different colon-cancer risks. Lancet 2(8029):110–1
132. Eisinger AL, Prescott SM et al (2007) The role of cyclooxygenase-2 and prostaglandins in colon cancer. Prostaglandins Other Lipid Mediat 82(1–4):147–154
133. Wang D, DuBois RN (2008) Pro-inflammatory prostaglandins and progression of colorectal cancer. Cancer Lett 267(2):197–203

134. Bennett A, Del Tacca M (1975) Proceedings: prostaglandins in human colonic carcinoma. Gut 16(5):409
135. Bennett A, Tacca MD et al (1977) Prostaglandins from tumours of human large bowel. Br J Cancer 35(6):881–884
136. Pugh S, Thomas GA (1994) Patients with adenomatous polyps and carcinomas have increased colonic mucosal prostaglandin E2. Gut 35(5):675–678
137. Bosetti C, Gallus S et al (2006) Aspirin and cancer risk: an updated quantitative review to 2005. Cancer Causes Control 17(7):871–888
138. Elwood PC, Gallagher AM et al (2009) Aspirin, salicylates, and cancer. Lancet 373(9671):1301–1309
139. Ju J, Nolan B et al (2008) Voluntary exercise inhibits intestinal tumorigenesis in Apc(Min/+) mice and azoxymethane/dextran sulfate sodium-treated mice. BMC Cancer 8:316
140. Martinez ME, Heddens D et al (1999) Physical activity, body mass index, and prostaglandin E2 levels in rectal mucosa. J Natl Cancer Inst 91(11):950–953
141. Abrahamson PE, King IB et al (2007) No effect of exercise on colon mucosal prostaglandin concentrations: a 12-month randomized controlled trial. Cancer Epidemiol Biomarkers Prev 16(11):2351–2356
142. Giovannucci E (2007) Metabolic syndrome, hyperinsulinemia, and colon cancer: a review. Am J Clin Nutr 86(3):s836–s842
143. Guo YS, Narayan S et al (1992) Characterization of insulinlike growth factor I receptors in human colon cancer. Gastroenterology 102(4 Pt 1):1101–1108
144. Koenuma M, Yamori T et al (1989) Insulin and insulin-like growth factor 1 stimulate proliferation of metastatic variants of colon carcinoma 26. Jpn J Cancer Res 80(1):51–58
145. Watkins LF, Lewis LR et al (1990) Characterization of the synergistic effect of insulin and transferrin and the regulation of their receptors on a human colon carcinoma cell line. Int J Cancer 45(2):372–375
146. Kaaks R, Lukanova A (2002) Effects of weight control and physical activity in cancer prevention: role of endogenous hormone metabolism. Ann N Y Acad Sci 963: 268–281
147. Goalstone ML, Wall K et al (1999) Increased amounts of farnesylated p21Ras in tissues of hyperinsulinaemic animals. Diabetologia 42(3):310–316
148. Leitner JW, Kline T et al (1997) Hyperinsulinemia potentiates activation of p21Ras by growth factors. Endocrinology 138(5):2211–2214
149. Stephens E, Thureen PJ et al (2001) Fetal hyperinsulinemia increases farnesylation of p21 Ras in fetal tissues. Am J Physiol Endocrinol Metab 281(2):E217–E223
150. Gunter MJ, Hoover DR et al (2008) Insulin, insulin-like growth factor-I, endogenous estradiol, and risk of colorectal cancer in postmenopausal women. Cancer Res 68(1):329–337
151. Limburg PJ, Stolzenberg-Solomon RZ et al (2006) Insulin, glucose, insulin resistance, and incident colorectal cancer in male smokers. Clin Gastroenterol Hepatol 4(12):1514–1521
152. Saydah SH, Platz EA et al (2003) Association of markers of insulin and glucose control with subsequent colorectal cancer risk. Cancer Epidemiol Biomarkers Prev 12(5):412–418
153. Schoen RE, Tangen CM et al (1999) Increased blood glucose and insulin, body size, and incident colorectal cancer. J Natl Cancer Inst 91(13):1147–1154
154. Giovannucci E, Pollak MN et al (2000) A prospective study of plasma insulin-like growth factor-1 and binding protein-3 and risk of colorectal neoplasia in women. Cancer Epidemiol Biomarkers Prev 9(4):345–349
155. Ma J, Pollak MN et al (1999) Prospective study of colorectal cancer risk in men and plasma levels of insulin-like growth factor (IGF)-I and IGF-binding protein-3. J Natl Cancer Inst 91(7):620–625
156. Kemmler W, Wildt L et al (2003) Acute hormonal responses of a high impact physical exercise session in early postmenopausal women. Eur J Appl Physiol 90(1–2):199–209
157. Morimoto Y, Hizuta A et al (1999) Functional expression of Fas and Fas ligand on human intestinal intraepithelial lymphocytes. Clin Exp Immunol 116(1):84–89

158. Ngo TH, Barnard RJ et al (2002) Effect of diet and exercise on serum insulin, IGF-I, and IGFBP-1 levels and growth of LNCaP cells in vitro (United States). Cancer Causes Control 13(10):929–935
159. Nicklas BJ, Ryan AJ et al (1995) Testosterone, growth hormone and IGF-I responses to acute and chronic resistive exercise in men aged 55–70 years. Int J Sports Med 16(7):445–450
160. Porch JV, Jain K et al (1997) Aging, physical activity, insulin-like growth factor I, and body composition in Guatemalan women. Am J Clin Nutr 66(4):874–879
161. Pyka G, Taaffe DR et al (1994) Effect of a sustained program of resistance training on the acute growth hormone response to resistance exercise in older adults. Horm Metab Res 26(7):330–333
162. Schmitz KH, Ahmed RL et al (2002) Effects of a 9-month strength training intervention on insulin, insulin-like growth factor (IGF)-I, IGF-binding protein (IGFBP)-1, and IGFBP-3 in 30–50-year-old women. Cancer Epidemiol Biomarkers Prev 11(12):1597–1604
163. Fairey AS, Courneya KS et al (2003) Effects of exercise training on fasting insulin, insulin resistance, insulin-like growth factors, and insulin-like growth factor binding proteins in postmenopausal breast cancer survivors: a randomized controlled trial. Cancer Epidemiol Biomarkers Prev 12(8):721–727
164. Beagley KW, Husband AJ (1998) Intraepithelial lymphocytes: origins, distribution, and function. Crit Rev Immunol 18(3):237–254
165. Tagliabue A, Luini W et al (1981) Natural killer activity of gut mucosal lymphoid cells in mice. Eur J Immunol 11(11):919–922
166. Ebert EC, Groh V (2008) Dissection of spontaneous cytotoxicity by human intestinal intraepithelial lymphocytes: MIC on colon cancer triggers NKG2D-mediated lysis through Fas ligand. Immunology 124(1):33–41
167. Taunk J, Roberts AI et al (1992) Spontaneous cytotoxicity of human intraepithelial lymphocytes against epithelial cell tumors. Gastroenterology 102(1):69–75
168. Lee YJ, Lee HR et al (2006) White blood cell count and the risk of colon cancer. Yonsei Med J 47(5):646–656
169. Voskuil DW, Monninkhof EM et al (2007) Physical activity and endometrial cancer risk, a systematic review of current evidence. Cancer Epidemiol Biomarkers Prev 16(4):639–648
170. Tardon A, Lee WJ et al (2005) Leisure-time physical activity and lung cancer: a meta-analysis. Cancer Causes Control 16(4):389–397

Chapter 8
Physical Activity, Weight Control, and Cancer Prognosis

Kathryn H. Schmitz, Melinda L. Irwin, and Rebecca M. Speck

Abstract There is a growing body of empirical evidence that both physical activity and body weight are associated with cancer prognosis and survival. The majority of evidence that physical activity may prevent recurrence or mortality of cancer is in breast and colon cancer. The evidence linking obesity at diagnosis to poorer prognosis is strongest for breast cancer, but there are studies supporting this link for other cancers as well, including colon, endometrium, kidney (renal cell), esophagus (adenocarcinoma), gastric cardia, pancreas, prostate, gallbladder, and liver. It is unknown if these associations are explained by factors that are already in place at the time of cancer diagnosis or factors that are amenable to intervention after diagnosis, or both. Research on this topic is emerging, and more discoveries are needed in this area. Additionally, evidence shows that physical activity and weight control may be useful for preventing or attenuating some persistent effects of cancer treatments. Oncologists are urged to prescribe exercise programs or refer patients to the increasingly available exercise programs specific for cancer survivors, as well as to advise weight loss or control as appropriate for each patient.

1 Introduction

A common definition of "cancer survivor" is any individual who has had a diagnosis of cancer, from the point of diagnosis and for the balance of life. Cancer survivors are a subset of the US adult population that is expected to grow substantively in the coming decades. More than 10 million people in the United States are cancer survivors, and more than 16% of adults older than age 65 are cancer survivors [1]. The increasing success of cancer treatments has required a shift in focus toward new outcomes, such as preventing recurrence and mortality and accommodating the

K.H. Schmitz (✉)
Division of Clinical Epidemiology, Department of Biostatistics and Epidemiology, University of Pennsylvania School of Medicine, Philadelphia, PA 19104-6021, USA
e-mail: schmitz@mail.med.upenn.edu

A. McTiernan (ed.), *Physical Activity, Dietary Calorie Restriction, and Cancer*, Energy Balance and Cancer 3, DOI 10.1007/978-1-4419-7551-5_8,

unique medical and psychosocial needs of cancer survivors. As such, the role of physical activity and weight control in improving outcomes for cancer survivors is likely to increase in importance as well.

Cancer treatment typically includes some combination of surgery, radiation therapy, and/or chemotherapy, and may also include hormonal therapies or other targeted therapies. Each of these therapies is associated with acute as well as persistent adverse physiologic and psychological effects. The terms "long term effects" or "late effects" [2] are used to distinguish two types of persistent effects according to the timing of their onset. Long-term effects are adverse effects or complications that appear during treatment and persist long afterward, for months, years, or the duration of life. An example of a long-term effect would be fatigue. Late effects are side effects or complications that are absent or subclinical at the end of therapy, but that emerge after compensatory systems fail or some second insult (e.g., deconditioning) occurs that results in a clinically significant diagnosis which can be traced back to effects of treatment. An example of a late effect would be the diagnosis of a cardiac arrhythmia years after treatment with a cardiotoxic chemotherapeutic agent such as adriamyacin [3]. Physical activity and weight control may be useful for preventing or attenuating some persistent effects of cancer treatments [4], and may also be useful for prevention of recurrence or cancer mortality among cancer survivors.

The acute effects of treatment on body weight and physical activity and the potential for positive effects of physical activity or weight control during active cancer treatment are beyond the scope of this review. Effects of physical activity during active cancer treatment have been reviewed elsewhere [5, 6]. The goal of this chapter is to review available scientific evidence regarding (1) associations between physical activity and cancer recurrence and mortality, (2) the effects of physical activity on persistent effects of cancer treatment, (3) associations between obesity, weight change, and cancer recurrence and mortality, and (4) the effects of obesity and weight change on persistent effects of cancer treatment. The end of the chapter includes a brief summary and statement of research needs on these topics.

2 Physical Activity and Cancer Recurrence and Mortality

The body of research and current understanding of the role of physical activity in reducing risk of cancer recurrence and mortality is more extensive in some cancers than others. The greatest evidence of the association is in breast cancer, with lesser data available on colorectal cancers. Further, the evidence and knowledge gained in theses studies has not been consistent across or within cancer sites. Additionally, there is variation across studies in the methods and data collection tools by which physical activity information has been obtained.

Twelve observational studies have examined physical activity or fitness in relation to breast cancer recurrence, breast cancer-specific mortality, or all-cause mortality [7–18]. Thus, these studies were not interventions or randomized controlled trials, but simply observational in that men and women completed physical activity questionnaires prior to or after diagnosis, and were then followed for up to 10 years to examine whether those reporting higher amounts of physical activity were less likely to experience a recurrence or death from cancer than those reporting lower amounts of physical activity. Studies vary in their physical activity type and time point of interest. Recreational or leisure time, occupational, household, routine activity, and transportation-related activity have all been examined. Time points for physical activity data collection have included prediagnosis, postdiagnosis, and lifetime. Eleven of the studies examined physical activity and breast cancer prognosis. There was only one study [15] that examined the association of cardiorespiratory fitness at study entry with breast cancer survival outcomes. Sample sizes of the 12 studies ranged from 412 to 14,811 (average = 2,696).

Seven of twelve studies [11–16, 18] have found statistically significant inverse associations between physical activity or fitness and survival. The average hazard ratio for breast cancer-specific mortality comparing the most active or most fit to least active or least fit individuals is 0.56 [11–13, 15]. The average hazard ratio for all-cause mortality for the most active or most fit women compared to the least active or least fit is 0.64 [11–15, 18]. In other words, breast cancer mortality and all-cause mortality is reduced by 44 and 36%, respectively, in women who report being physically active or fit prior to or after a breast cancer diagnosis. Only two studies [11, 13] examined breast cancer recurrence and observed a significant association with physical activity level, recurrence being 26–46% lower comparing women with the highest to the lowest category of activity.

The dose–response association of physical activity since diagnosis with overall and breast cancer-specific mortality, as well as recurrence, was explored using data from the Nurses' Health Study, which included 2,987 breast cancer survivors with over a median of 96 months of follow-up [13]. Results indicated a 29% decrease in overall mortality among women who did at least 3 MET-hours per week of aerobic activity after diagnosis (i.e., ~1 h/week of moderate-intensity physical activity such as brisk walking), with limited additional protection from increased levels of physical activity. In women completing at least 9 MET-hours per week of physical activity (i.e., ~2–3 h/week of moderate-intensity physical activity) compared to women who did less than 3 MET-hours per week, the decrease in breast cancer-specific mortality and recurrence were 50 and 43%, respectively. In another example, a prospective cohort study analyzed the intensity of lifetime recreational physical activity in 1,231 women diagnosed with breast cancer, who were followed a minimum of 8.3 years for cancer progression, recurrence or new primaries, and a minimum of 10.3 years for death [11]. Results found moderate-intensity recreational activity decreased the risk of a recurrence, progression, or new primary cancer, and decreased the risk of breast cancer-specific mortality and all-cause mortality among women. Vigorous-intensity recreational activity resulted in no such associations.

Given that women who are more physically active after diagnosis may have been similarly active before diagnosis, it is important to note that it is possible that physically active individuals develop tumors that are biologically less aggressive. Therefore, being physically active prior to diagnosis may have been associated with an earlier disease stage. Two studies that assessed physical activity in the year prior to diagnosis observed nonsignificant reduced risks of breast cancer death with higher levels of prediagnosis physical activity [12, 14]. However, one study examined change in physical activity from before to after breast cancer diagnosis, with an observed increased risk of death associated with decreasing physical activity [14]. Furthermore, compared with women who remained physically inactive both before and after diagnosis, increasing physical activity after diagnosis was associated with a reduced risk of death. This finding emphasizes the importance of maintaining or increasing physical activity levels after a diagnosis of breast cancer to gain the maximum benefits of physical activity on survival.

The evidence as to the role of physical activity in colon and colorectal cancer survival comes from four observational studies [19–22]. The Nurses' Health Study observed an inverse dose–response association of physical activity and colorectal cancer-specific mortality and all-cause mortality in 554 women with a previous diagnosis of colorectal cancer. A 61 and 57% reduced risk of colorectal cancer-specific and overall mortality, respectively, was observed in women engaging in at least 18 MET-hours per week of physical activity after diagnosis, compared to women who did less than 3 MET-hours per week [20]. A dose–response association of physical activity and colon cancer disease-free survival was also seen in a cohort of 832 male and female patients who participated in the Cancer and Leukemia Group B (CALGB) trial [21]. A 49% reduction in risk of recurrence was associated with 18 MET-hours per week, or 6 h of walking per week at 2.5 miles per hour. The Asia Pacific Cohort Studies Collaboration had 539,201 individuals with a median of 6.8 years of follow-up. Physical activity (yes/no) was associated with a 23% reduced risk of colorectal cancer death. Finally, colon and colorectal cancer death were evaluated in relation to cardiorespiratory fitness (CRF). Mortality was assessed in 38,801 men over 29 years of follow-up. A classification as "fit" (upper 80% of CRF) was associated with lower risk of mortality from colon (HR = 0.61, 95% CI, 0.37–1.00), and colorectal cancers (HR = 0.58, CI 95%, 0.37–0.92) [22].

In summary, these observational findings of postdiagnosis physical activity and improved survival suggest that exercise may confer additional improvements in breast and colon cancer survival beyond surgery, radiation, and chemotherapy. However, despite this growing body of observational evidence suggesting a strong link between physical activity and cancer survival, there is still the potential for confounding by unknown or poorly characterized variables. For example, physical activity may be a marker of overall health behaviors including adherence to adjuvant treatments. Thus, randomized controlled trials testing the effects of physical activity on cancer survival and/or surrogate/biological markers mediating the association between physical activity and survival are necessary and would provide critical information for cancer survivors about whether and how much lifestyle change can affect their prognosis. While a trial of physical activity on cancer survival has yet to be done, a small number of randomized trials of exercise on surrogate/biological markers of survival have been published. The effects of exercise on cancer bio-markers is reviewed in Chapter 7 of this text.

3 Effects of Physical Activity on Persistent Effects of Cancer Treatment

3.1 Aerobic or Cardiorespiratory Fitness

The effect of physical activity on cardiorespiratory fitness has long been established in the general population. However, given the cardiotoxic effects of many commonly used chemotherapeutic drugs as well as radiation treatment to the chest, it has additional meaning and importance to cancer survivors [3]. To date, 14 randomized controlled trials (RCTs) of physical activity interventions for cancer survivors after treatment have assessed aerobic or cardiorespiratory fitness [23–35]. The typical measures of cardiorespiratory function utilized have included VO_2 Max tests and timed distance walked tests. Thirteen of the fourteen studies reported positive improvement in cardiorespiratory function, and over half of the studies showed statistically significant results. Thirteen of the fourteen studies included breast cancer survivors, nine of which enrolled only breast cancer survivors. The studies examined a variety of fitness interventions, including home-based and monitored exercise programs in walking, yoga, tai chi chuan, aerobic, and resistance training.

3.2 Muscular Strength and Endurance

Cancer treatment may result in a decrease in activity, and deconditioning associated with disuse of muscles. Thus, it is important to determine whether exercise training improves muscular strength in cancer survivors. Common tests used to determine strength included one-repetition maximum tests, hand grip strength, and overhead or leg press. RCTs of physical activity interventions in cancer survivors have assessed changes in both upper and lower body strength. Four studies have measured upper and lower body strength in aerobic and nonaerobic physical activity interventions during treatment [36–39]. Nine randomized clinical trials have examined the effects of some form of resistance training, tai chi chuan, or yoga on muscle strength in cancer patients or survivors [31–33, 40–45]. The studies during treatment are split between breast and prostate cancer survivors, while all post-treatment studies enrolled breast cancer patients. The ability to generalize the findings of these studies is limited by their narrow focus on cancer type. All of the studies that assessed exercise level during and post-treatment observed positive effects of training, and four during treatment [36–39] and three post-treatment [40, 43, 44] studies reported statistically significant improvements in strength.

3.3 Flexibility

Decreased range of motion is a common result of cancer surgeries. Scarring or tissue damage may result in altered or compromised physical function. Eight randomized clinical trials have examined the effects of exercise training on flexibility in post-treatment cancer survivors. Four studies have assessed effects of aerobic exercise or yoga on lower body flexibility with the sit-and-reach test in breast and colon cancer survivors [25–27, 46]. All four studies observed improvements in flexibility, but only one [25] observed a statistically significant improvement comparing changes between treatment and control participants. Five other studies evaluated the effects of tai chi chuan, dance, and movement, or aerobic exercise and stretching on shoulder range of motion in breast cancer survivors [23, 41, 44, 47, 48]. Studies were not consistent in observing positive improvements, and only one study found significant between-group differences in shoulder range of motion [41].

3.4 Lymphedema

Lymph node removal as a procedure in breast cancer surgery or irradiation of lymph nodes during radiation therapy can result in damage to the lymphatic system. The damage can inhibit the lymphatic system from functioning properly in that the affected body part has difficulty in managing fluid balance and temperature regulation. Inhibition of the lymphatic system may impair immune response, wound healing, and general response to trauma or injury. Lymphedema-related swelling and pain can develop in the affected body part immediately after surgery or radiation treatment, or it could emerge years later. Thus, lymphedema is a long-term adverse effect of treatment among several types of survivors, including those with breast, head and neck, melanoma, genital, lower gastrointestinal tract, and bladder cancers. Evidence suggests lymphedema occurs in 6–50% of breast cancer survivors, depending on the number of nodes removed and the intensity of radiation treatment [49–51]. Six randomized clinical trials have examined the risk of lymphedema onset or symptom worsening among breast cancer survivors as a result of exercise training, by measuring changes in arm circumferences or volume [23, 40, 41, 45, 48, 52, 53]. None of the studies reported negative adverse effects to arm circumferences or symptoms as a result of aerobic or resistance exercise training. Lower-limb lymphedema occurs in 20–30% of cancer patients who have had lymph node removal or radiation in the groin or retroperitoneal lymph nodes [54–63]. To date, no studies have been conducted on the safety or efficacy of exercise for cancer survivors with or at risk for lower limb lymphedema.

3.5 Weight Change

A growing body of evidence has examined the effects of aerobic and resistance exercise training on body weight and body composition in cancer survivors. Fourteen randomized clinical trials have examined the effect of exercise on body weight and body fat percentage following cancer treatment [25–29, 31, 33, 34, 42–45, 64–68]. Half of the studies have observed positive change in body weight; however, only 2 of the 14 randomized clinical trials observed statistically significant improvement [43, 66]. A greater number of studies have reported positive and significant results for change in body fat percentage, with 71% of studies observing positive results [25, 27, 31, 34, 44, 45, 64, 66, 67], and 43% of studies finding significant results [25, 27, 31, 64, 66, 67]. Evidence suggests that exercise may decrease body fat percentage, but may not be influential in decreasing body weight in cancer patients or survivors, which is similar to observations in persons without cancer.

3.6 *Quality of Life*

Health-related quality of life and patient-reported outcomes is a growing area of research in cancer survivorship. Many investigators conducting physical activity interventions for cancer survivors both during and after treatment have incorporated quality of life measures into their studies. Since 2003, results have been published from seven randomized clinical trials in which overall quality of life was examined in physical activity interventions during cancer treatment [36, 38, 39, 69–72]. Fifteen studies have evaluated changes in overall quality of life in post-treatment physical activity interventions [25, 26, 28, 29, 31, 35, 43, 47, 48, 72–77]. All seven studies conducting physical activity interventions during treatment observed positive improvement in quality of life, and three studies reported statistically significant findings. Twelve of the fifteen studies reported positive effects on overall health-related quality of life as the result of a physical activity intervention after cancer treatment, and 60% of the studies reported statistically significant results. In addition to overall quality of life, investigators have specifically examined social, emotional, functional, physical, and mental quality of life. Though the majority of the research has occurred in breast cancer patients, the results appear to be consistent and that physical activity improves overall quality of life in cancer survivors.

3.7 *Fatigue*

Cancer-related fatigue is one of the most commonly reported side effects of cancer and the related treatments, and is not predictable by cancer site or tumor type. Cancer-related fatigue is unique from other types of fatigue in its persistence and severity [78]. The effects of physical activity interventions on cancer-related fatigue have been tested in 26 randomized clinical trials to date, 12 during treatment [36, 38, 39, 69, 70, 72, 79–84] and 14 post-treatment [24, 25, 27–30, 34, 35, 75, 77, 81, 85–87]. The majority of both during and post-treatment physical activity trials found positive improvements in cancer-related fatigue. One third of the during treatment interventions reported significant results in cancer-related fatigue, while half of the post-treatment studies observed statistically significant improvements. As with many physical activity interventions, the majority of studies were conducted in breast cancer survivors. Research that focuses on the mechanism by which physical activity affects cancer-related fatigue is necessary.

4 Obesity at Initial Diagnosis and Cancer Survival

The vast majority of observational studies that have looked at the relationship between weight at diagnosis and cancer outcomes have demonstrated an increased risk of cancer recurrence and death in men and women who are overweight or obese at the time of cancer diagnosis [88–91]. In a landmark study conducted by the American Cancer Society, obesity in adult men and women was associated with increased mortality from cancers of the colon, breast, endometrium, kidney (renal cell), esophagus (adenocarcinoma), gastric cardia, pancreas, prostate, gallbladder, and liver [88]. Estimates from this study suggest 14% of all cancer deaths in men and 20% of all cancer deaths in women from a range of cancer types are attributable to overweight and obesity. Furthermore, there was a 52 and 88% increase in the risk of all cancer death for men and women, respectively, who were severely obese (BMI $\geq$40 kg/m^2) compared with men and women who were normal body weight (BMI <25 kg/m^2).

The most frequently diagnosed invasive cancer among women is breast cancer, and rates of obesity continue to climb in the United States. As such, there has been significant research directed toward the relationship between obesity and breast cancer prognosis. A meta-analysis of 12 observational studies published by 2001 reported a 56% increased risk of breast cancer mortality among obese compared to nonobese women [92]. An earlier meta-analysis of observational studies completed in 1995 reported a hazard ratio for breast cancer recurrence at 5 years of 1.78 (95% CI 1.5–2.11) and for breast cancer death at 10 years of 1.36 (95% CI 1.19–1.55) for women in higher BMI categories compared with women at lower BMI categories [93]. The authors noted that the association of obesity with cancer mortality was apparent even after adjusting for stage at diagnosis and adequacy of treatment.

Multiple cohort studies in pre- and postmenopausal women observe higher rates of recurrence and mortality among women who are obese at diagnosis [94]. For example, Daling and colleagues [90] reported that women younger than 45 years of age who had invasive breast cancer and a BMI >25 kg/m^2 were 2.5 times as likely to die of their disease within 5 years of diagnosis compared with women with breast cancer and a BMI <21 kg/m^2.

For prostate cancer, there has been conflicting evidence regarding whether obesity was associated with increased risk for aggressive disease or worse outcomes following initial treatment. There is increasing evidence, reviewed elsewhere [95], that obesity increases risk for aggressive prostate cancer, while concurrently reducing risk for less aggressive cancer. Obesity also increases the risk for recurrence after prostatectomy. Given this, it is notable that there is still debate about the influence of obesity on prostate cancer mortality [95].

Pancreatic cancer is a highly fatal disease, with incidence rates nearly matching mortality rates. There is increasing evidence from recent cohort studies that obesity increases risk of pancreatic cancer incidence, and thus mortality [96].

There have been three studies that have investigated the association between BMI at diagnosis and risk of recurrent, second primary cancer, or mortality from colon cancer [97–99]. Dignam and colleagues investigated the association between

BMI at diagnosis and risk of recurrence, second primary cancer, and mortality in 4,288 colon cancer patients [97]. A BMI greater than 35.0 kg/m^2 at diagnosis was associated with a 38 and 49% increased risk of recurrence or death, respectively, as compared to a BMI less than 25 kg/m^2. Meyerhardt and colleagues observed an increase in overall mortality among women with stage II–III carcinoma in one cohort (2003) [98], but no association of BMI with any survival outcomes in a different cohort (2008) [99].

5 Weight Gain and Cancer Survival

Epidemiological studies have also shown that weight gain after a breast cancer diagnosis is associated with an increased risk for recurrence and death compared with maintaining normal weight after diagnosis [100]. This is especially worrisome given the fact that, among women treated for breast cancer, a majority of them gain a significant amount of weight in the year following breast cancer diagnosis, and return to prediagnosis weight is rare [101]. Analyses from the Nurses' Health Study showed that weight gain after diagnosis (~5–10 lbs) was related to approximately 50% higher rates of breast cancer recurrence and death [100]. The findings were especially apparent in women who never smoked, among women with earlier stage disease or those who were normal weight before diagnosis.

While these findings are intriguing, not all studies have observed an association between obesity or weight gain and poor survival. Caan and colleagues did not observe an association between postdiagnosis weight gain and breast cancer recurrence risk in the first 5–7 years postdiagnosis [102]. Meyerhardt and colleagues, using data from the Cancer and Leukemia Group B (CALGB) 89803 study of 1,053 patients who had stage III colon cancer, demonstrated no association between BMI or weight change and survival in colon cancer patients [99]. It is unknown if chemotherapy dose specifications may account for the differences between these studies and the studies showing an increased risk of death with higher BMI and weight gain. Thus, obesity may be associated with poor prognosis or may be associated with receiving inadequate chemotherapy dosage. Data addressing this issue is provided by Buist and colleagues, who examined the association between BMI and receipt of appropriate primary tumor therapy and adjuvant therapy in 897 women diagnosed with breast cancer. They found that receipt of appropriate primary therapy and adjuvant therapy was not associated with BMI in women treated for breast cancer [103]. This finding is consistent with the hypothesis that obesity is associated with poor prognosis, not inadequate chemotherapy dosage.

One final concern recently raised by Daniell and colleagues is that being obese, compared with being normal weight, prior to and at cancer diagnosis is associated with earlier tumor metastasis, or more rapid growth of node metastases before diagnosis, as well as differences in hormone receptor status [104]. Thus, these genetic differences in tumors among obese patients may have already influenced the growth of metastatic tissue before their initial diagnosis. Therefore, weight loss after diagnosis may not influence prognosis because of the already established genetic alterations. However, without a methodologically strong weight loss trial conducted in overweight and obese cancer survivors, we are unable to definitively know whether weight loss impacts survival or not. Regardless, obesity and weight gain still have adverse effects on risk of other new cancers and overall survival. Specifically, there is evidence that cancer survivors die of noncancer causes at a higher rate than persons in the general population (deaths being primarily from cardiovascular disease and diabetes) [3]. Therefore, surviving cancer requires not only treating the primary cancer but also avoiding second cancers for which patients are at increased risk. To improve overall survival, it is critically important for cancer survivors to prevent or attenuate weight gain and obesity.

6 Effects of Obesity and Weight Gain on Persistent Effects of Cancer Treatment

Historically, cancer has been associated with cachexia. Even now, for gastrointestinal cancer, weight loss is common and is predictive of survival [105]. But while some cancers and cancer treatments are associated with weight loss, there is also evidence that for other cancers weight gain is a persistent effect of treatment. There is also some evidence that obesity and weight gain after cancer diagnosis are associated with persistent effects of cancer treatment. Each of these topics is reviewed below.

There is evidence of an association of adult obesity and prior treatment for childhood cancers, including acute lymphoblastic leukemia, patients treated with glucocorticoids, and central nervous system cancer treated with cranial irradiation [106–108]. There is evidence that adult survivors of childhood obesity are less physically active and have reduced exercise capacity, which increases risk for obesity [109]. Hypothesized causes linking treatment for childhood cancer with obesity include low physical activity, low resting metabolic rate, and hormonal insufficiency [109].

There is also one paper showing that obesity is a common long-term effect of thyroid cancer [110], as a result of the temporary hypothyroid state that is essential to treating the cancer. This effect seemed to be a larger issue for younger patients.

Multiple reviews of the effects of breast cancer treatment suggest that at least half of women receiving chemotherapy gain weight. A review on this topic in 2001 by Partridge concluded that this common outcome was associated with menopausal status at diagnosis (more weight gain among premenopausal women), systemic therapies (e.g., hormonal or chemotherapy drugs), and dose of systemic therapies [111]. The average persistent weight gains at that time were 2.5–5.0 kg, with more significant weight gains of 10–20 kg reported in up to 20% of patients. Studies published since 2001 report average weight gains ranging from 1.7 to 10.85 kg, with length of follow-up varying from 6 months to 3 years post-treatment, in sample sizes ranging from 44 to 514 women [101, 112–114].

Mechanisms underlying weight gain after breast cancer treatment have been explored. Changes in dietary intake have not been supported [115–117], but there is evidence that there is a decrease in physical activity during therapy that might be contributory [115, 116, 118]. There is conflicting evidence regarding changes in resting energy expenditure or lean mass that could contribute to weight gain [112, 116, 119, 120].

Obesity may interact with the other effects of treatment to increase or decrease the risk of other persistent effects of treatment. The most obvious example of this is that for many cancer survivors treated with radiation and/or chemotherapy, there are increased risks for negative cardiovascular, pulmonary, and metabolic outcomes [1, 109]. Obesity is known to be associated with each of these body systems and may act synergistically with the toxic effects of radiation or chemotherapy to result in earlier or more severe adverse outcomes. Research in this area is scant and much needed.

One particular persistent effect of cancer treatment that is clearly associated with and made worse by obesity is lymphedema. Women who are obese at the time of breast cancer diagnosis or who gain weight after diagnosis generally have a higher risk of developing lymphedema [121, 122]. In light of this, it is disappointing that there has only been one small clinical trial, to date, that has explored whether a weight loss intervention would improve outcomes among cancer survivors with lymphedema. A pilot study in England that lasted 12 weeks showed significant reductions in interlimb swelling differences among breast cancer survivors who lost weight compared to those randomized to a control condition [123]. More research is needed on the potential for weight loss in cancer survivors to prevent, attenuate, delay, or improve lymphedema and other persistent effects of cancer treatment.

7 Overall Summary

Evidence that physical activity may prevent recurrence or mortality from breast and/or colon cancer is emerging. Further research on this topic is needed to draw conclusions regarding the benefit of exercise for cancer recurrence and mortality. That said, there are many other excellent positive effects of regular physical activity that have been demonstrated among cancer survivors. For example, strong evidence links increased physical activity in cancer survivors with improved quality of life and increased fitness. A 2006 publication from the American Cancer Society [91] states that although the current public health guidelines of 30–60 min of moderate-intensity aerobic exercise five times per week have not been studied systematically in cancer survivors, there is no reason to think that this also would not benefit survivors. Overall, results indicate that guidelines for cardiovascular exercise for cancer survivors who have completed treatment need not be different from those of the general population, and that particular physiologic and psychosocial effects of cancer and its treatments are positively affected by cardiovascular exercise, resistance training, and flexibility training. Clinical trials showing a benefit of physical activity interventions on reducing deaths, recurrences, and reducing the impact of late or long-term treatment effects also would make a valuable contribution to our understanding of the needs of this growing population.

The evidence linking obesity at diagnosis to poorer prognosis is strongest for breast cancer, but there are studies supporting this link for other cancers as well, including colon, endometrium, kidney (renal cell), esophagus (adenocarcinoma), gastric cardia, pancreas, prostate, gallbladder, and liver. The question of whether this is due to factors that are already in place at the time of cancer diagnosis or factors that are amenable to intervention after diagnosis has yet to be fully answered. If the link between obesity and cancer prognosis is due to mechanisms amenable to intervention after the initial diagnosis, it would be expected that weight change after diagnosis would be associated with cancer survival outcomes. Research on this topic is emerging; results conflict across the few completed studies, suggesting more work is needed in this area. Regardless of whether weight loss is associated with reduced risk for recurrence or mortality from cancer, there is also the potential for weight loss among cancer survivors to reduce other cancer burdens, the persistent effects of treatment. Research on this topic is particularly scant and much needed.

In conclusion, there is empirical evidence that both physical activity and body weight are associated with cancer prognosis and survival. Oncologists are urged to prescribe exercise programs or refer patients to the increasingly available exercise programs specific for cancer survivors, as well as to advise weight loss or control as appropriate for each patient.

References

1. Committee on Cancer Survivorship: Institute of Medicine and National Research Board (2006) From cancer patient to cancer survivor: lost in translation. National Academy of Sciences, Washington, DC
2. Aziz NM, Rowland JH (2003) Trends and advances in cancer survivorship research: challenge and opportunity. Semin Radiat Oncol 13:248–266
3. Carver JR, Shapiro CL, Ng A et al (2007) American society of clinical oncology clinical evidence review on the ongoing care of adult cancer survivors: cardiac and pulmonary late effects. J Clin Oncol 25:3991–4008
4. Schmitz KH, Capppola A, Stricker C et al (2007) The intersection of cancer and aging: establishing the need for breast cancer rehabilitation. Cancer Epidemiol Biomark Prev 16:866–872
5. Markes M, Brockow T, Resch KL (2006) Exercise for women receiving adjuvant therapy for breast cancer.Cochrane Database Syst Rev. Oct 18;(4): CD005001
6. Schmitz KH, Holtzman J, Courneya KS et al (2005) Controlled physical activity trials in cancer survivors: a systematic review and meta-analysis. Cancer Epidemiol Biomarkers Prev 14:1588–1595
7. Abrahamson PE, Gammon MD, Lund MJ et al (2006) Recreational physical activity and survival among young women with breast cancer. Cancer 107:1777–1785
8. Borugian MJ, Sheps SB, Kim-Sing C et al (2004) Insulin, macronutrient intake, and physical activity: are potential indicators of insulin resistance associated with mortality from breast cancer?. Cancer Epidemiol Biomarkers Prev 13:1163–1172
9. Dal Maso L, Zucchetto A, Talamini R et al (2008) Effect of obesity and other lifestyle factors on mortality in women with breast cancer. Int J Cancer 123:2188–2194
10. Enger SM, Bernstein L (2004) Exercise activity, body size and premenopausal breast cancer survival. Br J Cancer 90:2138–2141
11. Friedenreich CM, Gregory J, Kopciuk KA et al (2009) Prospective cohort study of lifetime physical activity and breast cancer survival. Int J Cancer 124:1954–1962

12. Holick CN, Newcomb PA, Trentham-Dietz A et al (2008) Physical activity and survival after diagnosis of invasive breast cancer. Cancer Epidemiol Biomarkers Prev 17:379–386
13. Holmes MD, Chen WY, Feskanich D et al (2005) Physical activity and survival after breast cancer diagnosis. JAMA 293:2479–2486
14. Irwin ML, Smith AW, McTiernan A et al (2008) Influence of pre- and postdiagnosis physical activity on mortality in breast cancer survivors: the health, eating, activity, and lifestyle study. J Clin Oncol 26:3958–3964
15. Peel JB, Sui X, Adams SA et al (2009) A prospective study of cardiorespiratory fitness and breast cancer mortality. Med Sci Sports Exerc 41:742–748
16. Pierce JP, Stefanick ML, Flatt SW et al (2007) Greater survival after breast cancer in physically active women with high vegetable-fruit intake regardless of obesity. J Clin Oncol 25:2345–2351
17. Rohan TE, Fu W, Hiller JE (1995) Physical activity and survival from breast cancer. Eur J Cancer Prev 4:419–424
18. Sternfeld B, Weltzien E, Quesenberry CP et al (2009) Physical activity and risk of recurrence and mortality in breast cancer survivors: findings from the LACE study. Cancer Epidemiol Biomarkers Prev 18:87–95
19. Huxley R (2007) The role of lifestyle risk factors on mortality from colorectal cancer in populations of the Asia-Pacific region. Asian Pac J Cancer Prev 8:191–198
20. Meyerhardt JA, Giovannucci EL, Holmes MD et al (2006a) Physical activity and survival after colorectal cancer diagnosis. J Clin Oncol 24:3527–3534
21. Meyerhardt JA, Heseltine D, Niedzwiecki D et al (2006) Impact of physical activity on cancer recurrence and survival in patients with stage III colon cancer: findings from CALGB 89803. J Clin Oncol 24:3535–3541
22. Peel JB, Sui X, Matthews CE et al (2009b) Cardiorespiratory fitness and digestive cancer mortality: findings from the aerobics center longitudinal study. Cancer Epidemiol Biomarkers Prev 18:1111–1117
23. Basen-Engquist K, Taylor CL, Rosenblum C et al (2006) Randomized pilot test of a lifestyle physical activity intervention for breast cancer survivors. Patient Educ Couns 64:225–234
24. Bennett JA, Lyons KS, Winters-Stone K et al (2007) Motivational interviewing to increase physical activity in long-term cancer survivors: a randomized controlled trial. Nurs Res 56:18–27
25. Burnham TR, Wilcox A (2002) Effects of exercise on physiological and psychological variables in cancer survivors. Med Sci Sports Exerc 34:1863–1867
26. Courneya KS, Friedenreich CM, Quinney HA et al (2003) A randomized trial of exercise and quality of life in colorectal cancer survivors. Eur J Cancer Care (Engl) 12:347–357
27. Courneya KS, Friedenreich CM, Sela RA et al (2003) The group psychotherapy and home-based physical exercise (group-hope) trial in cancer survivors: physical fitness and quality of life outcomes. Psychooncology 12:357–374
28. Courneya KS, Friedenreich CM, Quinney HA et al (2004) Predictors of adherence and contamination in a randomized trial of exercise in colorectal cancer survivors. Psychooncology 13:857–866
29. Daley AJ, Crank H, Saxton JM et al (2007) Randomized trial of exercise therapy in women treated for breast cancer. J Clin Oncol 25:1713–1721
30. Fillion L, Gagnon P, Leblond F et al (2008) A brief intervention for fatigue management in breast cancer survivors. Cancer Nurs 31:145–159
31. Herrero F, San Juan AF, Fleck SJ et al (2006) Combined aerobic and resistance training in breast cancer survivors: A randomized, controlled pilot trial. Int J Sports Med 27:573–580
32. Nieman DC, Cook VD, Henson DA et al (1995) Moderate exercise training and natural killer cell cytotoxic activity in breast cancer patients. International Journal of Sports Medicine 16:334–337
33. Nikander R, Sievanen H, Ojala K et al (2007) Effect of a vigorous aerobic regimen on physical performance in breast cancer patients – a randomized controlled pilot trial. Acta Oncol 46:181–186

34. Pinto BM, Frierson GM, Rabin C et al (2005) Home-based physical activity intervention for breast cancer patients. J Clin Oncol 23:3577–3587
35. Thorsen L, Skovlund E, Stromme SB et al (2005) Effectiveness of physical activity on cardiorespiratory fitness and health-related quality of life in young and middle-aged cancer patients shortly after chemotherapy. J Clin Oncol 23:2378–2388
36. Courneya KS, Segal RJ, Mackey JR et al (2007) Effects of aerobic and resistance exercise in breast cancer patients receiving adjuvant chemotherapy: a multicenter randomized controlled trial. J Clin Oncol 25:4396–4404
37. Schwartz AL, Winters-Stone K, Gallucci B (2007) Exercise effects on bone mineral density in women with breast cancer receiving adjuvant chemotherapy. Oncol Nurs Forum 34: 627–633
38. Segal RJ, Reid RD, Courneya KS et al (2003) Resistance exercise in men receiving androgen deprivation therapy for prostate cancer. J Clin Oncol 21:1653–1659
39. Segal RJ, Reid RD, Courneya KS et al (2009) Randomized controlled trial of resistance or aerobic exercise in men receiving radiation therapy for prostate cancer. J Clin Oncol 27:344–351
40. Ahmed RL, Thomas W, Yee D et al (2006) Randomized controlled trial of weight training and lymphedema in breast cancer survivors. J Clin Oncol 24:2765–2772
41. Kilgour RD, Jones DH, Keyserlingk JR (2008) Effectiveness of a self-administered, home-based exercise rehabilitation program for women following a modified radical mastectomy and axillary node dissection: a preliminary study. Breast Cancer Res Treat 109:285–295
42. Ligibel JA, Campbell N, Partridge A et al (2008) Impact of a mixed strength and endurance exercise intervention on insulin levels in breast cancer survivors. J Clin Oncol 26:907–912
43. Morey MC, Snyder DC, Sloane R et al (2009) Effects of home-based diet and exercise on functional outcomes among older, overweight long-term cancer survivors: RENEW: a randomized controlled trial. Jama 301:1883–1891
44. Mustian KM, Katula JA, Zhao H (2006) A pilot study to assess the influence of tai chi chuan on functional capacity among breast cancer survivors. J Support Oncol 4:139–145
45. Schmitz KH, Troxel AB, Cheville A et al (2009) Physical activity and lymphedema (the PAL trial): Assessing the safety of progressive strength training in breast cancer survivors. Contemp Clin Trials 30:233–245
46. Culos-Reed SN, Carlson LE, Daroux LM et al (2006) A pilot study of yoga for breast cancer survivors: physical and psychological benefits. Psychooncology 15:891–897
47. Cho OH, Yoo YS, Kim NC (2006) Efficacy of comprehensive group rehabilitation for women with early breast cancer in South Korea. Nurs Health Sci 8:140–146
48. Sandel SL, Judge JO, Landry N et al (2005) Dance and movement program improves quality-of-life measures in breast cancer survivors. Cancer Nurs 28:301–309
49. Mansel RE, Fallowfield L, Kissin M et al (2006) Randomized multicenter trial of sentinel node biopsy versus standard axillary treatment in operable breast cancer: the ALMANAC Trial. J Natl Cancer Inst 98:599–609
50. Paskett ED, Naughton MJ, McCoy TP et al (2007) The epidemiology of arm and hand swelling in premenopausal breast cancer survivors. Cancer Epidemiol Biomarkers Prev 16:775–782
51. Petrek JA, Naughton MJ, Case LD et al (2006) Incidence, time course, and determinants of menstrual bleeding after breast cancer treatment: a prospective study. J Clin Oncol 24: 1045–1051
52. Hayes SC, Reul-Hirche H, Turner J (2009) Exercise and secondary lymphedema: safety, potential benefits, and research issues. Med Sci Sports Exerc 41:483–489
53. McKenzie DC, Kalda AL (2003) Effect of upper extremity exercise on secondary lymphedema in breast cancer patients: a pilot study. J Clin Oncol 21:463–466
54. de Vries M, Vonkeman WG, van Ginkel RJ et al (2006) Morbidity after inguinal sentinel lymph node biopsy and completion lymph node dissection in patients with cutaneous melanoma. Eur J Surg Oncol 32:785–789

55. Haberthur F, Almendral AC, Ritter B (1993) Therapy of vulvar carcinoma. Eur J Gynaecol Oncol 14:218–227
56. Ingvar C, Erichsen C, Jonsson PE (1984) Morbidity following prophylactic and therapeutic lymph node dissection for melanoma – a comparison. Tumori 70:529–533
57. Karakousis CP, Heiser MA, Moore RH (1983) Lymphedema after groin dissection. Am J Surg 145:205–208
58. Karakousis CP, Driscoll DL, Rose B et al (1994) Groin dissection in malignant melanoma. Ann Surg Oncol 1:271–277
59. Okeke AA, Bates DO, Gillatt DA (2004) Lymphoedema in urological cancer. Eur Urol 45:18–25
60. Urist MM, Maddox WA, Kennedy JE et al (1983) Patient risk factors and surgical morbidity after regional lymphadenectomy in 204 melanoma patients. Cancer 51:2152–2156
61. van Akkooi AC, Bouwhuis MG, van Geel AN et al (2007) Morbidity and prognosis after therapeutic lymph node dissections for malignant melanoma. Eur J Surg Oncol 33: 102–108
62. Werngren-Elgstrom M, Lidman D (1994) Lymphoedema of the lower extremities after surgery and radiotherapy for cancer of the cervix. Scand J Plast Reconstr Surg Hand Surg 28:289–293
63. Wrightson WR, Wong SL, Edwards MJ et al (2003) Complications associated with sentinel lymph node biopsy for melanoma. Ann Surg Oncol 10:676–680
64. Irwin ML, Varma K, Alvarez-Reeves M et al (2009) Randomized controlled trial of aerobic exercise on insulin and insulin-like growth factors in breast cancer survivors: the Yale Exercise and Survivorship study. Cancer Epidemiol Biomarkers Prev 18:306–313
65. Matthews CE, Wilcox S, Hanby CL et al (2007) Evaluation of a 12-week home-based walking intervention for breast cancer survivors. Support Care Cancer 15: 203–211
66. Mefferd K, Nichols JF, Pakiz B et al (2007) A cognitive behavioral therapy intervention to promote weight loss improves body composition and blood lipid profiles among overweight breast cancer survivors. Breast Cancer Res Treat 104:145–152
67. Schmitz KH, Ahmed RL, Hannan PJ et al (2005a) Safety and efficacy of weight training in recent breast cancer survivors to alter body composition, insulin, and insulin-like growth factor axis proteins. Cancer Epidemiol Biomarkers Prev 14:1672–1680
68. von Gruenigen VE, Courneya KS, Gibbons HE et al (2008) Feasibility and effectiveness of a lifestyle intervention program in obese endometrial cancer patients: a randomized trial. Gynecol Oncol 109:19–26
69. Campbell A, Mutrie N, White F et al (2005) A pilot study of a supervised group exercise programme as a rehabilitation treatment for women with breast cancer receiving adjuvant treatment. Eur J Oncol Nurs 9:56–63
70. Courneya KS, Jones LW, Peddle CJ et al (2008) Effects of aerobic exercise training in anemic cancer patients receiving darbepoetin alfa: a randomized controlled trial. Oncologist 13:1012–1020
71. Demark-Wahnefried W, Case LD, Blackwell K et al (2008) Results of a diet/exercise feasibility trial to prevent adverse body composition change in breast cancer patients on adjuvant chemotherapy. Clin Breast Cancer 8:70–79
72. Mutrie N, Campbell AM, Whyte F et al (2007) Benefits of supervised group exercise programme for women being treated for early stage breast cancer: pragmatic randomised controlled trial. Bmj 334:517
73. Demark-Wahnefried W, Clipp EC, Morey MC et al (2006) Lifestyle intervention development study to improve physical function in older adults with cancer: outcomes from Project LEAD. J Clin Oncol 24:3465–3473
74. Demark-Wahnefried W, Clipp EC, Lipkus IM et al (2007) Main outcomes of the FRESH START trial: a sequentially tailored, diet and exercise mailed print intervention among breast and prostate cancer survivors. J Clin Oncol 25:2709–2718

75. Dimeo FC, Thomas F, Raabe-Menssen C et al (2004) Effect of aerobic exercise and relaxation training on fatigue and physical performance of cancer patients after surgery. A randomised controlled trial. Support Care Cancer 12:774–779
76. Ohira T, Schmitz KH, Ahmed RL et al (2006) Effects of weight training on quality of life in recent breast cancer survivors: the Weight Training for Breast Cancer Survivors (WTBS) study. Cancer 106:2076–2083
77. Vallance JK, Courneya KS, Plotnikoff RC et al (2007) Randomized controlled trial of the effects of print materials and step pedometers on physical activity and quality of life in breast cancer survivors. J Clin Oncol 25:2352–2359
78. Ryan JL, Carroll JK, Ryan EP et al (2007) Mechanisms of cancer-related fatigue. Oncologist 12(Suppl 1):22–34
79. Dimeo FC, Stieglitz RD, Novelli-Fischer U et al (1999) Effects of physical activity on the fatigue and psychologic status of cancer patients during chemotherapy. Cancer 85: 2273–2277
80. Headley JA, Ownby KK, John LD (2004) The effect of seated exercise on fatigue and quality of life in women with advanced breast cancer. Oncol Nurs Forum 31:977–983
81. Kim SD, Kim HS (2005) Effects of a relaxation breathing exercise on fatigue in haemopoietic stem cell transplantation patients. J Clin Nurs 14:51–55
82. Mock V, Dow KH, Meares CJ et al (1997) Effects of exercise on fatigue, physical functioning, and emotional distress during radiation therapy for breast cancer. Oncology Nursing Forum 24:991–1000
83. Mock V, Frangakis C, Davidson NE et al (2005) Exercise manages fatigue during breast cancer treatment: a randomized controlled trial. Psychooncology 14:464–477
84. Windsor PM, Nicol KF, Potter J (2004) A randomized, controlled trial of aerobic exercise for treatment-related fatigue in men receiving radical external beam radiotherapy for localized prostate carcinoma. Cancer 101:550–557
85. Berglund G, Bolund C, Gustafsson UL et al (1994) One-year follow-up of the 'Starting Again' group rehabilitation programme for cancer patients. European Journal of Cancer 30A:1744–1751
86. Milne HM, Wallman KE, Gordon S et al (2008) Effects of a combined aerobic and resistance exercise program in breast cancer survivors: a randomized controlled trial. Breast Cancer Res Treat 108:279–288
87. Pinto BM, Clark MM, Maruyama NC et al (2003) Psychological and fitness changes associated with exercise participation among women with breast cancer. Psychooncology 12:118–126
88. Calle EE, Rodriguez C, Walker-Thurmond K et al (2003) Overweight, obesity, and mortality from cancer in a prospectively studied cohort of US. adults. N Engl J Med 348:1625–1638
89. Chlebowski RT, Aiello E, McTiernan A (2002) Weight loss in breast cancer patient management. J Clin Oncol 20:1128–1143
90. Daling JR, Malone KE, Doody DR et al (2001) Relation of body mass index to tumor markers and survival among young women with invasive ductal breast carcinoma. Cancer 92:720–729
91. Doyle C, Kushi LH, Byers T et al (2006) Nutrition and physical activity during and after cancer treatment: an American Cancer Society guide for informed choices. CA Cancer J Clin 56:323–353
92. Ryu SY, Kim CB, Nam CM et al (2001) Is body mass index the prognostic factor in breast cancer?: a meta-analysis. J Korean Med Sci 16:610–614
93. Goodwin PJ, Ennis M, Wincour J et al (1995) Development of a weight management program in women with newly diagnosed locoregional breast cancer. In: Bitzer J and Stauber M (eds)Pschosomatic obstetrics and gynecology. Monduzzi Editore, International Proceedings Division, Bologna
94. Carmichael AR (2006) Obesity and prognosis of breast cancer. Obes Rev 7:333–340
95. Kristal AR, Gong Z (2007) Obesity and prostate cancer mortality. Future Oncol 3:557–567

96. Michaud DS (2004) Epidemiology of pancreatic cancer. Minerva Chir 59:99–111
97. Dignam JJ, Polite BN, Yothers G et al (2006) Body mass index and outcomes in patients who receive adjuvant chemotherapy for colon cancer. J Natl Cancer Inst 98:1647–1654
98. Meyerhardt JA, Catalano PJ, Haller DG et al (2003) Influence of body mass index on outcomes and treatment-related toxicity in patients with colon carcinoma. Cancer 98: 484–495
99. Meyerhardt JA, Niedzwiecki D, Hollis D et al (2008) Impact of body mass index and weight change after treatment on cancer recurrence and survival in patients with stage III colon cancer: findings from Cancer and Leukemia Group B 89803. J Clin Oncol 26:4109–4115
100. Kroenke CH, Chen WY, Rosner B et al (2005) Weight, weight gain, and survival after breast cancer diagnosis. J Clin Oncol 23:1370–1378
101. Irwin ML, McTiernan A, Baumgartner RN et al (2005) Changes in body fat and weight after a breast cancer diagnosis: influence of demographic, prognostic, and lifestyle factors. J Clin Oncol 23:774–782
102. Caan BJ, Emond JA, Natarajan L et al (2006) Post-diagnosis weight gain and breast cancer recurrence in women with early stage breast cancer. Breast Cancer Res Treat 99:47–57
103. Buist DS, Ichikawa L, Prout MN et al (2007) Receipt of appropriate primary breast cancer therapy and adjuvant therapy are not associated with obesity in older women with access to health care. J Clin Oncol 25:3428–3436
104. Daniell HW (2009) Weight loss after breast cancer diagnosis may not improve prognosis. J Clin Oncol 27:829–830 author reply 830–831
105. Persson CR, Johansson BB, Sjoden PO et al (2002) A randomized study of nutritional support in patients with colorectal and gastric cancer. Nutr Cancer 42:48–58
106. Gurney JG, Ness KK, Sibley SD et al (2006) Metabolic syndrome and growth hormone deficiency in adult survivors of childhood acute lymphoblastic leukemia. Cancer 107: 1303–1312
107. Reilly JJ, Ventham JC, Newell J et al (2000) Risk factors for excess weight gain in children treated for acute lymphoblastic leukaemia. Int J Obes Relat Metab Disord 24:1537–1541
108. Reilly JJ, Brougham M, Montgomery C et al (2001) Effect of glucocorticoid therapy on energy intake in children treated for acute lymphoblastic leukemia. J Clin Endocrinol Metab 86:3742–3745
109. Hewitt M, Weiner SL, Simone JV (2003) Childhood cancer survivorship: improving care and quality of life. The National Academies Press, Washington, DC
110. Mendoza A, Shaffer B, Karakla D et al (2004) Quality of life with well-differentiated thyroid cancer: treatment toxicities and their reduction. Thyroid 14:133–140
111. Partridge AH, Burstein HJ, Winer EP (2001) Side effects of chemotherapy and combined chemohormonal therapy in women with early-stage breast cancer. J Natl Cancer Inst Monogr (30):135–142
112. Harvie MN, Campbell IT, Baildam A et al (2004) Energy balance in early breast cancer patients receiving adjuvant chemotherapy. Breast Cancer Res Treat 83:201–210
113. Kumar N, Allen KA, Riccardi D et al (2004) Fatigue, weight gain, lethargy and amenorrhea in breast cancer patients on chemotherapy: is subclinical hypothyroidism the culprit?. Breast Cancer Res Treat 83:149–159
114. McInnes JA, Knobf MT (2001) Weight gain and quality of life in women treated with adjuvant chemotherapy for early-stage breast cancer. Oncol Nurs Forum 28:675–684
115. Demark-Wahnefried W, Hars V, Conaway MR et al (1997) Reduced rates of metabolism and decreased physical activity in breast cancer patients receiving adjuvant chemotherapy. Am J Clin Nutr 65:1495–1501
116. Demark-Wahnefried W, Peterson BL, Winer EP et al (2001) Changes in weight, body composition, and factors influencing energy balance among premenopausal breast cancer patients receiving adjuvant chemotherapy. J Clin Oncol 19:2381–2389
117. Goodwin PJ, Ennis M, Pritchard KI et al (1999) Adjuvant treatment and onset of menopause predict weight gain after breast cancer diagnosis. J Clin Oncol 17:120–129

118. Kutynec CL, McCargar L, Barr SI et al (1999) Energy balance in women with breast cancer during adjuvant treatment. J Am Diet Assoc 99:1222–1227
119. Campbell KL, Lane K, Martin AD et al (2007) Resting energy expenditure and body mass changes in women during adjuvant chemotherapy for breast cancer. Cancer Nurs 30:95–100
120. Del Rio G, Zironi S, Valeriani L et al (2002) Weight gain in women with breast cancer treated with adjuvant cyclophosphomide, methotrexate and 5-fluorouracil. Analysis of resting energy expenditure and body composition. Breast Cancer Res Treat 73:267–273
121. Meeske KA, Sullivan-Halley J, Smith AW et al (2009) Risk factors for arm lymphedema following breast cancer diagnosis in Black women and White women. Breast Cancer Res Treat 113:383–391
122. Werner RS, McCormick B, Petrek J et al (1991) Arm edema in conservatively managed breast cancer: obesity is a major predictive factor. Radiology 180:177–184
123. Shaw C, Mortimer P, Judd PA (2007) A randomized controlled trial of weight reduction as a treatment for breast cancer-related lymphedema. Cancer 110:1868–1874

Index

A. McTiernan (ed.), *Physical Activity, Dietary Calorie Restriction, and Cancer*, Energy Balance and Cancer 3, DOI 10.1007/978-1-4419-7551-5,

FSC
www.fsc.org
MIX
Papier | Fördert gute Waldnutzung
FSC® C083411

Kolibri 360 GmbH
Ferdinand-Jühlke-Straße 7
99095 Erfurt, Deutschland
produktsicherheit@kolibri360.de